D0581786

DIET AND ARTHRITIS

DIET AND ARTHRITIS

A comprehensive guide to treating
arthritis through diet

Dr Gail Darlington
and Linda Gamlin

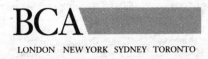

LONDON   NEW YORK   SYDNEY   TORONTO

To NORMAN
for unfailing support
and
to DAVID
as always

This edition published 1998
By BCA
By arrangement with Vermilion
An imprint of Ebury Press

CN 1235

Printed and bound in Great Britain by
Mackays of Chatham PLC, Chatham, Kent

CONTENTS

SECTION FOUR
Other Diets and Supplements

ACKNOWLEDGEMENTS

Dr Gail Darlington would like to thank Miss Patricia Street, of Epsom General Hospital, and Mrs Maggie Simkins of Eastern Surrey Health Promotion, for their advice on dietetics, and the librarians at Epsom General Hospital – Mr Gordon Smith, Mrs Marion Morrison and Mrs Fiona Rees – for their invaluable assistance.

Linda Gamlin would like to thank the following people for their help with the research on this book: Dr Olaf Adam of the University of Munich; Dr Jill Belch of the University of Dundee; Dr Jonathan Brostoff of the Middlesex Hospital, London; Dr Maciej Brzeski of Falkirk Royal Infirmary; Wynnie Chan of the Ministry of Agriculture, Fisheries and Food; Professor Robert Clark of the University of Newcastle; Professor Anders Green of Odense University; Mrs Janet Groves of Lanes Ltd; Dr Graham Hughes of St Thomas's Hospital, London; Dr John Hunter of Addenbrooke's Hospital, Cambridge; Dr Laura Itzhaki of the University of Cambridge; Dr Martin Leighfield of Queen Elizabeth Hospital for Children, London; Dr Mikko T. Nenonen of Kuopio University, Finland; Professor Richard S. Panush of St Barnabas Medical Centre, New Jersey; Dr Ray Rice of the Fish Foundation; Mrs Rebecca Sewell of the Dunn Nutrition Unit Library, Cambridge; Dr Bonnie Sibbald of the University of Manchester; Dr Lars Skoldstam of Kalmar Hospital, Sweden; Dr Norman Staines of King's College London; Dr G.R Struthers of Coventry and Warwickshire Hospital, and the many hundreds of other doctors and medical researchers whose published work has contributed to the information reported in these pages.

Many thanks also to Mary Verdut for translations from German, to Hayley Kerr for her excellent typing, to my agent Bill Hamilton for his continuing support and encouragement, and to Robert Sackville-West for keeping me afloat financially during this very long project.

Finally, a special thank-you to editor Joanna Sheehan for her tremendous patience, and her commitment to the highest possible standards in preparing this book for press.

FOREWORD

· *The Young Ballerina – How It All Began* ·

As a consultant rheumatologist, working at Epsom General Hospital in the south of England, I regard myself as an ordinary doctor practising in much the same way as other rheumatologists do. Where I differ from many orthodox rheumatologists is in using dietary treatments as well.

It all began in 1980, when a very pretty, fourteen-year-old girl came into my clinic with her mother, referred by the family doctor because she suffered from incipient rheumatoid arthritis. She was a graceful youngster, slim and dainty, with long chestnut-coloured hair. Her greatest love was ballet, and she could still dance beautifully at that time, but over the coming months her painful and swollen joints made dancing increasingly difficult, and she finally had to give up.

She had very severe rheumatoid disease and, in spite of my best efforts, I could only partially control her symptoms with the drugs available. There was a steady downhill progress, and it seemed that she would, before long, be seriously disabled. I felt greatly saddened by the fact that I could not help her more.

One day the girl's mother telephoned me and asked whether I would object to their seeing another doctor, one in private practice, who would try to treat the rheumatoid arthritis with a diet. I replied that, in my opinion, it wouldn't do any good, but that I was happy for her to try the diet as long as she kept on taking her drugs as well and for her to come back to see me if and when diet didn't help.

Three months later, to my great surprise, the girl returned – not entering my consulting room slowly and painfully as before, but breezing in, wearing jodhpurs and having just returned from a riding holiday. The contrast between her state of health then and three months earlier was astounding.

My orthodox training told me that she had gone into an episode of spontaneous remission, as sometimes happens in rheumatoid arthritis. Nevertheless, since she had been deteriorating steadily for the previous six months a spontaneous remission seemed unlikely, and I decided to find out more about the doctor who had treated her and the dietary treatment he had used. Meanwhile I suggested that the girl stay on the diet *and* keep to her drugs.

I telephoned Dr John Mansfield, who had put her on the diet, and asked for more information. With great professional generosity he invited me to a working lunch and explained his diet – an 'elimination diet' as he called it – in some detail. To my orthodox medical ears it sounded fairly strange but I was interested enough to try it with some of my patients. I arranged a pilot study in which twenty patients suffering from rheumatoid arthritis would go through his elimination diet and I would analyse the results using standard scientific methods. The results amazed me: of the twenty patients about a third showed a significant improvement, and in a very short space of time.

I have now been working with this particular form of diet for almost fourteen years, and have carried out scientific research, published in *The Lancet* and elsewhere, which confirms its benefit for a certain percentage of patients.

But in spite of my long involvement with studies of diet and arthritis, I am in no way a propagandist for the elimination diet. I merely think that it is an area which needs to be investigated in just as scientific a way as we look at Drug A versus Drug B. I shall continue to do that in the future, and to investigate other forms of dietary therapy, if these seem potentially worthwhile, so that patients may have well-researched guidance in their efforts to help themselves by dietary means.

Dr Gail Darlington
Epsom General Hospital

Note:
In this book 'we' is used in two different senses. For the most part it refers to the two authors, and expresses their joint opinions. However, in some parts of the book, where research carried out at Epsom General Hospital is being described, 'we' refers to Dr Gail Darlington, Dr Norman Ramsay, and others involved in the research.

The authors would be interested to hear from readers who have tried any of the dietary measures suggested in this book, with details of their response to the dietary change. Please write to Linda Gamlin, c/o Ebury Press, Random House, 20 Vauxhall Bridge Road, London SW1V 2SA. Doctors and medical researchers requiring referenced versions of any part of this book may write to the same address. Dr Darlington regrets that she cannot offer individual advice to readers, nor accept new patients.

INTRODUCTION

· *Why Choose This Book?* ·

If you are considering a dietary treatment for your arthritis, you will not be short of advice. A glance at the titles on sale in any bookshop reveals a bewildering range of dietary prescriptions, while family and friends will probably have their own well-meaning suggestions about what foods to avoid or what supplements to take.

Wherever there is a great human need or an unsolved problem, apparent solutions to that problem will spring up and be acclaimed a success – at least for a while. Miracle diets for arthritis, are, we would suggest, rather like treatments that supposedly prevent wrinkles, reverse the ageing process or cure baldness: however unlikely they are to work, people will go on trying them and believing in them. The fact that there are so many different popular diets for arthritis suggests that they cannot possibly all be right. Indeed, some give entirely contradictory advice.

The different kinds of arthritis

Common sense can help with assessing some of these conflicting claims. To begin with, if this book were called *How to Grow Vegetables* you would no doubt expect it to give specific advice on different kinds of vegetable crops – after all, cabbages, potatoes, beans, tomatoes, lettuces and carrots each have to be sown at specific times and require very different growing conditions. If the book spoke only of 'vegetables' all the way through, and gave the same blanket advice for all of them, anyone who knew even a little bit about gardening would regard it with scepticism.

There are almost as many different kinds of arthritis as there are vegetables – and they are very different in their origins, their causes and their response to diet – but strangely, most popular books on diet and arthritis speak simply of 'arthritis'. And they offer all arthritis sufferers the same dietary advice. This alone should be enough to make any reader wary.

This book is different. It gives specific advice for each of the many different forms of arthritis. It also aims to cover *all* the different kinds of arthritis and *all* the different types of diet – a very tall order!

But there are several things the book does not do. In particular, it does not make false promises. It does not imply that, whatever your type of arthritis, if you follow our dietary advice you will soon be completely cured. Any book which makes such promises is simply preying on the arthritis sufferer and selling false hopes, just as the sellers of patent medicines used to do in the nineteenth century.

The advice in this book, if followed carefully, could help some readers a great deal. Some people do reap enormous benefits from dietary treatment, returning to their former state of health and staying there – a change that can seem little short of miraculous, especially if they have been seriously disabled by their disease.

These are the lucky ones, and you *could* be among them. But it is certainly not going to happen for everyone. Other readers will feel a moderate benefit or a few small improvements. Some may find that they need to take fewer drugs. And finally, there will be some readers will have no change at all – but they will at least have the peace of mind of knowing that they have tried out dietary treatment in the best possible way.

This is an honest and realistic assessment of what you might expect to gain from following our advice. Beware of any book, practitioner or potion offering *all* arthritis sufferers a total, lifelong, guaranteed cure!

But I hate science!

Please don't be put off by the scientific content of this book. If you don't want to read it you don't have to – the book is designed so that the practical advice – all given in Chapters 2.2–2.8 (pp.143–272) – is virtually science-free.

So why is the science there in the rest of the book? Firstly, because some patients *do* want to know all the whys and wherefores of their disease, and of the dietary treatments available. Secondly, because science (sometimes of a very garbled kind) is commonly used to give a mantle of credibility to all sorts of unproven diets and other treatments. Most of the popular books on diet and arthritis use some scientific terms and ideas, usually in a very confused and misleading way. We are offering something better.

If you find yourself baffled by the talk of acids, calcification and antioxidants in other books and magazine articles, you can turn to these pages for the facts. (Unfortunately the facts tend to be rather more complex than the simplistic falsehoods served up elsewhere, but that is in the nature of facts.) But if you simply want straightforward advice, you can ignore these sections altogether.

· *Different Ways to Use This Book* ·

There are several different ways in which you can use this book. If you simply want practical advice on your diet, then turn straight to Section 2. Use the A–Z directory in Chapter 2.1 (see p.79) to look up the particular form of arthritis from which you suffer. (If you're not sure of the exact diagnosis, check with your doctor.)

There should be an entry that applies to you in the A–Z, however unusual your form of arthritis. (If there is not, then you should check with your doctor for a more accurate and up-to-date diagnosis.) You can, if you like, skip the first part of the entry (the symptoms and causes) and go straight to the last part of the entry, which lists the dietary measures recommended for this form of arthritis. That will guide you to the chapters in Section 2 that are relevant.

Section 1 of the book is for anyone who is interested in knowing more about diet and arthritis, particularly about why it is so controversial. It describes the new discoveries in this field, such as the elimination diet and the anti-inflammatory properties of certain oils. It looks at why there are so many different popular diets available and it tackles the question of why diet has yet to be accepted by most members of the medical profession as a valid treatment for some patients with arthritis.

Section 2, as we have already said, contains all the practical advice on treating arthritis by dietary means.

Section 3 looks at vitamins, minerals and other nutrients in some detail. It is a section that you can dip into as and when you need it.

Section 4 provides basic information on the many other dietary treatments and 'nutritional supplements' that you may read about in the press, come across in a health food shop, or be recommended by friends. It should help you to make an informed judgment about these diets and products, and decide whether you want to try them or not. It also details any risks that might be associated with these diets.

We must emphasise, at this point, that you should not start a diet without first talking to your doctor. If you intend to use this book as your guide, please read all the relevant chapters first and then ask your doctor's advice. It may help to show your doctor the diet guidelines included here. The reaction to your enquiry may be unenthusiastic, or even hostile, but if you have read Section 1 you will be in a good position to discuss the issues involved and to participate in an intelligent joint decision. *Should you be advised that a diet might damage your general health, please follow that advice and do not try the diet.*

New Light on Diet and Arthritis

Chapter 1.1

DIET AND ARTHRITIS: FACT, FICTION AND CONTROVERSY

'7.30 am: While still in bed, the patient should have a cup of milk, with a dessert-spoonful of whisky, brandy, or other stimulant, or with a small quantity of tea, cocoa, and a small piece of bread, toast, or biscuit.'

'8.30–9 am: Breakfast of milk, with a little tea, coffee, or cocoa, toast or bread and butter, bacon, ham, fish, or eggs.'

'11 am: A tumblerful of milk, a cup of broth or beef-tea, or a sandwich, and a glass of wine.'

'1–1.30 pm: A substantial meal of meat, poultry, fish, or game, with fresh vegetables, some light pudding or cooked fruit, and a glass of wine or malt liquor.'

'4 pm: A glass of milk with a small quantity of tea, coffee, or cocoa, and some bread and butter or a plain biscuit.'

'7 pm: Another substantial meal similar to the midday one.'

'9.30–10 pm: A cup of milk, or bread and milk, or milk with some farinaceous food.'

If the thought of this rich diet (recommended for rheumatoid arthritis sufferers in 1906) makes you feel a little queasy, then here is a more modern alternative, known as a 'living food' diet and likewise recommended for those with arthritis. The daily menu could include any of the following, prepared with a blender or liquidiser where necessary, but with no cooking or heating of any item:

Bread substitute made of sprouted wheat, apple and water.
Butter substitute made of almonds and the water from fermented cucumbers.
Cheese substitute made from fermented sesame seed, and sunflower seeds.

A yoghurt substitute made of fermented oats.
Fermented drink made of sprouted wheat, rye and water.
Lentil sprouts.
Buckwheat-beetroot cutlets.
Stew made of sprouted buckwheat, raw carrot, fermented cucumber and raw, red cabbage.
Soup made with cabbage juice, avocado, raw courgettes and comfrey leaves.
Seaweed rolls.

There is not much in common between these two diets and while they are extreme examples, they illustrate the point that just about *anything* in the dietary line has, at some time, been recommended for arthritic patients. Among the popular diet books that you might find on a library shelf today, one forbids all milk products on the grounds that they 'cause mucus formation and deposits of calcium' which 'lead to arthritis', while another book orders the arthritic to drink a glass of full-cream milk before every meal, and to eat plenty of butter, because milk-fat and butter 'lubricate the joints'.

Hardly surprising, then, that when most doctors are questioned about diet by an arthritic patient, they reply (often in an emphatic and exasperated tone) 'Nothing whatever to do with it – just eat a sensible, balanced diet'.

To describe the topic of diet and arthritis as a jungle is somewhat unfair to jungles. There is probably more controversy, mis-understanding and conflicting advice about this subject than any other medical issue. The 'diet jungle' is one that most orthodox rheumatologists stay out of because the tangled complexities are far too daunting, and besides, few previous explorers have returned with their medical credibility intact. Yet we believe there is a way through this jungle, and that many of the earlier discoveries and claims about diet – even if they seem to be totally at odds with each other – can now be reconciled and explained.

With that explanation there comes the possibility of effective dietary treatment at least for some arthritic patients. The main treatment in question, the elimination diet (which is described later in this chapter) has been shown to help a great many patients with rheumatoid arthritis. In our experience, about 36% of those patients may do so well with this form of dietary treatment that they are able to stop taking drugs for several years, some indefinitely (see p.33). That is a remarkable level of improvement by anyone's standard. It would be right to be sceptical of such claims if they were unsubstantiated –

but they are not. They are backed up by hard evidence, obtained from a well-conducted, rigorous scientific trial (described in full on pp.26–29).

Before going any further it is important to emphasise that *we are not talking about all types of arthritis here*. In this particular chapter, for the most part, we are only discussing rheumatoid arthritis (see p.129) and the condition known as episodic arthritis or 'palindromic rheumatism' (see p.122), in which there are fairly short episodes of arthritis separated by periods of good health.

Some of those with 'palindromic rheumatism' – roughly a third of patients – go on to develop rheumatoid arthritis. Moreover, people with 'palindromic rheumatism' tend to respond to our dietary programme in a similar way to patients with rheumatoid arthritis, so it is reasonable to bracket these two diseases together here. In this chapter, we will use the term **'rheumatoid-like arthritis'** for these diseases, and for cases where rheumatoid arthritis is suspected but has not yet been confirmed.

The possible relevance of diet to other forms of arthritis, and to simple arthralgia (joint pain with no definable cause) is discussed under the individual headings for those diseases in Chapter 2.1 (p.79).

· *Professor Epstein's Story* ·

'On November 21, 1968 the patient could not resist temptation, and ate about 30 gm of his favourite Cervelat sausage. Twenty-six hours later, slight discomfort appeared in the right heel, followed successively by considerable pain of the joints of the hands and feet, elbows and left calf.' So runs a slightly eccentric research paper, published in 1969 by Professor Stephan Epstein, then a dermatologist at the University of Wisconsin.

Professor Epstein was afflicted by 'palindromic rheumatism' which had begun when he was 65 and had continued for four years. Sometimes just a few joints were involved, with the pain moving from one joint to another. In more severe attacks, the majority of his joints were painful.

The attacks lasted between one and ten days, and had been increasing in duration and frequency. Professor Epstein suspected that foods were at the root of his attacks and embarked on a programme of detective work to see if he could identify the culprits. At first, a great many different meats and vegetables seemed to be responsible, but in time he realised there was a link between many of them: they tended to be foods containing nitrate, the traditional preservative used to make bacon, ham and frankfurters. Nitrates are also applied to fields as fertilisers, and they occur as pollutants in drinking water and sometimes as residues in crops such as tomatoes, spinach, lettuce and green beans. Eventually, he concluded that there were only two different substances which triggered his attacks: sodium nitrate and peppermint oil.

These were rather odd substances for anyone to be sensitive to, and Professor Epstein was cautious about his discovery. Being a scientist, he decided to go one step further and try his suspects 'blind'. He asked a pharmacist to prepare capsules containing sodium nitrate, capsules containing peppermint oil, and dummy capsules containing an inert substance. All the capsules looked the same and each bottle was labelled with a code number only, so Professor Epstein had no idea which was which. He took them in a random order, over a period of weeks, and noted his reaction to each. Once he had tested all the capsules, he asked the pharmacist to tell him which capsule had contained which substance. The answers confirmed that he had reacted only to nitrate and peppermint, not to the dummy capsules.

The object of blind testing (which is a part of any good scientific study) is to distinguish genuine reactions to food from **psychogenic reactions**. The power of the human imagination is such that, if someone believes they are sensitive to a particular food, they may react to it anyway, even if that belief is false. If the dummy capsules sometimes produce strong reactions, and the genuine capsules sometimes fail to provoke symptoms, then a psychogenic reaction must be suspected. (The technical name for the dummy capsules is a **placebo**, something which we will describe in more detail later.)

Professor Epstein knew that he, as much as anyone else, could be susceptible to psychogenic reactions, but the blind testing showed that his responses to nitrates and peppermint were genuine. Armed with this knowledge, he was able to overcome his palindromic rheumatism. By eating unfertilised garden-grown vegetables, avoiding bacon, ham and various types of sausage, and staying off peppermints, Professor Epstein suffered no further attacks of arthritis.

· *The Tale of a Cheese-aholic* ·

It is not often that the word 'passion' creeps into the austere pages of the *British Medical Journal*, but here it is, in a paper published in June 1981: 'Since her early 20s the patient had had a passion for cheese, consuming up to 0.4 kg (1 lb) a day.'

The patient in question had severe erosive rheumatoid arthritis affecting many joints. It had begun when she was 27, and had been getting steadily worse for the past eleven years. She was very pale, in constant pain, became exhausted quickly, and had morning stiffness of the joints lasting for several hours. Looking after her three children was becoming increasingly difficult.

A variety of drugs had been tried but the patient reacted badly to most of them. Only a corticosteroid was of any help, and even on this powerful drug her symptoms were getting steadily worse.

She was admitted to Hammersmith Hospital in West London for a while, and the doctors treating her there were struck by the enormous amount of cheese she was eating. While they were as sceptical as most doctors about any role for food in rheumatoid arthritis, they asked the patient, as an experiment, to stop eating cheese, milk, butter and any other dairy products. To their surprise, after three weeks she began to feel less pain, some of the joint swelling decreased, and her morning stiffness passed more quickly. Over the months that followed, the improvements continued. After five months she had almost fully recovered, could walk normally again and had only the slightest hint of arthritis left in her joints. She was able to stop taking corticosteroid drugs. This was a stunning improvement in someone who had been so severely ill. Laboratory tests also improved, confirming the recovery that was clearly visible to patient and doctors alike.

It is well known that rheumatoid arthritis is a fluctuating disease, and most patients have periods when they are somewhat better, and periods when they feel worse. Occasionally patients with rheumatoid arthritis do shake the disease off completely, for no apparent reason. This phenomenon, known as **spontaneous remission**, is more common among those with mild rheumatoid arthritis that has begun relatively recently. It is rarer among those with severe long-standing disease, such as this patient, although it can happen.

Had a spontaneous remission occurred in this patient, which just happened to coincide with her change of diet? A temporary setback in her recovery made this seem unlikely: she had been making steady progress, with all her joints improving, when she inadvertently ate some food containing milk. Within twelve hours her joints had become painful and swollen again.

This was interesting evidence, but the doctors needed to test their patient more formally. Once she had been consistently well for over five months the doctors asked if she would agree to be 'challenged' with cheese and milk. Admitted to hospital, the former 'cheese-aholic' was encouraged to go back to her old ways and over three days she consumed 1.4 kg (3 lb) of cheddar and drank seven pints of milk. The reaction began within 24 hours and built up to a severe attack of rheumatoid arthritis. Her joints became swollen and painful, her morning stiffness returned, and the laboratory tests all changed dramatically. Certain tests, which looked for **antibodies** (see p.412) to the foods, showed that she reacted to both cheese and milk, but far more strongly to cheese. The patient returned to her dairy-free diet thereafter, and within a few weeks the symptoms subsided.

This was not a 'blind' food challenge tests (see p.18), since the patient knew she was eating milk and cheese, but the study was accepted as a valid one despite this. There were several reasons for such acceptance. Firstly, the patient showed such a dramatic improvement on removing cheese and milk from her diet, despite the fact that she greatly missed these favourite foods – not a likely scenario for a psychogenic improvement. Secondly, she suffered such a severe and prolonged relapse, with clearly visible joint inflammation, when the foods were returned, that the response was unlikely to be a psychological one. Finally, and most convincingly, blood tests made after the food challenge revealed unusual antibodies to cheese and milk of a kind that are typical of allergic reactions, known as **IgE antibodies**. (The significance of these is discussed in more detail on p.40, but it is worth noting here that most arthritics who are food-sensitive do *not* show IgE antibodies to the culprit food.)

After publishing their research paper, the doctors decided to repeat their tests using cheese or milk contained in capsules, and the patient responded in the same way. There was no response to dummy capsules.

· *Another Three Cases* ·

Whenever scientific reviews are written on diet and arthritis they usually include the case-studies of Professor Epstein and the 'cheese-aholic' described above. These are known in the trade as **anecdotal evidence** – each is a one-off study of a single patient. Not much weight is attached to this kind of evidence because every patient is different, especially in a variable disease such as rheumatoid arthritis, so it is impossible to extrapolate from one patient to all other patients who nominally have the 'same' disease. Nevertheless, such case studies are of interest. There are about a dozen more in the scientific literature describing an improvement in rheumatoid arthritis when specific foods are omitted from the diet.

Unlike isolated case-studies, more thorough investigations, involving larger numbers of patients do carry some weight with doctors and medical researchers.

One such study involved patients who *believed* they were affected by food, and tested them with the suspect food in capsules to see how they reacted. The trial was carried out by Professor Richard S. Panush, then at the University of Florida, who had found that, among the patients in his rheumatology clinic, about 30% maintained that they were affected by certain foods. He selected a group of these who all had 'rheumatoid-like arthritis' (see p.17) and chose sixteen suitable candidates for further investigation.

Initially, they were fed an **elemental diet**, which is a powdered food that makes a meal-in-a-cup when mixed with water, and which provides all the calories, vitamins and minerals required. It is manufactured from natural foodstuffs, but these are treated so that the protein molecules in them (the parts most likely to spark off food sensitivity) break down into smaller fragments. In theory, when broken down, the molecules should no longer provoke the same reaction. By living solely on an elemental diet, someone who is sensitive to certain foods is given a 'holiday' from those foods. There is no need to know exactly which foods are causing problems as long as *everything* else is avoided – only the elemental diet is consumed. For those who are sensitive to food, symptoms usually clear up while they are on an elemental diet, and this happened for most of those studied by Professor Panush.

Once the patients were established on the elemental diet, Professor Panush then tested them with the foodstuff which they suspected of causing their arthritic symptoms. The food was always given in capsules so that the patient could not taste it, but enough capsules were given to provide a normal, meal-sized portion. At times, Professor Panush tested the patients with dummy 'placebo' capsules which contained an inert powder. The patients did not know which capsules were which, nor did those administering the capsules and assessing the patients' symptoms.

This type of study is known as a **double-blind trial** because both the patients *and* those directly studying them are unaware of which substance is which. As you might guess from this, doctors can be victims of their imagination, just as much as patients, and when assessing a patient's symptoms they could be influenced by their own expectations. The double-blind trial is intended to prevent any unintentional bias.

The power of psychogenic reactions (see p.18) was well illustrated by one of the patients in Professor Panush's study, who thought he was sensitive to milk. During testing with capsules, taken three times a day, he reported suffering far more severe morning stiffness on day one, day three and day five, with much less morning stiffness on the intervening days. After day five, his morning stiffness was greatly reduced. He reported most tender joints on the first day of testing, and felt generally better towards the end of the testing period. In fact he had been given nothing but dummy capsules for the first eight days of testing, followed by milk capsules only from days nine to eleven. It was during the earliest tests, when the patient suspected that he might be getting milk capsules and dummy capsules on alternate days, that he showed the greatest responses, whereas the least response came towards the end of the testing period when he really was being given milk capsules.

Of the sixteen patients tested, only three actually responded to their suspect foods, and all three were among those suffering from 'palindromic rheumatism'. One of these patients was affected by shrimps, a second by milk, and a third by nitrates. These three patients consistently responded to the test capsules and failed to show any reaction to the dummy capsules.

· *Rare or Common?* ·

If these three research papers identify food as a factor in five patients with 'rheumatoid-like arthritis', then why does the average family doctor or rheumatologist firmly reply '*Nothing* whatever to do with it!' when asked about diet and arthritis?

In part, it is because doctors believe that the five patients described in these papers are highly unusual cases – exceptions to the rule. Bear in mind, that the three patients with verifiable food problems in Professor Panush's study were the minority – for another thirteen who firmly believed they had a food problem, nothing could be confirmed by tests with food in capsules. (How this might have happened is discussed on p.34.)

Then again, the doctor has no idea what you mean by 'diet' when you pose your question. You might have been reading about a vegetarian or vegan diet, a no-nightshades diet, or the special diets proposed by Dr Collin Dong or Dr Giraud Campbell (all described in Section 4). These diets prohibit certain foods (they are 'avoidance diets') but the list of prohibited foods differs substantially from one diet to another.

On the other hand, the doctor might think that you mean the kind of diet that advocates taking cider-vinegar and honey, or blackstrap molasses, kelp, alfalfa tablets or cod liver oil. These we call 'supplemented diets'. Then there is a third type of diet that combines both approaches: the 'avoid-and-supplement' diets such as that of Sister Margaret Hills or Dr D. C. Jarvis (see Section 4).

Every one of these diets is radically different, and the 'explanations' of how they work, as given by their proponents, are frequently contradictory, and, in some cases, quite baffling and bizarre. Your doctor is unlikely to have the time or inclination to get into a discussion about these different diets.

As your doctor firmly dismisses the idea of diet and arthritis, he or she may be recalling Professor Panush's conclusion that, at the very most, only 5% of patients with rheumatoid-like arthritis can be helped by avoiding certain foods. (We will come back to the 5% estimate, and how it was arrived at, later.) Rather than have you waste time and money messing about with diets, and run the risk of malnutrition into the bargain, your doctor may think it better to assume that you are one of the 95% for whom diet is irrelevant.

If you refer back to the beginning of this chapter you will see that our claims are very different. We have stated that many patients with rheumatoid arthritis may be helped to some extent by a change of diet, with up to 36% being so much better that they may be able to come off all drugs. This is a key part of the controversy over diet and arthritis: is it unusual for patients with rheumatoid-like arthritis to improve when certain foods are removed from their diet, or is it a fairly common phenomenon? To put the question another way, are the cases described so far in this chapter exceptions to the rule – or the tip of an iceberg? We would suggest that food reactions are fairly common among patients with rheumatoid arthritis, but that they are rarely detected either by doctors or by the patients themselves.

Why should they so often go undetected? The answers to this question, based on many years' experience in the use of diets with arthritic patients, are as follows:

Firstly, most patients who can benefit need to avoid *more than one* food. A bad reaction to three, four or more foods is common, and some arthritics react to as many as 15 different foods. The patient who is only affected by milk and cheese, or only by shrimps, or by nitrates and peppermint is a rarity. Noticing sensitivity to one food is relatively easy, especially if it is something eaten as rarely as shrimps or peppermint. Noticing a sensitivity to several foods is far more difficult.

Secondly, the reactions in the joints are not instantaneous: someone who is affected by milk does not usually experience a reaction within minutes of drinking milk. The reaction can take hours to begin, sometimes a day or more. Remember that the Cervelat sausage took 26 hours to affect Professor Epstein (see p.17) – this is unusually slow, but it illustrates the point. Nor do the reactions fade quickly. They tend to reach a peak in about 24–48 hours and may then take several days to wear off.

Thirdly, foods eaten regularly or in excess are common offenders. Staple foods such as milk, wheat, eggs and oranges are very likely to be culprits, or it can be any other food that the individual is excessively fond of. The cheese-aholic (see p.24) was not unusual in apparently being 'addicted' to the food that caused her symptoms.

Fourthly, an adverse reaction to food tends to develop slowly, over a period of years. Notice that the cheese-aholic began her 'passion for cheese' in her early 20s, but did not develop rheumatoid arthritis until she was 27. Most people do not suspect a food of causing problems if they were previously eating it for years with impunity.

Put these four factors together and it is easy to see how sensitivity to food goes unnoticed. Imagine a patient with rheumatoid arthritis who is sensitive to three or more foods, common foods that are eaten every day or several times a day. The foods were part of their diet long before the rheumatoid arthritis developed. The symptoms that are now provoked by these foods appear some time after the food is eaten and last for many hours, maybe days. Clearly, the patient is in a state of reaction to the foods *for all or most of the time* – the effects of breakfast run together with the effects of lunch, and the effects of lunch with those of supper. The patient probably does not notice the link with food, and the doctor (who is sceptical about diet-and-arthritis anyway) certainly does not.

The isolated cases that surface in the medical literature tend to be those where someone reacts to a *single* food, and they are frequently patients with 'palindromic rheumatism', where the arthritis occurs in discrete episodes. Patients with palindromic rheumatism are obviously more likely to wonder if foods are connected with the episodes, and they have a far easier task in identifying the food.

The evidence for these claims is examined on pp.26–34. Before considering that evidence, it is necessary to explain how a link between food and rheumatoid arthritis, assuming one exists, can be revealed in the individual patient. Given the four factors that obscure this link, it is clearly not an easy matter to identify offending foods, and careful detective work is needed. That detective work follows a standard pattern, known as an **elimination diet**.

· *The Elimination Diet* ·

At present, the elimination diet is the only form of diagnosis that can reveal if someone's arthritis is related to food. It is important to stress that there are no alternatives – no short-cuts or quick diagnostic tests. Certainly there are other methods offered, at a price, by various practitioners. Some analyse hair samples or blood samples, others will take your pulse, test muscle reactions or even swing pendulums over a list of foods to discover which ones affect you! But the combined experience of doctors working in this field is that the quick tests either do not work at all, or are far too unreliable.

The idea of the elimination diet is simplicity itself: the patient stops eating almost everything they normally eat for a while and lives on a small range of rarely eaten foods (the **exclusion phase**). During the exclusion phase, which usually lasts 7–10 days, there should be some noticeable improvement in the arthritis if the patient is one of those affected by food. The patient then tests single foods, one by one, to see which ones cause symptoms (the **reintroduction phase**). For those patients who show no improvement at all and no marked reactions to foods during the first three weeks, the diet is abandoned without completing the reintroduction phase.

Any foods that provoke reactions during the reintroduction phase are identified as culprit foods and avoided thereafter. Years of work with rheumatoid arthritis patients have shown that the list of culprit foods is rarely the same from one patient to the next (although certain foods do crop up far more often than others – see p.71). In other words, everyone who successfully completes the elimination diet finishes up with a tailor-made personal diet. With other avoidance diets, such as the published form of Dr Dong's diet, the same diet is given to everyone. Those patients who recover on Dr Dong's diet (and other avoidance diets) are almost certainly avoiding some foods unecessarily, because the diet is a same-for-everyone diet, not a tailor-made one.

While the idea of the elimination diet is simple, in practice it requires some expert guidance – and it takes quite a bit of commitment, intelligence and resourcefulness on the part of the patient. *This is not an easy option.* If you are considering this diet, please do not embark on it half-heartedly or without forward planning. It would be helpful for you to read the rest of this chapter first, and Chapter 2.4 (p.170) *in full* before starting. You must also have your doctor's blessing because the diet is not advisable for everyone. It can be too arduous for those who are severely ill or underweight.

Putting the elimination diet to the test

In the rheumatology clinic at Epsom General Hospital in Surrey, England, the elimination diet has been part of our treatment programme for over 10 years. We use it mainly for those with rheumatoid arthritis although from time to time we have tried it with other forms of arthritis as well.

After a pilot study with twenty patients, it seemed essential to conduct a rigorous scientific trial of the treatment. Because the trial was dealing with such a controversial treatment, special care was taken to make it 'bullet-proof' – able to withstand the sternest scientific criticism. Two medical statisticians and one specialist in experimental design helped to check the plans for the study, and they confirmed that it was a good design. Dr John Mansfield, who has many years experience with elimination diets, assisted with the trial, as did Dr Norman Ramsey, a medical physicist, who gave invaluable help in recording and assessing changes in the patients' symptoms. The results were published in *The Lancet* in February 1986.

Forty-four patients, all suffering from rheumatoid arthritis, actually completed the full trial. All these patients carried out an elimination diet, although half of them underwent six weeks of a placebo treatment (see p.27) first, so that the results could be compared with the diet.

After the dietary treatment, 36% of patients described themselves as being 'much better', 39% rated themselves as 'better', while a quarter thought they were the same or worse. More specific and objective measurements confirmed these results. They showed that the diet produced a far greater improvement than the placebo treatment. It resulted in less pain, fewer inflamed joints, greater grip strength, and a far shorter period of morning stiffness. Several of the laboratory tests that assess disease activity also showed better results after the diet.

Understanding placebos

Psychogenic improvements are still an important part of medical treatment, but before the mid-nineteenth century, when medical knowledge was scanty and effective medicines few, they were probably the *major* part. In those days, doctors often prescribed useless sugar pills to keep their patients happy, with remarkably good effects, and such pills became known as placebos from the Latin word meaning 'I shall please'. Sugar pills pleased the patient and produced a modest, though temporary, improvement. When the **placebo effect** began to fade, as it does after a few months, sugar pills of a different colour might then be prescribed, producing a new surge of placebo effect.

Placebo reactions have now been extensively studied in the hope of improving the objective assessment of new treatments. It is important to show that a new drug has real merit in itself and is not just producing a placebo effect. Research has shown that capsules have a greater placebo effect than tablets, and injections are more powerful still. In the case of capsules or tablets, the colour and size make a difference. Of particular interest is the discovery that *any* kind of treatment (including going on a diet) has some placebo effect. Even seeing a doctor and simply talking gives some such benefit, provided the doctor is sufficiently kind and encouraging. Where the drug or other treatment is actually beneficial in itself, the placebo effect adds to that benefit.

In any rigorous scientific trial, a new treatment is compared with a **placebo treatment**, so that the placebo effect can be measured and then 'deducted' from the total benefit seen with the treatment. If the new treatment is a drug, then that drug and the placebo are packaged in identical capsules. There are usually two groups of patients, one taking the new drug, the other taking a placebo. The group taking the placebo is known as the **control group**, and the trial is called a placebo-controlled trial. When neither doctor nor patient know which capsule is which – see p.21 – then this is called a **double-blind placebo controlled trial**. It is the Gold Standard of medical research.

Suppose that, on a scale of one to ten, the average improvement of those receiving the new treatment scores five, while the average improvement of the group taking the placebo is two. Then the degree of improvement attributable to the treatment alone is rated at three. Complex statistical analyses are used to look at the scatter of individual values about the average for each group. By assessing this scatter, a statistician can then check whether the difference in averages between the patients taking the treatment and those taking the placebo is large enough to be taken seriously, or whether it is just a matter of chance. If there is a real difference the result is said to be 'statistically significant'.

In a scientific trial, treatments have to be as uniform as possible, so we standardised the programme for the elimination diet a little. Normally, patients who do not improve during the first three weeks of the elimination diet are advised to abandon it, but for this trial we asked everyone to carry out a full reintroduction phase, regardless of whether they were better or not.

We then considered the groups *as a whole* when assessing their improvement at the end of the elimination diet, rather than looking at how well individuals had done. In other words, we took a standard measurement such as grip strength, then worked out the average improvement in grip strength for the whole group on the diet, or the whole group on the placebo treatment.

This meant that we were lumping together those who did well on the diet with those who showed no benefit from it. This was to the disadvantage of the diet, because the pilot study had shown that it worked splendidly for some people and not at all for others. But we hoped that the diet could overcome this handicap – as indeed it did. The improvements were statistically significant when assessed for the group as a whole. (If we disregarded the quarter of patients who had not responded to the diet, and just analysed the average symptoms of those who were 'better' or 'much better', the improvement was even more striking.)

Lumping everyone together was a necessary step to compensate for the possibility of some patients experiencing spontaneous remissions (see p.19) or partial remissions during the time they were on the diet. We needed to show that any improvement in those on the diet was more than just a temporary, spontaneous improvement – an upswing that would have happened anyway and had nothing to do with the diet. One way to show this would be to monitor the patients for two years or more as we do with patients who attend the clinic ordinarily – some have now been followed up for twelve years and they remain well on their restricted diets (see p.33). However, in an experimental trial, long-term monitoring is very difficult and expensive – and it delays publication of the results. It made more sense for us to have a reasonably large number of patients in each group, and to average all their results together – that way, the spontaneous improvements of some patients should be outweighed by the spontaneous deterioration in other patients.

As a final check on the validity of the results, we looked at the question of weight loss. On average, the patients lost 4.7 kg (10.4 lbs). Losing weight takes the load off joints such as the knees and ankles, and can lessen the pain in these joints, but it is not thought to have any more general effects on rheumatoid arthritis.

Our study showed that the diet produced improvements in non-weight-bearing joints such as those in the hands (hence greater grip strength) as well as a general calming of the disease process (as shown by laboratory tests). So while it seemed most unlikely that weight loss explained all the improvements achieved by the diet, we needed to be absolutely sure that it did not do so. We, therefore, compared the weight loss of the three-quarters of patients who were better or much better, with the weight loss of the quarter who were the same or worse after the diet. There was no significant difference. Nor did the 36% of patients who felt very much better and had the greatest improvement in measurable symptoms – the '**good responders**' – show any excessive weight loss.

· *One Swallow Doesn't Make A Summer* ·

You may well ask why, if this trial produced such good results, the medical establishment has not been converted to the use of elimination diets for patients with rheumatoid arthritis? Well, just as 'one swallow doesn't make a summer', one research paper does not produce a medical revolution.

Rheumatologists and other doctors practising today have been trained to believe that the whole idea of diet affecting arthritis is nonsense – except in the very special case of gout (see Chapter 2.7–p.242). Ideas which are drummed in so firmly while at medical school are not likely to be ousted by a single piece of research.

An individually adjusted diet

One other trial has produced a very good result by means of an elimination diet, but unfortunately this fact has been overlooked because the research was published under the rather misleading title '*Controlled trial of fasting and one-year vegetarian diet in rheumatoid arthritis*'. The research team, led by Dr Jens Kjeldsen-Kragh of the University of Oslo, based their diet regime on one used by a Norwegian health farm which claimed success in treating rheumatoid arthritis. It is an excellent study, but the title does not really describe the diet fully.

Patients spent the first month of the trial at the health farm, and ate nothing for the the first 7–10 days, apart from herb teas and vegetable juices. After the fast, *one food item was introduced to their diet every two days*. If there was any increase in joint swelling, pain or stiffness the food was avoided thereafter. The only foods that were never reintroduced were meat and fish.

The patients were monitored for a full year, and compared with a control group who had spent the first month at a convalescent home (a placebo treatment intended to match the month-long stay at the health farm). The diet group (assessed as a whole) were significantly better than the control group in terms of pain, numbers of swollen and tender joints, grip strength and general well-being. Laboratory tests told the same story.

Some patients – 44% of the total diet group – had responded substantially better than others. These 'good responders' accounted for much of the overall improvement of the diet group.

There is no doubt in our minds that what this study used was an elimination diet, with the partial fast at the beginning equivalent to our exclusion phase. Indeed, Dr Kjeldsen-Kragh describes the ultimate diet of the patients as an 'individually adjusted diet' and states that his team's results 'corroborate the findings of Darlington et al. and Beri et al. who likewise used an individually adjusted diet.' Unfortunately, most doctors lack the time to study research papers in detail, so this part probably goes unread and the misleading impression given by the title of this paper is not corrected.

Ardent vegetarians will no doubt think that the permanent exclusion of meat was the crucial element in the success of this trial. There is evidence that this is unlikely, from several Swedish studies (see p.390), which have treated rheumatoid patients with a fast followed by a vegetarian or vegan diet. There was no testing of individual foods in these diet studies – and there was no lasting benefit beyond the initial improvement seen during the fast.

Other studies

The study referred to as 'Beri et al', by Dr Kjeldsen Kragh, was carried out in India by a team of researchers under Dr Deepa Beri. Although the diet differed in detail, the fundamental principle was the same as that of the elimination diet used in our trial.

In the New Delhi version of the diet, the exclusion phase (see p.25) consisted of a diet of fruit, vegetables, sugar and cooking oil. This was eaten for two weeks. At the end of the exclusion phase, each patient tested pulses (lentils, split peas, dry beans etc.) which they ate for two weeks, in addition to the previously allowed foods. If symptoms increased during this time, the patient stopped eating pulses and went back to the exclusion phase diet until they felt better.

The patients then tested wheat products (bread etc.) for two weeks, followed by rice for two weeks, yoghurt and other milk products for two weeks, then all other animal products (eggs, meat and fish) for two weeks. If any foods provoked symptoms, they were avoided thereafter, and no more testing was done until the symptoms had cleared.

Of the fourteen patients who completed the study, 10 showed significant improvement – a success rate of 71%. Unfortunately, there were another 13 patients who dropped out before the exclusion phase was complete. If we assume that none of these drop-outs had improved very much, then the overall success rate was 37% – ten 'good responders' out of a total of 27 patients.

The most common problem food was rice, which affected 60% of the patients with food reactions. Wheat came second with 50% and pulses third with 30%. This agrees with our observations that commonly eaten foods cause the most problems: rice and pulses form a much greater part of the diet in India than they do in Britain.

The patients' weight was monitored and five patients lost 9% of their starting weight. However, there was no difference in weight loss between good responders and poor responders, as in our study.

The main problem with this trial is that there was no control group, receiving a placebo treatment (see p.27), for comparison with the dietary treatment. This is perfectly acceptable for a 'pilot study', where a treatment is being tried out to see if a full placebo-controlled trial is worthwhile. However, results from a pilot study cannot be considered as good scientific proof that the diet works.

Three other double-blind placebo-controlled scientific trials of a similar kind have been carried out, all using elemental diets (see p.21) as sustenance during the exclusion phase. In one where elemental diet alone was given, 30% of patients improved markedly – a figure that fits in well with the 36% of good responders in the Epsom study, the 37% in the Indian study, and the 44% in the Norwegian study. A Dutch study with an elemental diet, where certain foods and drinks were allowed as well, (including some likely culprits) produced a smaller number of good responders (16%). Only one study has found no 'good responders'. This was carried out in Cambridge, and for the exclusion phase it used an elemental diet combined with a limited selection of foods such as chicken and rice, chosen because they were thought unlikely to provoke symptoms. While we would not be surprised if the inclusion of these foods reduced the percentage of good responders a little (because a few people might react to one or other of the foods), we would still expect there to be some good responders. The most obvious explanation for the complete lack of good responders is that the patients involved in this trial were not keeping religiously to the diet during the exclusion phase. Even eating a few mouthfuls of a 'forbidden food' can compromise the results during an elimination diet, and spoil a potential response.

Despite the lack of good responders, the Cambridge study did find a general improvement in the group on the elimination diet, compared to the placebo group. They had a greater grip strength and fewer tender joints after the exclusion phase, benefits which disappeared as foods were reintroduced. This suggests that some of them, at least, were responding quite well to the avoidance of certain foods.

Finally, there is one other study that should be mentioned because it is frequently quoted by doctors as showing that an elimination diet 'doesn't work'. This study was carried out at Northwick Park Hospital in Middlesex, England and used a straightforward avoidance diet (where all patients avoided the same foods throughout). The most serious criticism of this diet is that it did not exclude wheat, rye, oats or maize (corn), chicken, tea, coffee, tomatoes or potatoes. All these items, according to our results, are often identified as culprit foods by patients with rheumatoid arthritis. There were also very few patients in this study, reducing the chance of finding any who were sensitive to the foods which were excluded, such as milk and eggs.

Blind testing

To truly confirm the findings of an elimination diet, one should, ideally, carry out double-blind challenges with all the foods identified as symptom-provoking during the reintroduction phase. The difficulties of doing this for a large number of patients who have each identified several culprit foods, are colossal. The central problem is how to disguise the taste of the food. One method is to put the food into capsules (see p.18) but this is expensive, and requires the patient to swallow large numbers of capsules in order to obtain a meal-sized portion of the food. Most patients only respond to normal portions, not to tiny, capsule-sized amounts of the food. An alternative method is to disguise the food being tested in a richly flavoured soup or juice, which swamps the taste of the test food. This too has drawbacks, because the items in the soup or juice may provoke symptoms themselves.

Where double-blind tests can be carried out simply they have endorsed the results of the elimination diet. In the Cambridge study, for example, the researchers compared tap water with mineral water for the four patients who reported a reaction to tap water during the reintroduction phase. All four responded to tap water when given 'double blind', but did not react to mineral water.

Double blind challenge studies are currently taking place at Epsom General Hospital with patients who have successfully completed elimination diets.

Placebo effects and spontaneous remissions

When critics dismiss the good effects of the elimination diet they often suggest that the diet works purely by placebo effect (see p.27) or that patients just happen to go into spontaneous remission at the same time, and that this is being mistaken for a response to the diet. The scientific studies described above should dispel such criticisms, but in addition to these studies there are the long-term observations made in our rheumatology department. Among our patients we have a sizeable group who all showed a remarkable improvement in their rheumatoid arthritis when they embarked on the elimination diet, and who continue to do very well without taking any drugs. Some of these were severely ill before they began the diet and were getting steadily worse. To suggest that all these patients happened to go into spontaneous and sustained remission at exactly the same time as they began the elimination diet, is stretching coincidence to the point of incredulity. Remember that we set a very tight time-limit on the exclusion phase of the diet: if a patient does not improve within three weeks of beginning the exclusion phase, then the diet is considered to be ineffective for that patient. It is, of course, possible that a spontaneous remission, unrelated to the diet, could occur within those three weeks, but because it is such a narrow time-band the odds against this happening are high.

As for placebo effect, this is known to be a temporary phenomenon, an upsurge of well-being powered by the enthusiasm of the doctor and the high hopes of the patient. It invariably fades after a few weeks or months (see p.27). Some of the patients whom we first treated with an elimination diet in the early 1980s have remained well without any need for drugs for over 12 years. Any doctor who could generate this sort of placebo effect has missed their calling and should be practising as a faith healer!

Other patients have remained well for four or more years, but have then begun to be less careful about their diet, and have relapsed as a result. A few have also relapsed after as long as eight years of good health and no drugs, despite being scrupulous about their diets. The reasons for this are not clear, but may relate to changes in the gut flora (see p.37 and pp.39–40).

· *A Question of Numbers* ·

As already noted, the argument is not about whether specific food sensitivities can ever play a part in rheumatoid arthritis: no one who has looked at the scientific literature would deny that they can. The argument is about numbers – the percentage of rheumatoid arthritis patients affected. Is it 5%, as Professor Panush estimates, or 30–40% as most studies with elimination diets suggest?

First, let us look at how the 5% figure was calculated. Professor Panush asked 97 rheumatoid arthritis patients if they believed their symptoms were related to food: 29 of them (30%) said 'yes'. Of these 29 patients, 16 were studied, as described on p.21, and only three reacted to food in capsules. Professor Panush arrived at the 5% figure by assuming that there were no food-sensitive patients among the 70% who said 'no' at the outset, when asked if their rheumatoid arthritis was related to food.

His calculation went as follows: if 30% thought they were affected by food, and only 19% of them were right (3 out of 16 = 19%) then the percentage truly affected by food was 19% of 30%, or 5.6% of the total.

Given the difficulty of detecting food reactions in rheumatoid arthritis without a rigorous elimination diet, we would suggest that there may well have been others, among the 70% who answered 'no', who did in fact have food intolerance and were simply unaware of it. Furthermore, it seems likely that, among the sixteen patients tested, there were some who were food sensitive but who had misidentified their culprit food – again, without a rigorous elimination diet, accurate identification is not easy. For example, a patient who had regularly reacted to bread might think that wheat was their problem food, when in fact it was yeast. It is worth noting that almost all of the sixteen patients tested got better while eating nothing but an elemental diet: a good indication of food sensitivity. Professor Panush did not accept this as demonstrating food sensitivity, but relied solely on the response to food challenges in capsules. If the challenge was with the wrong food – with wheat instead of yeast, for example – then the patient's food sensitivity, though perfectly real, would have been considered disproved.

In our opinion, then, the 5% figure is based on various questionable assumptions, and is a serious underestimate. But even if it were an accurate estimate, there would still be a perfectly good case for trying an elimination diet. Suppose only 5% of rheumatoid arthritis patients are affected by food – that is still one patient in twenty. And the improvements seen among 'good responders' when the culprit food or foods are avoided is truly impressive. If you are currently suffering from rheumatoid arthritis, the elimination diet offers you *at least* a one-in-twenty chance of a substantial recovery from rheumatoid symptoms, to the extent that you may be able to return to a normal way of life and may no longer need drugs, or only need very few. The odds are a great deal better than the National Lottery, and the prize is surely just as desirable.

· *Two Major Questions* ·

In assessing the elimination diet, or any other new treatment, there are two crucial questions to ask. The first is 'Does it work?' and the second is 'How might it work?'.

The first question is obviously the most important. Before any treatment can be widely prescribed, there must be a firmly established scientific 'yes' to the first question. This should be based on a double-blind placebo-controlled trial (see p.27).

While it is helpful to be able to answer the second question, this is not essential. There are many drugs currently in use that certainly work, although no one knows exactly how. Other drugs, such as aspirin, were widely used for many years before their mechanism of action was discovered.

As far as the elimination diet goes, we consider that the scientific trial carried out in Epsom (see p.26) answers the 'Does it work?' question with a resounding 'yes' (in the sense that it works very well for *some* rheumatoid patients). Our ongoing experience with patients treated at the clinic corroborates this.

Having answered the 'Does it work?' question we should obviously address the 'How might it work?' question. Various ideas are considered on pp.39–42, but unfortunately there is no firmly established answer at the present time.

Doctors who reject dietary therapy out-of-hand tend to focus on the fact that no one can say for sure how it works. If the same argument were applied to drugs, hundreds of very useful and effective medicines would have to be removed from the pharmacy shelves immediately. That argument is not applied to drugs, nor to many other orthodox treatments, so there is no reason why it should be applied to the elimination diet.

Some myths about food and digestion

Certain established ideas about food and digestion often lead doctors to briskly dismiss dietary therapy for rheumatoid arthritis, but when carefully examined, these concepts turn out to be simplistic or mistaken. This is a subject we will look at before going on to 'How might it work?'. The first major misconception about food is that the digestive system breaks down all food molecules into small fragments before anything is absorbed. School biology textbooks still teach this, and one generation of students after another learns that starches (complex long-chain carbohydrates) are broken down into sugars, while proteins are broken down into amino acids. According to the standard texts, small molecules such as sugars and amino acids can be absorbed into the bloodstream, but the large intact molecules are kept within the digestive system.

If this were so, the immune system would only encounter large food molecules in the mouth, stomach or intestine. Proteins and peptides (short lengths cut from the protein chains consisting of six or more amino acids) are the main items recognised by the immune system. It is well known that single sugars and single amino acids are much too small to provoke an immune response, so any allergy or other immune reaction to food would take place in the digestive tract only. If the immune reaction produces symptoms, this is where the major symptoms should occur, although there might be some secondary symptoms elsewhere.

In a **true allergy** to food, this is exactly what happens (see p.83). The mouth, lips and throat are usually affected, while occasionally the allergenic food reaches the stomach or intestine before provoking a response. Other symptoms, such as a dramatic fall in blood pressure, are a result of the immune-system messengers such as histamine. These messengers are released during the allergic reaction in the lips, mouth and gut, and then travel around the body in the bloodstream.

If no intact food molecules were to get through the gut lining, it would clearly be impossible for food to provoke an immune response in distant parts of the body (such as the joints) without having first provoked a response in the mouth and gut. Although some rare forms of arthritis do seem to follow on from inflammation in the bowel (enteropathic arthritis – see p.98), in most rheumatoid arthritis patients there is no obvious underlying problem of this kind.

In fact the school textbook account of digestion is wrong: quite a few large molecules are absorbed intact, or in medium-sized fragments such as peptides. The research showing this has been published in the last 20 years, but has not yet been widely acknowledged. One study involved healthy adults drinking water that contained potato starch. When blood samples were taken, 15–30 minutes later, there were as many as 1500 starch grains in every teaspoonful of blood.

Following any meal, various undigested or partially digested food molecules appear in the bloodstream. Some of these originate from specialised zones in the gut wall which actively sample the gut contents. These zones, known as Peyer's patches, are a part of the immune system. They take in droplets of liquid from the gut which contain large undigested food molecules, and subject them to a form of 'inspection' by immune cells. In a healthy body, this process helps the immune system to distinguish food from invading microbes, and to mount attacks on the latter, but not on the former. (This process, in which the immune system learns to tolerate food, is called **oral tolerance**.)

The uptake of intact food molecules from the gut permits a range of reactions to food. For example, the immune system may make antibodies (see p.412) which bind to food molecule antigens in the blood. Antibodies and antigens can bind together in large numbers, rather like a rugby scrum. These large clumps are known as **immune complexes** and when they circulate in the blood they may cause symptoms in various ways. Whether these play a role in rheumatoid arthritis is something we will consider in the next section.

The extent to which food molecules pass through the gut wall – **gut permeability** – varies from person to person and from time to time. Some factors in the diet, and some drugs can increase gut permeabilty (see p.190–191).

Another major omission in basic textbooks is that digestion is described as a simple interaction between the human consumer and the food. The **gut flora** is rarely mentioned. This rather odd name describes the collection of bacteria and yeasts – billions of them – that live within our large intestine. Everyone has this flora, and healthy human beings coexist peaceably with their microscopic lodgers. The microbes benefit from food and a nice safe living space within the gut. In return, they play some part in digestion and in keeping the gut healthy. Most importantly, by taking up all the living space in the gut they crowd out disease-causing bacteria, making it far harder for them to find a foothold.

However, certain members of the gut flora can become too abundant and displace other, more useful kinds. It is also possible for certain useful types of bacteria to be lost, which might leave an imbalance in the gut flora as a whole. Various studies have suggested that the gut flora is altered in people with particular diseases, including patients with rheumatoid arthritis. These are largely uncharted waters for medical researchers, because it has always been extremely difficult, using traditional methods, to document the different species present in the flora and to measure their relative abundance. But recently scientists have begun using a sophisticated technique called gas-liquid chromatography to analyse bacterial products and so create an impressionistic profile of the gut flora. It does not reveal which species are present, but it does show when the composition of the gut flora changes. This streamlined technique is expected to revolutionise research in this area. Early studies with this technique have shown that a change of diet can alter the composition of the gut flora (see p.40).

These discoveries point to a novel way in which food can affect human health, by first affecting the gut flora. If foods favour certain microbe species – species that either release toxins or provoke the immune system in some way – this could cause long-term ill-health. Such possibilities introduce a whole new dimension into the relationship between food and disease, one which we have yet to understand fully, but which could, perhaps, be the key to explaining how dietary treatments for rheumatoid arthritis work.

So much for the misconceptions about digestion. A third mistaken belief concerns history and the human diet. Doctors often take the view that foods which have been consumed for hundreds or even thousands of years cannot possibly do any great harm, as long as they are part of a sensible balanced diet. The thinking behind this is that, if common foods led to serious disease in certain people, this would have been noticed long ago.

The story of coeliac disease puts paid to this idea. This severe and unpleasant bowel disorder stems from an unusual reaction to the proteins found in wheat and related cereals, called gluten. The abnormality which makes gluten such a damaging food seems to be present from birth, and those suffering from this abnormality are known as coeliacs. Today coeliacs are put onto gluten-free diets and generally they suffer few further symptoms. Before the 1940s, however, coeliac disease was considered mysterious and incurable. It was only during the famine in the Netherlands at the end of World War II, when bread was unavailable and people survived by eating tulip bulbs, that an observant doctor noticed his coeliac patients were far healthier than before, and decided to find out why. Wheat has been eaten for about 10,000 years, but its ill-effects on certain people were not noted until the 1940s!

A second example comes from the island of Guam, where the seeds of the false sago palm have long been eaten. There had always been a high incidence of senile dementia on Guam, but no one had ever linked this with false sago palm. Again, World War II caused a change in diet, the island being occupied by Japanese troops, causing a food shortage that forced the islanders to rely far more heavily on false sago palm. There was a delay before the effects of this were seen, but a steep increase in cases of senile dementia began in the 1950s and the epidemic continues today.

Even so the link with eating false sago palm seeds was not apparent to the islanders because of the time-lag: it took a detailed scientific study to pinpoint the cause of the epidemic. Clearly, the ill-effects of food can go unnoticed if they are not instantaneous effects and if the food is part of everyone's daily menu.

How might the elimination diet work?

Having disposed of the myths about food that often lead to an unthinking rejection of dietary therapy, we can look at the difficult question of how the elimination diet might work for arthritic patients.

The key event in rheumatoid arthritis is the abnormal and excessive growth of the synovial membrane or synovium (see p.421), which expands into the joint space and may begin to destroy the articular cartilage (see p.413). It is clear that the immune system, whose proper job is to defend against infection, is involved in this, because there is a stampede of immune cells into the synovium and the joint space. Indeed, the immune system is the major player in rheumatoid arthritis (see p.129).

Two major theories dominate speculation about the causes of rheumatoid arthritis (see pp.130–131). To summarise, there is the **auto-immune hypothesis** in which the immune system attacks the body itself through a breakdown in normal control mechanisms, and the **infective hypothesis**, in which a long-standing infection by a microbe, somewhere in the body (but not in the joints themselves) results in arthritis.

Food does not currently feature in either the auto-immune hypothesis or the infective hypothesis, because the discovery that avoiding certain foods can help some patients with rheumatoid arthritis is still ignored by much of the scientific community.

Can we make sense of the discoveries about diet in terms of either the auto-immune hypothesis or the infective hypothesis? Alternatively, can new theories be developed for the role of food? There seem to be four possibilities at present:

1. A food version of the infective hypothesis
Particular foods might nourish certain species of bacteria or yeasts that are a natural part of gut flora (see p.37), making them more common than they normally are. Or species that do not normally form part of the gut flora might benefit from these foods and become

established. These might then cause a reaction by the immune system, which leads to rheumatoid arthritis. The nature of such a reaction is however, unknown.

The idea that particular foods nourish particular microbes in the gut flora is at present speculative, but it has recently been shown that various changes in diet – including the elimination diet – produce a general change in the gut flora.

As for the second part of the theory – that bacteria in the gut might be linked with symptoms in the joints – this is based on parallels with reactive arthritis (see pp.126–8) and on recent studies of the gut flora of patients in the early stages of rheumatoid arthritis: these show that there are significant differences from the normal gut flora. Additionally, the Norwegian patients who underwent a combined elimination diet/vegetarian diet (see p.29) showed a change in their gut flora, and the 'good responders' showed a different gut flora change from those who did not respond to the diet.

It seems unlikely that changes in the gut flora alone can explain all the effects seen in food-related rheumatoid arthritis. When challenged with offending foods, some patients begin reacting within an hour, long before the food could have begun to influence the gut flora. On the other hand, in cases where the response to food is very slow, and continues long after the food has been withdrawn again, a gut-flora response fits the bill very nicely.

2. A true allergic reaction to the food

If there were a true allergy to food it would have to somehow cause rheumatoid arthritis *without* any notable effects on the mouth or gut, unlike normal food allergy (see p.83). Despite this problem, the possibility of true allergy has led researchers to look for the allergy antibody, IgE (see p.416) in patients with obvious sensitivity to foods. The Hammersmith Hospital 'cheese-aholic' (see p.18) was tested for antibodies to the proteins in cheese and milk, as already described, and her blood showed IgE specific for both. However, these antibodies were absent from the synovial fluid of her joints, which makes it doubtful that a true allergic reaction was directly involved in the arthritis. Furthermore, she was not typical in having IgE: three other rheumatoid arthritis patients with proven food sensitivity did not have IgE specific for their culprit food. However, one of these patients did have high levels of IgG4 antibodies to her problem food – IgG4 is thought to trigger mast cells in a similar way to IgE. It is not clear if IgG4 was playing a part in her rheumatoid arthritis. We can conclude that true allergy might play a minor role in some patients, but not in all.

3. Immune complex deposits
In this scenario, intact food molecules are absorbed into the bloodstream (see p.36) bind to antibodies and so form immune complexes. These might then deposit in the small blood vessels of the joints' synovial membranes (see p.421) and spark off inflammation there. A few patients with proven food reactions have been tested for an increase in CICs (circulating immune complexes – that is, immune complexes in the bloodstream) after eating their culprit foods. Two showed a small increase, but these were nothing exceptional; healthy people can show the same degree of increase in CICs after a meal.

To achieve high levels of CICs it is necessary to produce plenty of antibodies to the food concerned, but in fact, most patients show no clear-cut evidence for increased antibodies to culprit foods. Two patients studied by Professor Panush showed high levels of IgG antibodies (these are 'ordinary' antibodies, not the allergic kind) to their offending foods (shrimp and milk), but some healthy people who were studied for comparison showed similar levels of IgG antibodies to foods. Doctors in Israel, studying people whose rheumatoid arthritis was triggered by milk, found exactly the same. The only case in which abnormally high antibody levels were found was in a young patient with juvenile rheumatoid arthritis.

4. Some other type of immune reaction to food
This would be an immune reaction that was neither a true allergy nor a result of CICs. Two very interesting results exist which suggest that something abnormal happens, immunologically speaking, when rheumatoid arthritis patients try their culprit food.

The cheese-aholic (see p.18) showed a striking change in a test which looks at the efficiency of the reticuloendothelial system. This cumbersome name describes certain immune cells which clear dead cells and other debris from the blood. They are, in effect, the rubbish-disposal units of the body. The test involves extracting some red blood cells from the patient, heat-treating them so that they are damaged, then reinjecting them. The speed with which the heat-damaged red blood cells are removed from the bloodstream shows how well the reticuloendothelial system is working. It is known that patients with rheumatoid arthritis generally have slow rates of clearance. What was striking about the cheese-aholic was that her clearance rate dropped dramatically, from 15 minutes before the food test, to over 100 minutes shortly after the test. It was still at this slow rate *twelve days later*. How did the food do this? We simply do not know, but it is something that deserves further investigation.

Seven Australian rheumatoid arthritis patients, with known sensitivity to foods, were tested for a chemical in the bloodstream called 5-H-T or serotonin. This is a chemical messenger which has various effects on the body, and may help to promote inflammation by encouraging immune complexes (see p.41) to deposit from the blood. The researchers found that, when the patients were challenged with their culprit foods, tiny blood cells called platelets released serotonin into the bloodstream. They suggested that this might help to produce the joint symptoms in some way.

More than one mechanism?

In considering these puzzles, we need to bear in mind that two or more of the theories could eventually prove correct. It is entirely possible that different sets of mechanisms operate in different patients, or that their relative importance differs. Rheumatoid arthritis is, after all, a distinctly variable disease. The mechanism proposed by the gut flora theory might turn out to be the prime cause in some patients, with the symptoms being aggravated by other mechanisms, such as circulating immune complexes or a mild allergic reaction to certain foods. For other patients, a completely different mechanism could be the main cause. Medical researchers might wish that matters were simpler, and, therefore, easier to investigate, but it seems likely that the truth about rheumatoid arthritis will turn out to be very complex indeed.

· *The Wider View* ·

Many people who try an elimination diet for rheumatoid arthritis find that other medical problems improve during the diet, and return when they test certain foods. Headaches, migraine, mouth ulcers, sinusitis and diarrhoea are typical symptoms provoked by foods in the rheumatoid arthritis patients we have studied at Epsom. Indeed, the elimination diet was first developed as a treatment for symptoms of this kind. It evolved slowly in the 1920s, among US doctors, and was developed and applied extensively during the 1940s, by Dr Theron G. Randolph of Chicago. At the outset, in the 1920s, very little was known about allergy, and the word was used to mean any unusual reaction to a harmless substance. As more was learned about the immune system, some doctors began to use 'allergy' in a more restrictive sense, to mean only those reactions involving the immune system. In time, this tighter definition became the medical norm, although there were many doctors working on the fringes of conventional medicine who continued to use 'allergy' in the same general way as before. They included doctors working with elimination diets, mostly rather unconventional doctors who tried out elimination diets for a wide range of problematic diseases from asthma to ulcerative colitis, discovering that dietary change could be very useful for some disorders, but not for others.

A rift developed between the 'orthodox' medical world – doctors and scientific researchers who used the word allergy in the narrow sense – and the fringe element, who used the word allergy in the looser sense and whose ideas and discoveries came to seem highly unorthodox. Some in the latter group were, indeed, very unscientific in their methods and outlandish in their claims. Others, including Dr Randolph, were dedicated doctors with a firm grasp of scientific principles, even if they lacked the research funds to study their treatments objectively.

The two traditions, as regards the word allergy, continue to this day. Most alternative practitioners and writers of popular medical books use allergy in the old, broad sense. So do many doctors in private practice who work in this field. Conventional doctors, however, use 'allergy' in the narrower, immunological sense. With the discovery of the allergy antibody, IgE, in the 1960s, some narrowed the definition even further, so that allergy could only mean reactions involving IgE.

All this is not just history for history's sake: the disagreement about basic terminology fuels the controversies about dietary treatment, and makes it yet more difficult for the elimination diet to be taken seriously by mainstream doctors. It is important that we try to establish some consensus about what the words mean.

Firstly, we believe the word 'allergy' should be restricted to reactions that definitely involve the immune system, because that is now the established use in mainstream medicine. Continuing to use allergy in the broader sense simply fosters misunderstanding. We also believe that the term 'true food allergy' is useful in describing those immediate and violent reactions to food that are produced by IgE. (The modern medical terminology for these is a 'Type I hypersensitivity reaction to food'.) As for idiosyncratic reactions that do not seem to involve a direct attack by the immune system on food molecules, yet are definitely physical in origin rather than psychological, we feel the term **'food intolerance'** is useful in describing these. (For those interested in definitions, there is more on the meaning of 'food intolerance' on p.83.)

Because a major research programme cannot be carried out on every individual patient, there will often be cases where it is impossible to say if the immune system is involved in producing a food-induced symptom or not. An educated guess may be necessary, on the basis of the symptoms and the likely mechanism behind such symptoms. So if someone suffers headaches in response to a particular food, doctors would generally describe this as food intolerance, since it is unlikely that any reaction by the immune system would produce headaches as an isolated symptom. If, however, someone regularly suffers from nettle-rash or urticaria – a typical allergic symptom – after eating a particular food, most doctors would probably describe this as food allergy.

Unfortunately there are a great many reactions to food that refuse to fit into this seemingly neat allergy/intolerance classification. Suppose a patient suffers both asthma (which is thought of as an allergic reaction) and migraine, and suppose *both* clear up on avoiding milk. Should this to be called allergy or intolerance? In such cases, we favour the name 'food sensitivity' which, by our definition, is an umbrella term including both food allergy and food intolerance.

Cases of rheumatoid arthritis that respond to food elimination are another example of the problems of terminology. On the one hand, rheumatoid arthritis is a disease in which the immune system is clearly a major player. On the other hand, the absence of IgE antibodies to culprit foods in most patients (see p.40), and the absence of excessive anti-food antibodies of other kinds (see p.41), make it doubtful that there is a direct immune attack on food molecules. There may be some small immune response to the food, but it looks as if, for most patients, it only plays a minor role in the disease process. At the moment, therefore, it seems appropriate to describe the reactions of rheumatoid arthritis patients as 'food intolerance'.

What exactly is food intolerance?

Doctors working with elimination diets have claimed success with a surprising range of symptoms and diseases, and some of these claims have now been scientifically tested.

There is an excellent double-blind placebo-controlled trial of children with severe migraine, which showed over 80% of the children improving on the elimination diet and responding to specific food challenges. Similar trials have confirmed the success of elimination diets in treating irritable bowel syndrome (irregular bowel action usually with intestinal pain) and Crohn's disease, a severe inflammatory disorder of the bowel (see pp.98–99).

Successes have been claimed, but not objectively tested, with straightforward joint pain (arthralgia), mouth ulcers, unexplained nausea and vomiting, stomach ulcers, duodenal ulcers and constipation. A triad of symptoms that often responds to elimination diet is migraine, non-specific joint pain (arthralgia) and diarrhoea (or irritable bowel syndrome). Most controversial of all are the claims that fatigue, depression and anxiety sometimes clear up during an elimination diet, and return when various foods are tested.

In a sense there is very little in common between these different disorders, and it is reasonable to suppose that the mechanism behind each of them would be different. This would mean that food intolerance was just a convenient term that included many disparate reactions to food. Yet there are certain common findings in different patients which seem to connect all the different types of food intolerance together. One is that staple foods are the most frequent offenders. In the West this means wheat, corn, milk, eggs and oranges come near the top of the list, whereas in Asian countries rice is a more common culprit. A second characteristic feature is that there are rarely any marked associations between a particular food and a particular symptom or disease. A third unifying factor is the strange phenomenon of food 'addiction' in which patients develop passionate cravings for the very food that is the source of their problems. This certainly does not happen with every patient, but it is common enough to merit an explanation. We have already described one case in a patient with rheumatoid arthritis (see p.18).

A fourth unifying factor is the speed with which these different forms of food intolerance respond to an elimination diet: all do so within 3 weeks, and usually in 7–10 days. It is also common for there to be 'withdrawal symptoms' – a general deterioration during the first few days of the diet.

· *The Next Step* ·

If you suffer from rheumatoid arthritis, palindromic rheumatism, or simple unexplained joint pain, then we would suggest that it is worth trying an elimination diet, although you must try it with an open mind and remember that it does not work for everyone. The diet may also be worth trying for some people with osteoarthritis (see p.117–8). Detailed instructions for carrying out the diet are given in Chapter 2.4. Please read these in full, and talk to your doctor, before starting an elimination diet.

Chapter 1.2

SOOTHING OILS: FISH, OLIVES AND EVENING PRIMROSES

The Faroe Islands lie midway between Iceland, Norway and Scotland, specks of land in the midst of a cold and stormy sea. Inhospitable as the waters of the North Atlantic might seem they abound with fish, and the people of the Faroes have harvested these waters for generations. Fishing is a way of life here, and fish are a major part of the Faroese diet. By comparison with other parts of Europe, far less meat is eaten and fewer dairy products.

In the summer of 1988, a team of medical researchers began working on the island of Bordoy, one of the larger Faroe Islands. They aimed to survey the whole population of one county on the island, looking exclusively for disabilities affecting the hands and fingers. The study revealed a very high rate of osteoarthritis, particularly among men, and affecting the right hand more than the left – almost certainly due to heavy physical work in cold conditions. By contrast, rheumatoid arthritis was no more common than in other parts of the world – about 1% of the population was affected.

What was most interesting was the relatively mild form of rheumatoid arthritis found here. Among those suffering from this disease, relatively few had nodules (small lumps beneath the skin, often close to the arthritic finger joints). Nor did many have erosions of the bone around the arthritic joints, as revealed by X-rays. Nodules and erosions both tend to indicate more severe and rapidly progressing rheumatoid arthritis.

Over 90% of those Faroese with long-term rheumatoid arthritis remained able-bodied, and half still worked full-time. Again, the figures would generally be much worse in other parts of the world.

What could account for the mild nature of rheumatoid arthritis in these islands? One possible candidate is diet or, more specifically, the large amount of oily fish eaten by the Faroese. The Faroese research, in itself, offers absolutely no evidence for any connection between the two, but other research does point to oily fish as being important in rheumatoid arthritis.

· *Observing Lent* ·

At about the same time as the Faroese study, another group of medical researchers was at work over two thousand miles away, in Greece. Their aim was to compare the average diet of patients attending a hospital clinic for rheumatoid arthritis with the diet of patients coming to the hospital for a range of other diseases, and to see if they were the same.

Two major differences were found. Firstly, patients with rheumatoid arthritis used less olive oil, on average, than those without. Secondly, they were less likely to follow the dietary rules for Lent, laid down by the Greek Orthodox Church. These rules are stringent, and they apply for several weeks before Christmas, Ascension Day and Easter, and on the Wednesday and Friday of all the remaining weeks: in total they cover more than six months of each year. Most of this time is 'strict Lent' when meat, fish, eggs, milk, yoghurt and cheese are all forbidden, although shellfish, squid and octopus can be eaten. This holds for nineteen weeks of the year. For a further seven weeks, fish is allowed, but not meat, eggs or dairy products. During these periods of Lent, people mainly eat vegtables, oil, bread and fruit.

One factor in the Lenten diet emerged as being the most important: the amount of fish eaten. The higher the consumption of fish, the less likely a person was to need hospital treatment for rheumatoid arthritis. However, fish alone did not account for the effects of Lent food restrictions on rheumatoid arthritis. It was the Lenten diet *as a whole* that made a difference: the researchers suggest that the effect is probably due to a combination of eating more fish and shellfish, more fruit and vegetables, more olive oil and less meat and dairy produce. Unlike fish, olive oil alone could make a difference. (Other research tends to suggest that fish alone might make a difference in northern latitudes, because fish from colder seas are richer in some important constituents – see p.51.)

Whether this diet actually helps to *prevent* rheumatoid arthritis, or merely makes it *less severe*, is debatable, as the researchers themselves pointed out. The patients studied had all been referred to a large hospital in Athens for their rheumatoid arthritis, so they were undoubtedly a group with more severe symptoms than most. Patients with milder rheumatoid arthritis would mostly be treated by their local doctor. Perhaps the effect of olive oil and the Lenten diet is simply to make rheumatoid arthritis a relatively mild disease which tends to keep those patients eating such a diet away from the hospital – if *all* the patients with rheumatoid arthritis in a particular area had been studied, perhaps their average diet would have been much the same as the average diet of the population at large.

· *How it Began* ·

Both the Faroese study and the Greek study were inspired by the very promising results from medical research elsewhere in the world, using different kinds of oils as an experimental treatment for inflammatory diseases. In these experiments, the oils were given in capsules, as a supplement, to people eating a typical Western diet. Such studies had begun about a decade earlier, in the late 1970s, first with an oil derived from the seeds of a garden plant, evening primrose, and later with special oils derived from fish, called **omega-3 oils** (often written *w*-3 or n-3). The details of these studies are described later in this chapter (see pp.52–54).

But what had prompted researchers to look at these oils in the first place? It was the discovery of various messenger substances within the body that are affected by these oils. The next part of this chapter outlines the chemical processes that generate these messengers in the body, and the way these oils affect such processes. If it all seems too technical, you can go straight to the section headed Feeding Oils to Patients on p.52.

· *Short-lived Messengers* ·

Interest in evening primrose oil and fish oil was prompted by discoveries about two groups of chemical substances. The first group includes the **prostaglandins**, **thromboxanes** and **prostacyclins**. The second group is known collectively as **leukotrienes**. These substances are all made by our bodies and act as messengers, carrying instructions from one part of the body to another. They are basically fatty substances and they are made from fats in the body – hence the connection with oils in food.

In a sense leukotrienes, prostaglandins and their relatives are like hormones, in that they carry messages and instructions around the body. But unlike most hormones, they are extremely short-lived and localised messengers: they may be produced by one cell to influence the behaviour of another cell that is only a microscopically small distance away, and they are destroyed within minutes of being formed. (Imagine a group of construction workers building a house: the plans drawn by the architect and the instructions of the foreman would correspond to the messages carried by major hormones such as testosterone or adrenaline, whereas the shouts from one worker to another – 'Is that straight?', 'Watch out!', 'Can you mix some more cement?' – would correspond to the sorts of short-lived messages delivered by leukotrienes, prostaglandins and their kind.)

Leukotrienes, prostaglandins and their relatives are being made and destroyed all the time, throughout the body. Their effects differ depending on exactly where they are: in the stomach, for example, prostaglandins regulate the digestive process and help to maintain a protective layer that shields the stomach lining from acid and digestive enzymes. In the bronchi (the passages leading to the lungs) prostaglandins play a part in regulating the muscles that control the diameter of these airways. When there is a wound or an infection anywhere in the body, prostaglandins and leukotrienes are involved in regulating the response by the immune system, while prostacyclins and thromboxanes control the clotting of the blood.

Inflammatory diseases, such as rheumatoid arthritis, involve a damaging over-reaction by the immune system (see pp.65–6) and prostaglandins and leukotrienes, as key players in any immune response, are instrumental in keeping the inflammation going. This is why aspirin and other non-steroidal anti-inflammatory drugs (NSAIDs), are thought to be helpful in rheumatoid arthritis. They work by reducing the quantity of prostaglandins, prostacyclins and thromboxanes (but not leukotrienes) made by the body. NSAIDs achieve this by blocking the action of an enzyme whose job is to manufacture prostaglandins and their relatives. (For an explanation of what enzymes are, and what they do, see p.415.)

By silencing, or at least reducing, the messages conveyed by prostaglandins and their kin, NSAIDs damp down the whole inflammation process. (To use the house-building analogy again: if the workers were forbidden to talk to each other it would slow down the progress of the work considerably.) Clearly, however, NSAIDs are not precision drugs of the 'silver bullet' kind: in turning off prostaglandin production they have a lot of different effects on the body, including some non-beneficial ones on the stomach lining.

The enzyme which NSAIDs switch off, is called either cyclooxygenase or prostaglandin synthase, or simply **PGHS**. All enzymes need a raw material to work on: a substance which they change into the end product required. For PGHS, the usual raw material is **arachidonic acid** – at least, this is the raw material for Westerners eating a typical diet. The raw material can change with a different diet, as we shall see later.

Arachidonic acid is a fatty acid (see p.415), and an important component of cell membranes, with various jobs to do besides being a raw material. When needed for the production of prostaglandins, prostacyclins or thromboxanes, it is released from a cell membrane and chemically transformed by PGHS into the desired product. If leukotrienes are needed, arachidonic acid is the raw material once again, but it is worked on by a different enzyme, called lipoxygenase.

The role of food

What has all this to do with the food we eat? The answer to this question is complex, and we will deal with it in stages.

Firstly, arachidonic acid is found in food, and so is another fatty acid called **linoleic acid**, which acts as a raw material for the manufacture of arachidonic acid. Linoleic acid is found in a huge variety of foods, including meat, eggs, milk, butter, nuts, seeds and beans. It is particularly abundant in vegetable oils and margarine. Arachidonic acid is found in eggs, certain meats and freshwater fish (see p.155 for a full list).

Whether the production of prostaglandins can be affected by changes in the amounts of linoleic acid and arachidonic acid in our food is an intriguing question, but one that relatively few researchers have investigated. All the useful evidence on this topic is described on pp.55–57, but to summarise, it seems that eating more arachidonic acid than usual boosts production of prostaglandins, whereas eating more linoleic acid probably does not have much effect because there are strict limits on how much linoleic acid is converted to arachidonic acid, and thus to prostaglandins. Cutting out both linoleic acid and arachidonic acid entirely (something that can only be done for a short time, because linoleic acid is essential for health) reduces the production of prostaglandins considerably. The effects of cutting out arachidonic acid alone have never been studied.

The oils found in fish

Arachidonic acid is not the only substance that can be converted to prostaglandins, prostacyclins, thromboxanes and leukotrienes. An alternative raw material is a fatty acid found in oily fish, called eicosapentaenoic acid or **EPA**.

EPA is not made by the fish themselves but by tiny one-celled plants or algae that float at the surface of the sea and provide food for fish. Fish accumulate the EPA from their food, and it is those fish living in cold northern waters that tend to have the largest amounts in their bodies.

EPA only differs from arachidonic acid in one small chemical detail, but neither can be converted to the other. EPA belongs to the group of fatty acids known as omega-3 fatty acids, while linoleic acid and arachidonic acid belong to the group known as omega-6 fatty acids.

When leukotrienes, prostaglandins and their relatives are made from EPA, rather than arachidonic acid, most of them are subtly different: although they usually have a similar *type* of effect, the *size* of the effect may be greater or smaller. Several of them are less inclined to promote inflammation, and their overall effect on the blood is to make it clot far less readily. But to describe EPA as 'anti-inflammatory', as popular articles about fish oil often do, is simplistic and misleading.

EPA affects the immune system in many different ways, and it can make some inflammatory conditions worse – notably asthma for those patients who are aspirin-sensitive and asthmatic. For a full list of those conditions that may be made worse by omega-3 oils see Table 4 on p.152.

Evening primroses and 'starflowers'

Evening primrose oil supplies a fatty acid known as gamma-linolenic acid or **GLA** which the human body can convert to another fatty acid called **DGLA**. They are relevant to inflammatory diseases because DGLA is another replacement for arachidonic acid, as a raw material for the production of prostaglandins.

GLA is found in large quantities in evening primrose oil, as researchers discovered in the 1970s. More recently, it has also been found in the seeds of two other plants, blackcurrant and borage. (The latter has been renamed 'starflower' by some inventive marketing department, in an effort to give it a romantic note that can rival 'evening primrose', but its true name, used for at least 600 years, is 'borage'.) Neither GLA nor DGLA occur in significant amounts in anything normally eaten as food.

GLA and DGLA both occur in the body, but in tiny amounts: taking evening primrose oil boosts these amounts enormously to levels that would never be found in the human body naturally. DGLA is an omega-6 fatty acid like arachidonic acid, and very similar to it chemically, but when it acts as the raw material for PGHS, a particular kind of prostaglandin is produced which has low inflammatory potential. No leukotrienes, prostacyclins or thromboxanes are made from DGLA. It was these unusual effects that made researchers first take an interest in evening primrose oil as a potential remedy for inflammatory diseases.

If you have been struggling with the many different names and technical complexities of the last few pages, you will be horrified to know that this is an extremely simplified account of the interactions that occur between fatty acids such as arachidonic acid, EPA and DGLA, and enzymes such as PGHS. A complete description of these interactions, and of all the different effects that prostaglandins, prostacyclins, thromboxanes and leukotrienes have on the body, would easily fill a book this size. But this simple outline is enough to allow us to understand why, in the late 1970s and early 1980s, researchers began investigating the possibility of using evening primrose oil and omega-3 fish oil for inflammatory diseases such as rheumatoid arthritis.

· *Feeding Oils to Patients* ·

The first study of omega-3 fish oil as a potential treatment for rheumatoid arthritis was carried out in the city of Albany, in upstate New York, in the early 1980s. The researchers divided a set of rheumatoid arthritis patients into two groups. The first group took several capsules of omega-3 fish oil every day, and were asked to eat plenty of fish as well. They were also told to limit their intake of saturated fats, by restricting meat and dairy products. The second group took capsules containing an indigestible paraffin wax – a 'placebo' (see p.26) – and ate a diet that was rich in saturated fat but low in cooking oil and other sources of polyunsaturated fats.

This study only lasted for 12 weeks, and we now know that fish oil does not always show its full effects in this timespan. The patients taking fish oil did not improve during the 12-week period, but the group on the high-saturated-fat diet began to suffer more inflamed joints, and longer periods of stiffness in the morning. These symptoms improved within 2 months of stopping the high-saturates diet. By contrast, the group taking fish oil and a low-saturates diet deteriorated rapidly when their diet period ended, suffering more pain and feeling worse generally. This was a surprise to the researchers.

So many different aspects of the diet were changed in this study that it was very hard to interpret the results. All subsequent studies have been much simpler – they have merely looked at the effect of giving capsules of omega-3 fish oil in addition to the normal diet, comparing this with a placebo capsule (usually paraffin wax, or an oil that was thought to have no effect on the immune system). In almost every study to date – and there have been over fifteen of them – omega-3 fish oil has shown some small benefits for patients with rheumatoid arthritis. It usually produces a reduction in pain, and in the number of swollen and tender joints. Many researchers have also found reductions in morning stiffness and increases in the grip strength of the hands. There is no sudden or dramatic change, but a gradual improvement that is often sufficient for patients to reduce their dose of non-steroidal anti-inflammatory drugs.

Most of the studies have continued for longer than 12 weeks, with the longest ones lasting a year. It has become clear that omega-3 fish oils take at least 12 weeks to build up to their maximum effect, but that they usually continue to give benefits after the oil capsules have been discontinued, sometimes for as long as four or five months afterwards. The initial delay is probably related to the need for EPA to be absorbed by immune cells and accumulated in special storage compartments within the cell, before it can be used as a raw material in prostaglandin and leukotriene production. These stores of EPA last a long time, which accounts for the persistence of good effects after the omega-3 oil has been stopped.

None of these trials has observed a sudden deterioration after discontinuing omega-3 supplements, so this finding from the first fish oil trial (see p.52) remains a mystery. It looks as if this effect had nothing to do with the fish oil supplement. Perhaps the patients in the fish oil group, having been asked to avoid cheese, ice cream, butter, sausages, bacon and fatty meats for 12 weeks, went on a binge as soon as the restrictions were lifted, and ate large amounts of these foods. They might then have suffered the same kind of deterioration as experienced by the patients on the high-saturates group.

Unfortunately, this type of study has never been repeated, so there is no direct evidence for the role that a high intake of saturated animal fats might play in rheumatoid arthritis. Several studies have looked at much smaller increases in saturate consumption and these seem to have no effect. Only one subsequent experiment has involved a really high intake of saturated fat, and this used fat derived from coconut for five weeks only. There were no apparent effects on rheumatoid arthritis, which may be because the study was too brief, or, perhaps, because coconut fat, being of a different composition from saturated animal fats, might have different effects.

Feeding GLA oils to patients

Evening primrose oil, blackcurrant-seed oil and borage ('starflower') seed oil all contain gamma-linolenic acid or GLA (see p.51). (You will recall that GLA is converted to DGLA by the body, and DGLA can replace arachidonic acid as a raw material for prostaglandin production.) To make life easier, we will refer to these plant oils collectively as '**GLA oils**'. The earliest trials – indeed most of the trials to date – have been done with evening primrose oil, but more recent studies have shown that blackcurrant seed oil and borage seed oil have much the same effect. All the GLA oils are given in capsules, as supplements to an ordinary Western diet. Their impact on rheumatoid arthritis is modest, as with omega-3 fish oil, but many patients seem to experience some noticeable improvements in morning stiffness, pain and the number of swollen and tender joints.

The improvements come on slowly, if anything more slowly than with fish oil: in one experiment it took nine months for the maximum effect to be achieved, although the improvement had begun after three months.

Several of the studies involving GLA oils have shown that some patients can reduce their dose of NSAIDs (see pp.418–9) after taking the oil for some months. Indeed, several people reduced their NSAIDs step by step and finally stopped taking them altogether; they reported feeling better for having done so.

· *The Olive Oil Story* ·

Olive oil has had a Cinderella role in these studies of oil and rheumatoid arthritis. For many years it was one of the oils used as a placebo (see p.27) in experiments with fish oil and evening primrose oils. It was assumed to be of no use whatever in the treatment of an inflammatory disease. This was because olive oil did not seem to have any constituents that might be useful: no omega-3 fatty acids for example, and no GLA. Its main ingredient is a mono-unsaturated fatty acid (see p.357) called oleic acid. However, this is certainly not unique to olive oil – it is also found, in fairly large amounts, in meat, fish, eggs, milk, avocado pears, nuts, vegetable oils, butter, lard and margarine. Oleic acid belongs to a group of fatty acids called the omega-9s, none of which can be converted to leukotrienes or prostaglandins. Olive oil also contains some linoleic acid (see p.50), the major ingredient of other vegetable oils.

Olive oil, then, seemed to be an inert oil with no possible value against rheumatoid arthritis. But it had surprises in store. When we and other researchers used it as a placebo in our experiments, we frequently saw some improvements in those taking olive oil. These effects were too large and occurred too frequently to be dismissed as 'placebo effect' – the psychological benefit derived from any medicine. What is more, some of the experiments showed changes in the behaviour of certain immune cells, suggesting that olive oil was actually reducing inflammation.

No one had suspected that olive oil was capable of producing effects such as these. Indeed, for a long time researchers went on using olive oil as a placebo, convinced that it could not have any real effects, despite the mounting evidence to the contrary.

The clinching evidence was the study of Greek rheumatoid arthritis patients described at the beginning of this chapter. With the publication of this research in 1991, olive oil finally achieved proper recognition as an oil that could produce benefits for those with rheumatoid arthritis.

Yet the mystery remains as to how olive oil works. No one knows whether it is the oleic acid that is influential, or some other mystery ingredient. To the best of our knowledge, no research has been carried out in this area.

. *Unanswered Questions:* . *Arachidonic Acid*

It would be very useful indeed to know what effect there is from arachidonic acid in food. Might eating more or less of this fatty acid – found in eggs, some fish and several kinds of meat – affect rheumatoid arthritis in some way? The reasons for thinking that it might are partly theoretical ones, based on what is known about prostaglandin production (see pp.48–50), and partly the results of one experiment carried out in the 1970s.

This experiment suggested that eating more arachidonic acid *does* boost production of prostaglandins considerably, and that this affects small cells in the blood known as **platelets**. These are involved in the clotting of the blood and in the inflammation process.

The experiment used four healthy volunteers who ate 6 gm of arachidonic acid daily in addition to their normal diet. One way to assess how active the platelets are is to see how easily they aggregate in response to a standard chemical stimulus. Platelet aggregation – clumping together – is part of the process of clot formation in the blood. After just two weeks on the arachidonic acid supplement, the platelets of the experimental subjects began to aggregate far more readily. In fact, for two out of the four subjects the platelets' behaviour had changed so much that the researchers became alarmed and stopped the supplement earlier than planned. This dramatic and worrying response is one reason why no further experiments on arachidonic acid supplements have been carried out.

How relevant is this experiment to real-life diets? The 6 gm dose of arachidonic acid used is about twenty times the amount of arachidonic acid in an average diet. While very few people are likely to eat 6 gm of arachidonic acid daily, someone who consumed a lot of meat, especially kidney, liver, veal, turkey or venison, could be eating 0.6 gm daily, 10% of the dose in the experiment. Whether this would have an effect on platelet aggregation is a question that no one has yet investigated. Given the striking effect of 6 gm per day, it is possible that 0.6 gm would make some impact. Do platelets that clump together more readily also have a more energetic response to signals from the immune system, and therefore promote inflammation? There is no evidence that they do, but it seems possible. Whether such effects on the platelets would translate into actual effects on rheumatoid arthritis is another question that we cannot currently answer, but this again seems plausible.

What would be the effect of going to the other extreme and cutting out arachidonic acid entirely? This experiment has been tried, unintentionally, in studies of vegan diets which are devoid of arachidonic acid (except for the small amounts in seaweed, if this is eaten). It is clear that vegan diets alone do not have any significant beneficial effects on rheumatoid arthritis (see p.390) so cutting out arachidonic acid is apparently not helpful in itself. However, there is some limited evidence that reducing the intake of arachidonic acid while simultaneously taking supplements of omega-3s, may be of value (see p.391).

A few studies have looked at diets from which both linoleic acid and arachidonic acid were absent, using healthy volunteers and measuring their prostaglandin levels. Such diets substantially reduced production of prostaglandins. This effect occured very promptly – within 3 days – and was reversed promptly when linoleic acid was eaten once again.

Note that these were healthy people, and not arthritis sufferers. If people with rheumatoid arthritis followed such a diet, would they get the same fall in prostaglandin production, and, more importantly, would this produce any change in symptoms? Only one research paper that we have been able to find addresses this question. It showed that on a totally fat-free diet, patients with rheumatoid arthritis improved substantially. Unfortunately, this was not a double-blind trial, and it was very small-scale, so the result has to be treated cautiously, but it is in line with some of our observations at Epsom General Hospital: after an elimination diet (see p.25) some patients find that fatty food of any kind sparks off their symptoms again.

Even if this finding is correct, the practical applications are very limited, because a diet without any linoleic acid can only be followed for a short while: as already noted, linoleic acid is an essential fatty acid (see p.353) and when bodily stores run low a deficiency disease results. There would also be deficiencies of fat-soluble vitamins.

Something that urgently needs scientific study is the effect on rheumatoid arthritis of a diet which has no arachidonic acid and is very low in linoleic acid, containing just enough to avoid a deficiency disease, but no more. This could be a diet that contains little fat in total (although such a diet may be bad for the nervous system even if it is not deficient in linoleic acid) or a diet where almost all the fat comes from sea-living fish, which contain little linoleic acid. Both of these are, of course, very extreme diets, and few people would want to undertake them unless the benefits were substantial and proven.

Looking again at the Greek Orthodox Lenten diet (see p.47) it is worth noting that it excludes meat and eggs for half the year – so there is little arachidonic acid in the diet at such times but some omega-3s from fish and shellfish (the levels of omega-3s in oily Mediterranean fish tend to be lower than in cold-water fish but there are still significant amounts.) Might this be contributing to the success of the Lent rules in either averting rheumatoid arthritis, or keeping the disease relatively mild? Of course, the Lenten diet is also low in saturated animal fat, which may also influence rheumatoid arthritis (see pp.52–3). Perhaps all these factors are at work, along with the effects of olive oil, and the high intake of antioxidants (see p.339) from vegetables, nuts and seeds – all combining to produce an 'anti-inflammatory diet'.

· *What is DHA?* ·

If you have ever looked at fish oil supplements, you will have seen that one of the ingredients listed on the label is DHA or docosahexaenoic acid. This is another omega-3 fatty acid found in fish, and it is an essential fatty acid, as explained on p.355, with important functions in the brain. Recent research has also shown that DHA is a vital part of cell membranes in the heart, and protects against cardiac arrhythmias (irregular heartbeats). This accounts for part of the protection that omega-3 fish oils give against heart disease.

Whether DHA is of any use in alleviating rheumatoid arthritis is an unanswered question: some studies have suggested that it can be converted to EPA and, thus, boost the supply of EPA available for conversion to prostaglandins and leukotrienes (see p.51). If so, then the DHA would probably be useful in rheumatoid arthritis. DHA may also have some direct effects on the PGHS enzyme (see pp.49–50), reducing total production of prostaglandins.

When measuring the value of a fish oil, it is accepted practice to add the EPA content to the DHA content and to talk of the total content of omega-3s. This is certainly valid for heart disease, where DHA has a special therapeutic role. In the case of rheumatoid arthritis, it is probably better to assess an oil by looking at its EPA content alone (see below).

· *How Much Omega-3 is Required?* ·

Doctors would like to know exactly how much omega-3 is required to give benefits in rheumatoid arthritis. Unfortunately, this question is far from settled. The doses of omega-3 fatty acids used in the scientific trials of supplements range from 1.3 gm per day to 5.7 gm per day. One trial showed that there is definitely more to be gained from taking 2.6 gm of omega-3 per day than 1.3 gm per day but another did not show any substantial difference when the dose was doubled again, to around 5 gm per day. Most researchers have settled on an ideal dose of about 3–3.5 gm per day.ΩΩ

These figures are for total omega-3 fatty acids, ie. for EPA and DHA combined. The recommended dose can also be given as EPA alone, and 3 gm of total omega-3s corresponds to 1.8 gm of EPA per day. This holds true for any fish-oil supplement, because all the supplement manufacturers have set the ratio of EPA to DHA at the same level as that in MaxEPA, the supplement used in all the scientific trials to date. When comparing different supplements it makes no difference whether one compares the EPA content or the total omega-3 content.

But when it comes to comparing fish oil capsules with whole fish from the fishmonger, it does make a difference, because fish usually contains more DHA and less EPA than the fish oil used in supplements. Since the usefulness of DHA in rheumatoid arthritis is not absolutely certain (see p.58), the best way to assess the usefulness of whole fish, and to compare whole fish with fish oil capsules, is by EPA content.

Practical advice on the dose of fish oil capsules, or the amount of fish to eat, can be found in Chapter 2.2 (p.143).

· *Is Cod-Liver Oil Useful?* ·

It is a time-honoured belief that cod-liver oil relieves 'arthritis' (as with most traditional remedies, the type of arthritis is not specified). The new discoveries about omega-3s have revived scientific interest in cod-liver oil and prompted researchers to ask if it might contain enough omega-3s to help with rheumatoid arthritis. The answer is 'probably not'. A teaspoonful of cod-liver oil contains about half the EPA of a teaspoonful of omega-3 oil, which is made from the *flesh* of oily fish, rather than the liver. Cod-liver oil also has one big drawback: it contains large amounts of Vitamins A and D, and there is a danger of toxicity from these vitamins if too much is taken. This means that the maximum dose of cod-liver oil is much lower than the maximum dose of fish flesh oil (whose Vitamin A and D content is usually negligible). So the maximum amount of omega-3 fatty acid obtainable from a safe dose of cod-liver oil is only about 0.75 gram whereas the dose thought to be useful in rheumatoid arthritis is about 3 gm – four times as much. It seems unlikely, therefore, that taking cod-liver oil (or other fish liver oils) would be useful in rheumatoid arthritis.

One experiment has looked at the effects of a daily dose of cod-liver oil on people with osteoarthritis (see pp.61–2).

· *Is Linseed (Flax-seed) Oil Useful?* ·

This oil contains an omega-3 fatty acid known as alpha-linolenic acid that can, in theory, be converted to EPA by the body. (The same fatty acid is also found in soybean oil and blackcurrant seed oil.) Some researchers have suggested that linseed oil might be useful to vegetarians who do not wish to take fish oil, but who want to benefit from EPA. Sadly, it turns out that only a little of the alpha-linolenic acid is actually converted to EPA.

A recent experiment in which linseed oil was given to patients with rheumatoid arthritis for three months showed no benefits, and there was no increase in the amount of EPA in their bodies (as there would be if taking fish oil). These discouraging results suggest that there is little to be gained by rheumatoid arthritis patients from taking linseed oil. (However, it may be of some use to strict vegetarians in avoiding deficiency of DHA – see p.356.)

Another fatty acid that can, in theory, be converted to EPA is stearidonic acid. This is found in blackcurrant seed oil. No studies have been made to show how much is actually turned into EPA by the body, but it is probably very little.

· Oils and Other Arthritic Diseases ·

Far less attention has been paid to the effects of oils on other arthritic diseases, but we will summarise what little information is available.

Systemic lupus erythematosus

Supplements of omega-3 fish oils seem to produce a short-lived improvement in systemic lupus erythematosus. After three months on the oil, some patients do feel better, but the benefits disappear again by six months. One study continued with supplements for a year, and found that patients got significantly *worse* in the months after they stopped taking the fish oil. As well as a deterioration in symptoms, there was a slight rise in levels of the anti-DNA antibodies, which are characteristic of systemic lupus erythematosus. This is alarming, and we would suggest that no one with systemic lupus erythematosus should take supplements of omega-3 oil, nor embark on a daily diet of oily fish.

Neither olive oil nor GLA oils has been tried for systemic lupus erythematosus.

One rather unusual study asked patients with lupus to cut polyunsaturated fats out of their diet as much as possible, eating mainly saturated fats (see p.139). The results seem to be very different from the effects of saturated fat on rheumatoid arthritis, but this was only a pilot study and no firm conclusions can be drawn.

Raynaud's phenomenon (Raynaud's syndrome)

Fish oil supplements seem to affect Raynaud's phenomenon in various ways. One study showed an effect that could perhaps make the circulatory problems worse, rather than better, and for this reason we would not recommend fish oil to those with Raynaud's phenomenon.

Evening primrose oil at a dose of 600 mg per day appears to produce substantial benefits for about half of those with Raynaud's phenomenon, and lesser benefits for some other patients, although a few patients do not benefit at all. If there is an improvement, it comes on quite quickly – within four weeks. No one has tested other GLA oils (see p.54) to see if they work equally well.

Systemic sclerosis

Evening primrose oil improves the circulation in the fingers for those who suffer from Raynaud's phenomenon as part of their systemic sclerosis. Olive oil may have similar effects, although this has not been tested as thoroughly.

Psoriatic arthritis

Trials of fish oil supplements among patients with the skin disease, psoriasis, have had rather mixed results but the general conclusion is that fish oil might have some small benefits. One experiment involved patients who had painful joints as well (psoriatic arthritis) and the majority improved while taking fish oil. However, this was only a pilot study, and the result needs to be confirmed by a full scientific trial. There is a good deal of ongoing research into psoriasis and fish oil, and the benefits – or lack of them – may become better established in the near future.

Sjögrens syndrome

Evening primrose oil has been tried out for Sjögren's syndrome, but it does not seem to be effective.

Osteoarthritis

Inflammation is only a small part of the problem in most cases of osteoarthritis (see pp.67–8), so oil treatments are not expected to be effective against this disease. But because cod-liver oil has traditionally been used for osteoarthritis, one research group in London looked at its effects, when taken daily for six months. The researchers found no improvement, but they suggested that this might be because all the patients were taking NSAIDs (non-steroidal anti-inflammatory drugs – see p.418) which would damp down the small degree of inflammation present in the joints, perhaps leaving no scope for improvement by the oil. If this was indeed the case, then cod-liver oil might be useful for patients *not* taking NSAIDs. However, they are more likely to benefit from omega-3 fish oil (see below).

Olive oil was used as a placebo in this trial and proved equally ineffective. However, the dose was quite low, compared to the amount of olive oil that is known to be effective against rheumatoid arthritis. Olive oil has not been tested at a higher dose.

The experiment with cod-liver oil described above was preceded by a pilot study, in which the same research team studied omega-3 fish oil. In the pilot study, patients with osteoarthritis seemed to improve considerably after six months of omega-3 fish oil: they reported a lot less pain and less interference with their daily activities. The amount of EPA taken daily was 1.5 gm – twice as much as in the trial of cod-liver oil described above. Although this was only a pilot study, it did include a placebo group, and this group did not improve as much. It is tempting to think that there might be some value in taking omega-3 oil – or eating a daily portion of oily fish – for those with osteoarthritis. A full-scale scientific trial of omega-3 oil is needed.

Evening primrose oil and other GLA oils have not been tested in relation to osteoarthritis. Practical advice on taking oils for osteoarthritis is given on p.159.

THE MANY DIFFERENT KINDS OF ARTHRITIS: A RECIPE FOR CONFUSION

If you have read the first two chapters of this book, you will have noticed that we are always careful to be clear about which type, or types, or arthritis are under discussion. By comparison, most popular books on this subject are extremely vague, and use the word 'arthritis' indiscriminately, as if all forms of arthritis were much the same.

They most certainly are not. The different forms of arthritis are as different in their basic causes as insect bites, nettle stings, boils, warts and pimples – the fact that all produce bumps on the skin does not mean that they all orginate in the same way, nor that they can be prevented or treated in the same way.

Chapter 2.1 (p.79) looks at the many different arthritic diseases individually, and gives specific advice on dietary treatment for each one. In this chapter, we describe five larger categories, the main 'families' of arthritis. These are family groups into which the many different arthritic diseases can be classified.

This classification is useful when thinking about the possible effects of diet on arthritic diseases. Table 1 (see p.69) shows how the individual diseases (as listed in Chapter 2.1) slot into the five families described in this chapter.

The five main families are: infective arthritis, reactive arthritis, inflammatory arthritis, crystal arthritis and degenerative arthritis.

· *Infective Arthritis* ·

The first family of arthritic diseases includes all those caused by bacteria, viruses or other microbes invading the joints directly. This happens relatively rarely, but when it does it produces a severe reaction which requires urgent medical attention. Antibiotics are essential for the treatment of infective arthritis, and diet is entirely irrelevant.

What is inflammation?

Inflammation is a familiar process to anyone who has cut their finger or suffered a sore throat – the redness and swelling that occurs around the cut is due to inflammation, as is the prickly, hot feeling in the sore throat. Both are sensible and necessary reactions by the body, which is defending the cut, or the throat, from infection by microbes (bacteria or viruses). The defensive action is mounted by cells known as **immune cells** (see p.146) that wander round the body, in the blood and the lymphatic fluid (see p.147) rather like policemen on patrol, looking for invading microbes. When they locate an invasion, they attract and excite other immune cells. It is the influx of millions of these fighting cells that helps to produce the redness, warmth and swelling of inflammation. Tiny blood vessels in the vicinity grow wider to allow more blood to reach the battle zone, causing the redness and swelling. The blood vessels also become more leaky, so that immune cells can leave the bloodstream and advance towards the battlefront as rapidly as possible.

There are control mechanisms which damp down the reaction once the battle is won. After the wound has healed over, and any remaining bacteria have been killed, these controls come into force. The swelling and redness gradually disappear and everything returns to normal.

Like any police force, the immune system has to be constantly regulated and kept under control so that it does not cause more problems than it solves. However, the controls sometimes break down, and the immune system then runs amok, causing excessive inflammation where it is not needed.

This is what happens in the early stages of inflammatory arthritis: there is rampant, damaging, runaway inflammation in the synovial membrane (see p.421) of certain joints, often finger joints. All the players that perform in useful inflammation are there, some of them in enormous numbers. These immune cells produce cytokines, or chemical messengers (see p.415), to add to those already present. The type of cytokines which excite immune cells are produced in abundance, and they seem to overwhelm the cytokines that can calm down inflammation. Their many effects on the inflamed joint include stimulating cell proliferation, increasing the production of inflammatory chemicals called prostaglandins (see pp.48–9) and encouraging the breakdown of bone and cartilage.

· *Reactive Arthritis* ·

The second family of arthritic diseases includes all those that are an indirect response to infection. The microbes are not inside the joint itself, but elsewhere in the body, such as the digestive tract. Something about the particular microbes involved, or the way the body reacts to them, produces pain in the joints. This may persist for some time after the infection has cleared up. One of the most common types of reactive arthritis is Reiter's syndrome (see p.127).

Uncontrolled inflammation is an important factor in reactive arthritis, and it seems to be sparked off by some unusual interaction between the bacterium or virus and some component of the immune system: this would explain the association between Reiter's syndrome and the gene for HLA-B27 (see p.128).

Because an infection is clearly at the root of reactive arthritis, the effects of diet have not been studied. In theory, there might be certain ways in which diet could affect this family of arthritic diseases (see pp.126–7), but these are only possibilities: they have not been scientifically tested, and we cannot make any positive recommendations at present.

If some of the current theories about bacteria in rheumatoid arthritis (see pp.130–131) and ankylosing spondylitis (see pp.87–8) prove to be correct, then these may have to be reclassified as forms of reactive arthritis.

· *Inflammatory Arthritis* ·

The third group of joint diseases, the inflammatory kind, are far more varied and complex. They include rheumatoid arthritis, ankylosing spondylitis, psoriatic arthritis and many other much rarer diseases (a complete list is given in Table 1 – see p.69).

In all these conditions there is damaging inflammation (see p.64) inside the joint. The inflammation particularly affects a membrane, called the **synovium** or the **synovial membrane** (see Figure 4 p.42), which produces the essential lubricating fluid for the joint (the synovial fluid) and is vital to its functioning. The inflamed synovial membrane may become enlarged, and the inflammation process can begin to destroy the articular cartilage which protects the ends of the bones and reduces friction within the joint. When inflamed, the synovial membrane often over-produces synovial fluid, and this causes swelling and stiffness of the joint.

Once the disease process has begun in inflammatory arthritis, it seems to be self-perpetuating, although there may be periods when the inflammation dies down (remissions) and times when it gets much worse (exacerbations or relapses).

Sometimes this runaway inflammation begins because the immune system attacks the innocent cells of its own body – a phenomenon known as **auto-immune disease.** One of the auto-immune diseases that can affect the joints is systemic lupus erythematosus. Auto-immunity is also thought to be involved in some other types of inflammatory arthritis, but its relative importance in these diseases is far from certain, particularly in the case of rheumatoid arthritis (see p.130).

If auto-immunity has not sparked off the inflammation, then what has? This is a difficult question, and there is no single answer which applies to all the different forms of inflammatory arthritis. For most of the diseases in this family, the original cause of the inflammation is a mystery. However, for a certain number of patients with rheumatoid arthritis, it seems that a bad reaction to particular foods could be among the initiating causes of the inflammation – the case of the 'cheese-aholic' described on pp.18–20 is a good example.

For such patients, detecting the culprit foods by an elimination diet (see Chapter 2.4–p.170) and then avoiding them, can produce a striking improvement. For many others with rheumatoid arthritis, there may be some more limited benefits from avoiding certain foods – again, the elimination diet is the best way to identify such foods.

With other forms of inflammatory arthritis, the extent to which food intolerance might play a part in the disease is largely unknown, but where information *is* available about individual disorders, it is given in Chapter 2.1 (p.79).

The various oils that can have a calming effect on inflammation, described in Chapter 2.2 (p.143), are among the potential dietary treatments for rheumatoid arthritis and some other forms of inflammatory arthritis. Certain vitamins and other nutrients which act as antioxidants (see p.339) may also be helpful in inflammatory arthritis, and should be considered.

In addition to these general dietary treatments, there are a number of more particular dietary changes that can specifically affect certain forms of inflammatory arthritis. These are described in Chapter 2.1 (p.79), under the individual entry for each disease.

· *Crystal Arthritis* ·

The fourth family of arthritic diseases includes those caused by tiny crystals which form in the joint and provoke a reaction by the immune system: this involves severe pain and swelling. (This is only a brief outline of the process, which is described in more detail on p.104.) There are two main types of crystal arthritis, gout and pseudogout.

Exactly what leads to the formation of crystals in gout varies from one person to another. For many gouty patients, but by no means all, it is an over-rich diet washed down with plenty of alcohol.

The link between diet and gout has been obvious to doctors for centuries, and an abstemious lifestyle used to be the only treatment. Losing weight and cutting out alcohol may still be recommended as an initial treatment for those who are overweight, but there are now some highly effective drugs so that other diets (those low in purines) are rarely necessary. Nevertheless, a low-purine diet may be useful to certain people with gout (those who dislike taking drugs, for example, or who suffer with side-effects) and there are further details in Chapter 2.7 (p.242).

In the case of pseudogout (see p.123), diet is unlikely to help.

· *Degenerative Arthritis* ·

The fifth category of arthritis includes a single major disease – osteoarthritis. This common affliction of the elderly is called a degenerative disease because the main problem is that the cartilage in the joints is wearing out more rapidly than it can be repaired.

When osteoarthritis occurs in younger people, it is often the result of repeated small injuries to the joints, as in 'wicket-keepers' hands': the price some cricketers pay for having caught too many fast balls. Fortunately, osteoarthritis does not progress very rapidly, and most sufferers can continue to live quite normal lives.

As regards diet, losing weight helps if the hip, knee, ankle or finger joints are affected by osteoarthritis, but only for those who are overweight to begin with. Beyond that, there is probably very little that diet can do to actually reverse the degenerative process of osteoarthritis.

Sometimes, however, the pain and damage of osteoarthritis are being made worse by inflammation in the joints (although the inflammation is much less than in a disease such as rheumatoid arthritis). Consequently, some of the oils which calm down inflammation may produce a small improvement in osteoarthritis (see p.62).

Vitamins may also have a role to play in the treatment of osteoarthritis and, very occasionally, there are benefits from an elimination diet (see pp.117–9).

· *When Joint Pain is not Arthritis* ·

To earn the name 'arthritis', there has to be some recognisable disease process going on in the joints. Joint pain alone is not arthritis.

Unexplained joint pain may sometimes be the first symptom of some more serious disease, a forewarning of true arthritis. But it may simply be a pain for which the doctor cannot find an explanation, which comes and goes for many years, possibly getting a little worse, but never developing into arthritis.

Conventional medicine is not much concerned with joint pain of this kind, and anyone suffering from it will probably just be told to take painkillers. Yet it evokes rather more interest from doctors who have experience of treating arthritis with diet, because they have seen such joint pain clear up completely when patients try an elimination diet (the treatment described in Chapter 2.4–p.170). In such patients there are usually other symptoms as well, not just joint pain. A very common pattern is migraine, diarrhoea (or irritable bowel syndrome) and joint pain. Patients with these three symptoms often respond well to an elimination diet, with all three problems clearing up simultaneously.

Anyone with unexplained joint pain is strongly urged to try this particular diet, as their chances of benefit are high.

· *Bone Disorders* ·

Finally, there are certain diseases that do not belong to any of these five families, and mainly affect the bones, although there may be symptoms in the joints as well. These diseases include rickets and osteomalacia, both of which originate with a poor diet, and require specific dietary treatment.

Osteoporosis is also a disease of the bones. It is included in this book because people with inflammatory arthritis are more susceptible to osteoporosis than healthy people. Dietary treatments, along with exercise, are highly relevant to osteoporosis (see Chapter 2.3–p.161).

Table 1: The major families of arthritic diseases

Inflammatory arthritis
Ankylosing spondylitis
Behçet's syndrome
Arthritis accompanying coeliac
    disease
Arthritis accompanying Crohn's
    disease
Enteropathic arthritis
Enteropathic spondylitis
Felty's syndrome
Inflammatory polyarthropathy
Juvenile chronic arthritis
Palindromic rheumatism
Inflammatory polyarthropathy
Psoriatic arthritis
Rheumatoid arthritis
Sarcoidosis
Scleroderma
Sjögren's syndrome
Systemic lupus erythematosus
Systemic sclerosis
Arthritis accompanying ulcerative
    colitis
Seronegative arthritis
Seronegative spondylarthritides

Crystal arthritis
Gout
Pseudogout

Infective arthritis
'Septic arthritis'
Gonococcal arthritis
Meningococcal arthritis
Tuberculous arthritis
Some viral diseases causing arthritis
Lyme disease (may be a reactive
    arthritis in later stages)

Reactive arthritis
By-pass arthritis
Reiter's syndrome
Rheumatic fever
Arthritis following salmonella
    poisoning
Sexually Acquired Reactive Arthritis
    (SARA)
Whipple's disease
Some viral diseases causing arthritis

Degenerative arthritis
Osteoarthritis

Bone disorders
Osteochondritis
Osteomalacia
Osteoporosis
Paget's disease
Rickets

Chapter 1.4

WRONG TURNS AND
BLIND ALLEYS

Most of the popular diets currently recommended are reviewed in some
detail in Section 4. Here we intend to present a broad overview of these
diets, and suggest how such a jungle of conflicting advice may have
sprung up.

Many of the most popular diets are relatively new, and a number
originated in a similar way: with the personal recovery of the author
through dietary experimentation. This is the story behind Dr Dong's
diet, Sister Hills' diet and Dr Childers' diet, all of which require
avoidance of some foods.

We would suggest that each of these authors was suffering from
food-sensitive rheumatoid-like arthritis (as described in Chapter 1.1)
and that they happened, by chance, to devise a diet that omitted their
culprit foods. This would have accounted for their remarkable
recovery, something that is quite often seen with patients going
through the elimination diet. In the case of Dr Dong, his own account
supports this interpretation very strongly (see p.364).

Having hit upon a diet that omitted their culprit foods (and, quite
possibly, some other foods which were *not* culprits) these recovered
arthritics concluded that the same diet would automatically help others
so afflicted – or, indeed, anyone with any kind of arthritis. They began
to spread the word about their 'miracle diet'.

In doing so they felt obliged to explain how the diets worked. The
explanations varied but they generally invoked mechanisms in which
all arthritis was a result of the same kind of reaction to the *same*
offending foods – the reaction being attributed to 'toxins' or 'acids' in
food, for example, or to a lack of basic nutrients in processed foods.
(The most common explanations are discussed in detail in Chapter
4.9–p.403.) None of the explanations described the reaction to food as an
idiosyncratic one: none emphasised the fact that the individual patient
with rheumatoid arthritis could react to particular foods, foods which
might be perfectly harmless for someone else with the same form of

arthritis. Dr Dong, Dr Campbell and Dr Childers do all seem to have recognised the phenomenon of individual sensitivities to particular foods, but they disregarded this phenomenon when explaining how their diets work, and none of them put any emphasis on it in their books.

Similarly, most of the explanations were exceedingly general about 'arthritis' and did not allow for the fact that there are many different kinds of arthritis (see Chapter 1.3–p.63).

Spreading the word with enthusiasm, or treating patients directly in some cases, these recovered arthritics could have achieved success with other sufferers in three ways. Firstly, for some people with food-related rheumatoid arthritis, the list of prohibited foods just happened to include their culprit foods, so they experienced the same dramatic benefit as the originator of the diet. It is notable that *all* the diets prohibit some of the foods that are regularly identified as culprits by the patients studied at Epsom General Hospital. We have compiled a 'top twenty' list of offending foods – see Table 2 below – and compared the popular diets with this list. The Dong diet prohibits 11 out of the 20, and Dr Campbell's diet also prohibits 11 (but not the same ones, though there are a few overlaps), while Sister Hills' diet prohibits 8 out of the 20.

Secondly, a new and unorthodox treatment promoted by someone who was a walking advertisement for its benefits would have an extra-powerful placebo effect (see p.27) and there is little doubt that many arthritics responded well to this, even if the diet itself had little real benefit for them.

Table 2: Foods most likely to evoke symptoms in those rheumatoid arthritis patients who respond to an elimination diet

Food	Patients affected by food (%)	Food	Patients affected by food (%)
Corn	57	Malt	27
Wheat	54	Cheese	24
Bacon/pork	39	Grapefruit	24
Oranges	39	Tomato	22
Milk	37	Peanuts	20
Oats	37	Sugar (cane)	20
Rye	34	Butter	17
Eggs	32	Lamb	17
Beef	32	Lemon	17
Coffee	32	Soya	17

Thirdly, some people going into a phase of spontaneous remission or partial remission could have attributed the effects to trying the diet. Given that all the proponents *set no time limit* for the expected effects of the diet – indeed they usually insisted that the diet must be maintained for many months to see any benefit – the chances of this third factor coming into play at some stage were moderately high. (Steps are taken to compensate for this third factor in scientific trials – see p.28.) Furthermore, it was a logical conclusion from most of the explanations that improvement would be slow – the build-up of 'acid' had to be eroded, for example, or the 'toxins' gradually eliminated – so even a small improvement would be regarded as an indication of the diet 'beginning to work'. This would result in modest placebo effects or small spontaneous improvements, unrelated to the diet, being considered as promising signs of success.

We do not mean to imply that the originators of these diets were dishonest, only to show how readily they could have been misled into thinking that their diet was beneficial for everyone with arthritis. The fourth factor, common to all alternative therapies (and indeed to conventional medicine if patients are free to 'shop around' for treatment) is that those who get better tend to come back (or to write letters of eternal gratitude) while those who fail to improve are generally not heard from again. This can easily create an exaggerated impression of success in the mind of the diet's originator.

In the case of diets that rely solely on supplements (such as cider vinegar and honey, or blackstrap molasses) and do not prohibit any foods, it is still possible for placebo effect, spontaneous remissions or improvements, and wishful thinking on the part of those recommending the supplements, to produce an apparent cure for arthritis.

Other sources of real effects in some of the diets could be the inclusion of oily fish in the diet (see p.53), the reduction in saturated fat (see p.52) or the increased intake of antioxidants (see p.345) with a greater consumption of vegetable foods. The high fish content and reduced saturated fat of the Dong diet would probably be beneficial in the long term, for example, and so might the reduction in saturated fat on Sister Hills' diet.

A third source of real effects might be weight loss which can be very beneficial for those with osteoarthritis who are overweight. Many of the diets tend to be weight-reducing, although this is not their stated objective nor any part of the explanations given for their success.

Having carefully considered the explanations given by the proponents of each diet – explanations that invoke widespread malnutrition due to modern eating habits, poisoning by food additives, calcification of soft tissues or acid build-up in the tissues – we can find little in them that is in any way plausible or convincing. We consider such explanations in detail in Chapter 4.9 (p.403). Most of these explanations either invoke mechanisms for rheumatoid arthritis that were investigated thoroughly and discounted many years ago (eg. malnutrition) or mechanisms that fly in the face of the known facts about the disease (see pp.373–4).

· *The Traditional Diets* ·

Long before Dr Dong and Sister Hills entered the scene, there were diets handed on by word-of-mouth that supposedly cured arthritis. We would suggest that the same process of personal experimentation by people with food-related rheumatoid arthritis, as described above, could have led to some of these diets. But in the past there were other factors at work. Until the late nineteenth century the various forms of arthritis had not been differentiated by doctors. Gout, rheumatoid arthritis and osteoarthritis were all lumped together and seen as one rather variable disease.

In this situation, gout confused matters enormously. The link between diet and gout is indisputable and readily observed – the gouty individual, a fat, florid gentleman with a glass of port in his hand, is featured in many an eighteenth-century cartoon. Gout is caused in a very different way from rheumatoid arthritis or osteoarthritis (see Chapter 1.3–p.63) and the dietary link is entirely different from that in rheumatoid arthritis. When all forms of arthritis were viewed as one, however, gout must have reinforced the impression that diet was a major factor in arthritis. The fact that the traditional diets for arthritis tend to prohibit red meat and wine reinforce this impression that they were based, at least in part, on gouty patients, for such foods can indeed aggravate gout (see p.105).

Many authors of popular books today find it convenient to fall back on the medical innocence of former centuries and profess that there is no difference between the various types of arthritis. 'Folk medicine does not recognise a difference among bursitis, gout, rheumatoid arthritis, osteoarthritis and muscular rheumatism' declares Dr D C Jarvis, author of *Arthritis and Folk Medicine*. Dr Dong takes the instance of gout and says 'If one kind of arthritis is caused by food then why not other forms of arthritis?' This apparent naivety, in medically qualified authors, is puzzling, to say the least.

· *But it Worked for Me!* ·

There will, of course, be readers who have already tried one or more of the diets described in Section 4, or who know other arthritics who have tried them. If this is the case, then this last part of this chapter is for you.

A diet that you tried produced a prompt, substantial and lasting improvement

If you improved substantially on the diet, then food intolerance is the most likely explanation, but you may now be avoiding some foods unnecessarily. If you are finding the diet restrictive, you could try reintroducing foods singly to see how you react, following the basic procedures described in Chapter 2.4 (p.170). Begin with those foods least likely to evoke symptoms (see pp.182–5). If you have been avoiding these foods for more than six months, then you need to allow a longer test period, because your intolerance of the food might have lessened so that you do not react promptly. Eat each food every day for two weeks (or until symptoms recur), and do not reintroduce any other foods during that time. Even if the food produced no symptoms, cut it out of your diet temporarily after the two-week testing period, and move on to testing another food. Proceed with caution, and do not go back to eating any food that you strongly suspect of causing symptoms.

A diet apparently helped you, to some extent, but the benefit has been lost – what should you do now?

Firstly, it is possible that the good effects of the diet were illusory in some way. The ways in which a diet can seem to work when it is not actually doing any real good include:

1. Placebo effect (see p.27) thanks to the optimism with which the diet is tried.
2. A spontaneous remission (see p.19) or partial remission, happening by coincidence, some time after the diet began.
3. Weight loss, which may take the pressure off hip, knee and ankle joints. In the case of osteoarthritis, losing weight seems also to be more generally beneficial, for reasons that are not understood, and the finger joints may improve. (In this case the diet *has* done some good, but any weight-reducing diet would have done the same.)

If you began the diet with high hopes and there was an initial improvement which wore off after a few weeks or months, then placebo effect is a likely explanation. If the improvement was comparable, in degree and duration, with spontaneous improvements that you have experienced in the past, then the second factor might be at work. Rather than persist with the diet, you may find more benefit in trying an elimination diet (see Chapter 2.4–p.170) or an anti-inflammatory diet (see Chapter 2.2–p.143).

A diet helped, but the improvement was small

Assuming that the diet you tried prohibited certain foods, then a small improvement might indicate that you have food intolerance and that the diet happened to prohibit some of your culprit foods. If you are only partially better, then there may be other culprit foods which the present diet does not prohibit. The elimination diet would probably detect these.

TREATING YOUR ARTHRITIS WITH DIET

Chapter 2.1

FINDING THE RIGHT DIET: AN A–Z DIRECTORY OF THE DIFFERENT TYPES OF ARTHRITIS

Summary of contents:

To use this directory, look for your diagnosis (or symptoms) in the checklist below.

· *Introduction* ·

One of the entries listed above should correspond to your type of arthritis. If you are uncertain which one applies, check with your doctor. When you have an exact diagnosis you can look it up in the pages that follow, to find out more about the illness and whether any dietary treatments may help.

There may still be uncertainty about the diagnosis, especially if your arthritis has begun fairly recently. Or you may have been told that you have one condition, only to be given a different diagnosis some months later. Do not lose confidence in your doctor if this happens – the various kinds of arthritis are sometimes hard to tell apart in the early stages. The distinctive characteristics of the disease may only become apparent as it develops.

If you are in this early stage, where the exact diagnosis is uncertain, there is probably no harm in trying an elimination diet (see Chapter 2.4–p.170), as long as you are not underweight to begin with. If food reactions are playing a part in your disease, there is a good chance that cutting out the culprit food will be more effective at this early stage, before the disease process has become fully established. Needless to say, you should ask your doctor's advice – and follow it.

There are certain other symptoms and diseases that are relevant to arthritis and can help the doctor in reaching a diagnosis. Be sure to mention any recent problems, particularly rashes, other aches and pains, diarrhoea, sore throats or eye inflammation. Recent infections are also of interest, particularly sexually transmitted diseases – it may seem embarassing to mention these, but it is essential that you do so because they can be at the root of some forms of arthritis.

· *A – Z DIRECTORY* ·

· *AIDS* ·

Arthritis is sometimes the first symptom of infection with HIV (Human Immunodeficiency Virus), preceding other signs of AIDS (Acquired Immune Deficiency Syndrome). Doctors are still not sure whether this results from HIV increasing susceptibility to Sexually Acquired Reactive Arthritis (see p.136) or if HIV affects the joints directly as some other viral infections do (see p.142).

Many people who have long-standing rheumatoid arthritis, and then become infected with HIV, find that their rheumatoid arthritis goes into complete remission (the symptoms disappear) as AIDS develops. It seems that the parts of the immune system which are overactive in rheumatoid arthritis become disabled by the HIV virus.

Can diet help with HIV-related arthritis?

Diet is of no relevance in these cases.

· *Allergy and Arthritis* ·

Some allergic diseases seem to produce a brief attack of arthritis as well, usually during a severe but short-lived allergic reaction.

True allergies

Before dealing with this topic it is important to be absolutely clear about the meaning of 'allergy'. In this book, we use 'allergy' to mean one of the classical allergic diseases, such as hayfever: these are unusual reactions to harmless substances, reactions in which the immune system (p.416) is demonstrably involved. Unusual reactions that do not apparently involve the immune system are not allergies, according to this definition. (Some doctors define allergy even more narrowly and insist that it must involve the production of a special type of antibody (p.412) known as IgE (see p.416). The medical term for this particular reaction is Type I hypersensitivity; we refer to it as a true allergy.)

There are various tests which can show that the reaction is an allergy. The simplest is the **skin-prick test** where a small amount of the suspect substance is introduced into the skin – a red, itchy swelling confirms the diagnosis of allergy to that substance, although the test is not infallible. Laboratory tests include looking at a blood sample for IgE. If IgE against house-dust mite is found, for example, then the patient is clearly reacting to allergens (see p.412) produced by the mite.

Other classical allergic diseases include eczema and asthma when induced by an allergen (both can arise in other ways). Urticaria or nettle-rash is another condition that may be allergic or non-allergic in origin.

It is crucial to define the terms here, because there are different ways of using the word allergy. In common parlance it simply means an unusual reaction to anything. This much looser definition is also used by a few doctors working in this field (see p.43), by many alternative therapists, and in some popular books on health topics. This creates a great deal of confusion, especially in connection with food.

'Food allergy', in medical terms, is a prompt and often dramatic reaction to food by the immune system. In the more severe cases, there is swelling of the lips, mouth and tongue, 'nettle rash' all over the body, and a sudden fall in blood pressure. If there is swelling of the throat, this may cause suffocation. The fall in blood pressure alone can lead to a fatal collapse, so food allergy is doubly dangerous. (Fortunately, these effects can be reversed if the patient receives treatment promptly.) This is a true allergy, involving IgE.

Sometimes children 'grow out of' a food allergy, but if it persists beyond childhood the allergy is usually a lifelong condition. Fortunately, true food allergy is not particularly common.

Food intolerance is not allergy

Because food allergy is such a serious and potentially dangerous condition, many doctors are irritated by people using the term 'food allergy' to describe other reactions to food which are not life-threatening and which produce a completely different set of symptoms. The name generally used for these is food intolerance (p.44) and we employ this term for people with rheumatoid arthritis who respond well to an elimination diet. Food intolerance is only an umbrella term, and it undoubtedly includes a great many different kinds of reaction to food, but it remains a useful term despite this limitation.

It is part of the definition of food intolerance that it is *not* a true allergy to food. Although there may be some involvement by the immune system in food intolerance, the allergy antibody, IgE, is probably not involved, or involved on a minor scale only – someone who is intolerant of milk will not give a positive skin-prick test with milk, nor have IgE to milk in their blood.

Being precise about terminology is important because this part of the book (pp.82–85) does not refer to food intolerance, which is dealt with in Chapter 1.1. We are only discussing true allergies here.

Arthritis related to allergy

Arthritis is certainly not a common feature of true allergic reactions. It is rare, and the evidence that it exists is entirely anecdotal – based on the accounts of individual doctors about individual cases. This is not considered sound scientific evidence, but sometimes it is the best that medical science has to go on, especially with unusual forms of disease.

On the basis of anecdotal evidence, we can say that some people with hayfever also get joint pains during the pollen season, but not at other times of the year. This seems to be part of their allergic reaction to pollen.

A few people with true food allergy – who suffer symptoms such as swelling of the mouth, urticaria and water-retention (angioedema) after eating particular foods – may also have painful, swollen joints at the same time. The joint symptoms usually subside, as do the other reactions to the food, after a few days. The hands and wrists are the most commonly affected joints. Allergic reactions to drugs can also produce inflamed joints, although again this is rare.

Notice that, in all these cases, the joint pain is a short-lived reaction. This is very different from a long-term, ongoing joint disease such as rheumatoid arthritis. However, prompted by case-reports such as these, some doctors have looked again at rheumatoid arthritis, to see if it is more frequent in people with an allergic disposition. The answer seems to be 'no'. Furthermore, patients with rheumatoid arthritis are no more likely than other people to suffer from allergies.

Very occasionally, patients with food-related rheumatoid arthritis will show IgE antibodies to the culprit food. In such cases, it might be appropriate to regard them as having an unusual form of food allergy, rather than food intolerance, but this is a fairly academic distinction – what matters is that they get better when they avoid the culprit food.

Can diet help in arthritis associated with allergies?

In practical terms, if you have a true allergic reaction, and you experience joint symptoms at the same time, there is probably very little that you can do beyond following your doctor's advice for the allergic condition.

In the case of true food allergy, the advice to avoid the offending food should always be followed absolutely, even if your symptoms are fairly mild at present. Food allergy usually gets worse with each exposure to the food, and it can sometimes progress rapidly, from a minor reaction (such as tingling of the mouth and lips) to a serious collapse the next time the food is eaten. Reading the labels on prepared food is essential (see pp.194–204 for synonyms for common ingredients) and you should be wary about restaurant meals or bakery products which might contain the offending food in hidden form.

If you suffer from hayfever and simultaneous joint pains, talk to your doctor about the medicines you are taking for your hayfever. It may be worth trying a different type of hayfever drug to see if this helps your joints as well. Antihistamines are sometimes effective against the joint pain. Diet is unlikely to make any difference, but if there is a food which you only eat during the pollen season (such as cherries or strawberries), try cutting that food out next summer to see if the joint pains clear up. Any food which makes your tongue and mouth tingle should be avoided anyway – there is probably a cross-reaction occurring between the pollen and the food and this can develop into a full-blown and potentially damaging food allergy. The most common cross-reaction is between birch pollen and apples.

Anyone with unexplained joint pain and recurrent bouts of urticaria could be suffering from a reaction of some kind to food, either an allergy or an intolerance. An elimination diet (see Chapter 2.4–p.170) would probably be worth trying. If this is not helpful, then antihistamines may be effective – ask your doctor about these.

Finally, if you are of an allergic disposition or if allergies run in the family (again we are talking about true allergies here), and if you also have rheumatoid arthritis, it is well worth trying an elimination diet. Some Italian researchers have found that those with an allergic disposition have a greater chance of improving in response to such a diet than the average person with rheumatoid arthritis.

· *Ankylosing Spondylitis* ·

Ankylosing spondylitis is a disease that produces inflammation of the joints, rather like that of rheumatoid arthritis, but it mainly affects the spine or backbone and the larger joints such as hips and knees, whereas rheumatoid arthritis usually involves small joints, notably those in the fingers and wrists.

Far more men than women suffer from ankylosing spondylitis. In the past the ratio was put at 9:1 in favour of men, but recently doctors have recognised that more women have ankylosing spondylitis than was previously thought. Women often have a mild form of the disease, and this was sometimes mistaken for ordinary backache. Currently, the ratio of male to female sufferers is thought to be about 4:1 or 3:1.

Ankylosing spondylitis begins with stiffness and pain, usually in the back and the hips. At this stage the disease can seem like nothing more than a 'bad back', but there are certain crucial differences: the symptoms are worst in the morning, or after a prolonged rest, whereas they improve with exercise. There may be other tell-tale symptoms, such as pain in the chest, poor appetite and tiredness. About 20–25% of patients also have pain in their knees, ankles or other joints, including the hip joint. Sometimes the eyes are affected. However, the symptoms in the spine are usually the predominant ones.

To understand the effects of ankylosing spondylitis, it is useful to know something about the structure of a normal spinal column. The spine is made up of 33 very similar small bones, called **vertebrae,** one stacked on top of the other like building blocks. There are wing-like extensions on each of the vertebrae called 'articular processes', which stick out at an angle and meet the articular processes of the adjacent vertebra. These meeting points act as joints, allowing some bending of the spine but controlling the direction and extent of the movement. They are small synovial joints (see p.421), so there is a capsule around each joint and a synovial membrane or synovium inside.

Between the vertebrae lie **intervertebral discs**, pads made of fibrous cartilage with a softer, jelly-like centre. These discs cushion the vertebrae and protect them from rubbing against each other. The whole spine is also encased in ligaments (strips of tough, rubbery material) and there are muscles that can bend or straighten the spine. The muscles are attached to the vertebrae by tendons which are rubbery and flexible like ligaments.

Inflammation in the spine of someone with ankylosing spondylitis causes four important changes (not necessarily in the order given here). Firstly, the points where the ligaments and tendons are attached to the vertebrae become inflamed, and may even grow hard and inflexible as calcium salts, normally found only in the bones, become deposited there. Secondly, the synovial joints between the articular processes may suffer inflammation in the same way as any other synovial joint (see p.64), losing much of their mobility and, in the worst cases, seizing up completely. Thirdly, abnormal bony spurs grow from the vertebrae, and those from adjacent vertebrae can meet and gradually fuse together. Finally, calcium salts may be deposited at the edges of the intervertebral discs, which then grow hard and rigid. The discs can even become joined to the vertebrae by the calcium deposit.

Another change occurs in the joint between the sacrum (the triangular bone at the base of the spine) and the ileum (the bone at the back of the hip girdle). This joint, known as the sacro-iliac joint also becomes inflamed.

In time, the various changes in the spine, especially the deposits of calcium salts in the intervertebral discs, can produce complete fusion of the vertebrae, so that the spine is locked rigid. (This is what 'ankylosing' means: stiffening or loss of movement.) The spine may also become curved in the process. Fortunately this fusion and curvature can usually be prevented by keeping mobile and taking sensible exercise, combined with the careful use of drugs. Once the early stage of ankylosing spondylitis has passed, there is usually much less pain, and with proper treatment very few people become severely disabled by the disease.

Inheritance plays a very important part in ankylosing spondylitis. At least 90% of those with the disease carry a genetic marker known as HLA-B27 which they have inherited from one of their parents. HLA molecules are found in everyone, but they are of different types, just as there are different blood groups. Some types of HLA are associated with particular diseases.

There are other forms of arthritis which are linked to HLA-B27. Anyone with HLA-B27 is a hundred times more likely to suffer from Reiter's syndrome (p.127) following an infection of the uro-genital tract.

The vulnerability of HLA-B27 individuals to reactive arthritis (arthritis in response to an infection – see p.126) is an interesting piece of evidence. It leads on to an obvious question: could ankylosing spondylitis itself be a reaction to infection? If so, what is the microbe concerned, and where is it in the body?

Recent research may provide an answer to these questions. Dr Alan Ebringer of King's College, London has found that patients with active ankylosing spondylitis have high levels of antibodies to a bacterium called *Klebsiella*. The *Klebsiella* is thought to be living in their gut. Remember that it is entirely healthy and natural to have bacteria and other microbes in the gut – they are known as the gut flora (p.37). Sometimes, however, certain bacteria become over-plentiful, or abnormal bacteria invade the gut flora, and these can produce illness. *Klebsiella* is not a normal part of most people's gut flora, and it is sometimes implicated in outbreaks of diarrhoea in hospitals. However it is found in about 5% of healthy individuals, either in the gut or the lungs, so it can inhabit the human body without causing symptoms. In patients with ankylosing spondylitis it is present in fairly high numbers in the gut but does not cause any obvious reaction, such as diarrhoea. Only recently has anyone suspected that it might be involved in ankylosing spondylitis.

Klebsiella produces a protein which has some resemblance to the HLA-B27 molecule – in fact a short section of the protein is absolutely identical with HLA-B27. It is possible that this resemblance could provoke an auto-immune reaction, in which antibodies to the *Klebsiella* protein also bind to HLA-B27. The result could be an inappropriate reaction by the immune system.

Although this theory is very attractive, it still needs to be tested more fully, and such work is now going on at several hospitals. While *Klebsiella* and HLA-B27 might interact to produce ankylosing spondylitis, there must be other factors involved as well. This is clear because a minority of those with ankylosing spondylitis do not have HLA-B27 but have other HLA types. It is also important to remember that only 8% of men with HLA-B27 suffer from ankylosing spondylitis, and even fewer HLA-B27 women, so it is not at all a foregone conclusion that someone carrying this marker will suffer from the disease. (Nevertheless the disease does 'run in families' so low back pain in a relative of someone with ankylosing spondylitis should always be investigated carefully. Children in such families should be taken to the doctor if they develop any swelling of the joints, or symptoms in the eye.)

Can diet help in ankylosing spondylitis?

Encouraged by the new theory about *Klebsiella*, some doctors have been trying out special diets for ankylosing spondylitis. If *Klebsiella* really is to blame, and if a change in diet can reduce the numbers of *Klebsiella* in the gut (both fairly big 'ifs' at present) the inflammation in the joints should be reduced. However, such diets involve drastic changes to eating patterns, and they have not yet been subjected to full scientific testing (double-blind, placebo-controlled trials, as described on p.27) so we cannot at present recommend them.

Another group of researchers, working in Belgium, have tried out a milk-free diet for patients with ankylosing spondylitis. Their reasoning was that many bacterial fragments remain in milk, even though the bacteria themselves have been killed by pasteurisation. It is possible that these bacterial fragments provoke an ongoing reaction by the immune system, which then leads to some kind of reaction producing inflammation in the joints (as described above for *Klebsiella*).

When 25 patients with ankylosing spondylitis were told to avoid milk and milk products, 13 of them showed a marked improvement, with eight well enough to stop taking NSAIDs (non-steroidal anti-inflammatory drugs). Another four patients were a little better. Most of those who experienced a substantial improvement kept up their diet afterwards, and were still well two years later, suggesting that the improvement really was due to the diet, not just the random up-and-down variations of the disease.

Unfortunately, this was not a double-blind placebo-controlled trial, so we cannot recommend this diet unreservedly. However, there is little harm in cutting out milk products for a while and seeing if this helps – as long as your doctor agrees.

You should take a calcium supplement while on the diet, or eat some other food rich in calcium (eg. tinned sardines, eating the bones as well as the flesh of the fish; if you dislike fish, see p.317 for other foods rich in calcium). If there is going to be a response it should be obvious within six weeks.

A high intake of Vitamin E may be beneficial in ankylosing spondylitis (see p.305).

Other antioxidants (see p.339), such as Vitamin E and carotenoids, are also thought to be important in reducing the damaging effects of inflammation. Intake of these antioxidant nutrients can be boosted by eating more of certain foods, and such dietary changes, described in Chapter 2.8 (p.252), will have more general health benefits as well.

Those with ankylosing spondylitis are more likely than other people to develop osteoporosis, or thinning of the bones (see p.120). It is advisable to follow a diet that reduces the risks of this disorder, which can lead to fractures of the vertebrae, hip and wrist. A suitable diet is described in Chapter 2.3 (p.161).

Ensuring a high intake of Vitamin K may be particularly important in preventing osteoporosis among those with ankylosing spondylitis (see p.307).

· *Arthralgia* ·

The term arthralgia simply means 'joint pain'. Doctors generally use it to describe any joint pain that is just a pain, with no hint of inflammation (no swelling, stiffness, warmth, or tenderness when touched), and no signs that would suggest a diagnosis of osteoarthritis.

The possibility of injury should always be considered: overuse or misuse can readily lead to joint pain, especially in the hands (from typing for example) or the knees. Anyone playing a lot of sport may be at risk of damaging particular joints – footballers quite often injure their knees. Some joint pain of this type is actually bursitis (see p.95).

Another form of arthralgia is seen in some people with food intolerance (see p.44). Exactly why food should cause joint pain in certain people is unknown.

Can diet help with arthralgia?

If there is no reason to suspect injury, overuse, selenium deficiency (see p.335) or any known disease as a cause of the joint pain, then food intolerance is a prime suspect and an elimination diet is certainly worth trying: see Chapter 2.4 (p.170) for details. Experience suggests that a fair proportion of people with simple, unexplained arthralgia respond well to an elimination diet. In general, the pain disappears more quickly than that of rheumatoid arthritis – within a week of starting the elimination phase for some patients.

When food intolerance is at the root of the problem there are likely to be other symptoms besides joint pain. These may include migraine or frequent headaches, diarrhoea or irritable bowel syndrome, general feelings of malaise and possibly fatigue. Anyone with a collection of symptoms such as these should certainly try an elimination diet. It would be wise to seek your doctor's advice first, especially if your joint symptoms have never been properly investigated, or if you are seriously ill or underweight. Bear in mind, however, that your doctor may be dismissive of the idea of food intolerance as a source of your symptoms. In these circumstances, ask whether the diet would be harmful in any way, given your medical condition, and follow the advice you receive. It may be helpful to show your doctor the guidelines for the elimination diet given in Chapter 2.4 (p.170).

· *Arthritis* ·

Arthritis means an inflammation of one or more joints: 'arthr-' means 'joint', while '-itis' means 'inflammation'.

'Arthritis' is not a diagnosis in itself, because inflamed joints are a feature of many quite distinct diseases, such as rheumatoid arthritis, ankylosing spondylitis and Reiter's syndrome. The term 'arthritis' should not be used where there is no evidence of inflammation, such as swelling of the joint, redness or warmth. Simple joint pain, without inflammation, is generally referred to as 'arthralgia' (see p.89).

Note that 'osteoarthritis' is a misleading name, because inflammation is not a primary feature of this disease, though it may develop secondarily (see p.115). Many doctors and researchers would like to see a change in the name of this disease (possible alternatives are 'osteoarthrosis' or 'degenerative joint disease'), but there is always resistance to changing names that have been in use for a long time.

Can diet help with 'arthritis'?

It all depends on what sort of arthritis is involved: there is no general dietary advice that applies to all kinds of arthritis. You need to obtain a more exact diagnosis and then look up the entry for that disease.

· *Arthropathy* ·

This term means 'a disorder of the joints'. It is intended to include any disorder, whether caused by inflammation, wear-and-tear or other means. The term is a useful replacement for 'arthritis' in a disease which does not primarily involve inflammation, such as the mis-named 'osteoarthritis'. However, it is not widely used. To locate the dietary advice appropriate for your condition you will need a more precise diagnosis.

· *Back Pain* ·

Most back pain is due to strain, injury, a sagging mattress or an awkward posture that has to be maintained while working.

In rare instances, back pain turns out to be the first sign of ankylosing spondylitis (p.85). Often this goes undiagnosed for some time, because the symptoms can be very similar to those produced by back strain.

Can diet help with back pain?

There are three case reports of patients with severe back pain who responded well to an elimination diet. All these patients had several other symptoms as well. In one patient these included muscle aches, headache, joint pains, tiredness and constipation, while another patient suffered from blurred vision, migraine, tiredness and irritable bowel syndrome (diarrhoea with abdominal pain). The third had abdominal pain and a constantly blocked nose, in addition to backache.

Disabling back pain was the main symptom for these patients, however, and it cleared up simultaneously with the other symptoms on an elimination diet. This is only anecdotal evidence (individual case studies) and the link with food cannot be considered proven. But the fact that the patients had been thoroughly investigated for many years before trying dietary treatment, that nothing had previously helped them, whereas the diet produced a profound and lasting improvement, is interesting enough to encourage further research in this field. Nevertheless, most doctors would be sceptical about the idea of food playing any part in back pain and scientific confirmation is required.

For someone who has back pain, and other unexplained symptoms of the type described above, an elimination diet is worth considering (see Chapter 2.4–p.170). It is vital to obtain the approval of your doctor first since some back pain may be a symptom of more serious disease requiring prompt investigation.

· *Behçet's Syndrome* ·

This is a rare condition named after a Turkish physician, Dr Hulusi Behçet, who first identified it. There are more cases in Turkey and elsewhere in the eastern Mediterranean than in most other parts of the world, although Japan also has a high frequency of this disease. To give just one comparison, Behçet's syndrome is eighty times more common in Japan than it is in Minnesota. The reasons for this odd pattern of distribution are not understood, but it may be due to inherited factors, or to something in the environment (such as food, or microbes) or, quite possibly, to a combination of these factors.

The disease is mainly characterised by ulcers of the mouth and genitals, and inflammation of the eye (uveitis). Some patients (about 10% of the total) also suffer from arthritis. There may also be skin rashes and a variety of other symptoms, including psychiatric effects. There tend to be periods when the disease gets worse, and others when it grows milder.

The exact cause of Behçet's syndrome is unknown but the immune system is almost certainly involved in some way. It is possible that there is an unusual reaction to a particular virus infection. Drugs that suppress the immune system, such as corticosteroids, are used to treat the condition.

Can diet help with Behçet's syndrome?

The medical literature includes just one paper on this topic. Doctors in the United States investigated nine patients with Behçet's syndrome. They had been impressed by the fact that six of these patients avoided eating walnuts, having found that these nuts made their symptoms far worse. (One man dated the origin of his illness to a time when he had worked in a sawmill, sawing up walnut timber and inhaling a great deal of the dust.)

The researchers began by testing the effects of walnut extracts on certain immune cells (see p.416), called lymphocytes. They used lymphocytes from healthy people and from patients with Behçet's syndrome. Regardless of their origin, the lymphocytes reacted to walnut extract in exactly the same way – with a burst of unusually frenzied activity. (Such reactions are not unknown with plants and plant products, as quite a few contain chemicals, called mitogens, that act as aggravators to the immune system.)

Next, the researchers fed walnuts to five healthy people and five of the Behçet's syndrome patients who generally avoided walnuts. All those with Behçet's syndrome showed a marked and severe increase in symptoms, lasting for several weeks after eating the nuts.

The researchers then took samples of lymphocytes again, and retested them with walnut extract and several other mitogens. Eating the nuts had affected how the lymphocytes behaved. Everyone's lymphocytes were far less responsive than before, but whereas those from healthy people regained their former zest within a week or so of giving up walnuts again, the lymphocytes from those with Behçet's syndrome seemed to take longer to recover.

Exactly what this all means is hard to say, and unfortunately no one has pursued this line of investigation, which took place over 20 years ago. It seems clear that the six patients with Behçet's syndrome who avoided walnuts were right to do so. However, their Behçet's syndrome did not clear up completely when they avoided walnuts, so this was obviously not the whole story. Furthermore, for the other Behçet's patients in the set studied, walnuts did not influence their symptoms. In Japan, walnuts are not grown, and little eaten, yet Behçet's syndrome is relatively common.

With these facts in mind, the researchers suggested that there might be other foods, or even microbes, that could either trigger off Behçet's syndrome, or make it considerably worse. To be susceptible to one of these triggers, they speculated, the patient must have some particular quirk of the immune system, which made it develop a damaging and self-perpetuating reaction in response to the trigger. The quirk would probably be an inherited characteristic, which would explain why the disease is so much more common in some parts of the world than in others. It seems plausible that, if there is more than one trigger for Behçet's syndrome, there is more than one inherited quirk producing susceptibility.

Quite apart from the effects of walnuts, all of the nine Behçet's syndrome patients in this study found that certain foods aggravated their disease. Foods such as lemons, grapefruit, oranges and tomatoes were a particular problem, and this may have been nothing more than the acidity making their mouth ulcers more painful. However, chocolate was also identified as a problem food; and some patients were affected by other types of nuts, not just walnuts.

To the best of our knowledge there have been no other studies of Behçet's syndrome and food – such research is always very difficult with rare diseases because researchers cannot find enough patients locally to make the experiments valid. Neverthless, the research described above is intriguing, and it would seem worthwhile for anyone with Behçet's syndrome to try cutting out walnuts for a few months, along with pecan nuts and hickory nuts (which are from closely related trees) and any cakes, biscuits, cookies or other foods that might contain these nuts. Indeed, eliminating all nuts for a time might be a good plan. Chocolate could be left out at the same time, as well as foods such as citrus fruits and tomatoes.

It would be interesting to know if there might be a more general link between Behçet's syndrome and food. From experience with food intolerance causing other symptoms (see pp.44–45), it is clear that a food which is eaten every day, such as wheat or milk, can often be the culprit, yet it is difficult to establish the connection between food and symptoms except by carrying out an elimination diet (see pp.24–5. Given the possible role of food, an elimination diet might be worth trying for Behçet's syndrome, although the lack of research in this field makes it impossible for us to positively recommend such treatment. It is essential to seek your doctor's advice before trying this. Instructions for an elimination diet are given in Chapter 2.4. (p.270)

A study of patients with Behçet's syndrome in Japan showed that their antioxidant levels in the blood were unusually low, a common reaction to generalised inflammation. Supplements of Vitamin E seemed to reduce the inflammation, in so far as they produced improvements in several laboratory tests (such as C-reactive protein or CPR test) used for Behçet's syndrome and other inflammatory diseases. Rather than just taking Vitamin E, it would seem sensible to increase consumption of all the major antioxidants — detailed advice on this is given on pp.257–9. Boosting antioxidant levels is something that can be done in combination with other dietary treatments, such as avoiding a problem food.

While experimenting with any of these treatments, you should continue taking the drugs prescribed at the full dose. If you do improve, and wish to reduce your drug intake, you must get your doctor's agreement first.

· *Bursitis* ·

A 'bursa' is the biological equivalent of a small inflatable cushion. Rather than being inflated with air, a bursa is filled with fluid. There are about 150 of them, conveniently sited in the human body at spots where one part needs to be protected from another part by a little padding. There are, for example, several bursae around the elbow, the shoulder and the knee. They protect muscles or tendons, where they would otherwise rub against bones, or protect the skin where a hard bony area such as the elbow lies close beneath the surface.

A bursa has some similarities to a joint capsule – the ball of fibrous tissue that encloses the bones of a joint. The outer wall of the bursa is made of fibrous material which is lined with a synovial membrane. This membrane produces the fluid within the bursa which is very similar to the synovial fluid of a joint.

In bursitis, the membrane inside the bursa becomes inflamed and excess fluid is produced. The bursa becomes painful, warm, and expanded by fluid. The most common cause of bursitis is repeated friction and pressure to a particular joint. The knee can be affected, for example, by too much kneeling – the condition once known as housemaid's knee, but now more likely to afflict carpet-layers.

Bursitis can also occur in rheumatoid arthritis. The inflammation should subside at the same time that the inflammation in the joints responds to treatment.

Can diet help with bursitis?

It is unlikely to help, except perhaps in someone with rheumatoid arthritis whose joint symptoms respond to an elimination diet or an oil supplement (see Rheumatoid Arthritis – pp.129–3) in which case bursal inflammation might also be reduced.

· *By-pass Arthritis* ·

An intestinal by-pass operation is sometimes used to treat obesity. This surgical treatment reduces the amount of useful bowel by cutting it at two points and rejoining the cut ends. This leaves a fairly long piece of the bowel that is isolated from the rest and no longer receives any input of food. The surgeon seals up both ends of this piece, but it remains in the body. The purpose of the operation is to produce weight loss by ensuring that fewer nutrients are absorbed from food.

About 25% of patients who have had this operation go on to develop arthritis, mainly in the joints of the wrists, hands, knees and ankles. If the by-pass operation is reversed, and the bowel reinstated as before, the arthritis quickly clears up. Sometimes, a course of antibiotics will also clear the arthritis, suggesting that bacteria are playing a part. Indeed, there is evidence that a 'population explosion' of certain bacteria in the isolated section of bowel is responsible for the symptoms in the joints. The blood of patients with this problem contains many circulating immune complexes (see p.416), made up of bacterial antigens bound together with antibodies which the body has produced in reaction to those antigens. It is thought that circulating immune complexes can easily be deposited in the small blood vessels around a joint and spark off arthritis.

Can diet help with by-pass arthritis?

A change of diet will not affect by-pass arthritis, which should be treated with antibiotics or with surgery to reverse the original operation.

The reason for the interest in this condition by rheumatologists is that it shows the influence which the bacteria living in the gut (the gut flora – see p.37) might have on the health of the joints. Note that the bacteria themselves never penetrate the joints, nor even enter the bloodstream – it is just the antigens from the bacteria producing these effects. These antigens circulate in the blood and can then cause inflammation in the joints. This ability of the gut flora to produce arthritis 'at a distance' might explain some of the observed effects of diet on certain arthritic diseases (see pp.39–40).

· Capsulitis ·

This condition affects the shoulder joints (producing 'frozen shoulder') or, more rarely, the hip joints. The ball of ligaments which encloses the joint – the joint capsule – becomes inflamed and may tighten around the joint, either due to contraction or thickening.

Pain and restricted movement are the immediate consequences of capsulitis. In the case of frozen shoulder, there is usually only one shoulder joint affected, and the problem may follow an injury to the upper arm, or from a disease that affects the region around the shoulder. Diabetes or the use of barbiturate drugs may also be factors.

In the case of the hips, capsulitis may occur spontaneously, sometimes due to barbiturate usage; only one joint is usually affected in this case. Capsulitis of the hips can also occur as a result of an underlying problem within the joints, such as rheumatoid arthritis.

Treatment may involve drugs such as corticosteroids, either injected into the joint or taken by mouth, to calm the inflammation. Exercises and physiotherapy are also very important, particularly for frozen shoulder, and exercise programmes should be followed carefully.

Can diet help with capsulitis?

This has never been investigated but it seems unlikely. You could try one of the oils that soothe inflammation, as described in Chapter 2.2 (p.143).

· *Carpal Tunnel Syndrome* ·

This condition causes tingling, numbness and/or pain in certain of the fingers, sometimes wi h loss of movement as well. It is due to pressure on a nerve where it runs through a 'tunnel' between the bones of the wrist. This pressure can be created by swelling of soft tissues within the carpal tunnel, or by the retention of fluid.

Carpal tunnel syndrome may accompany rheumatoid arthritis or other diseases, but it sometimes occurs independently of any other disorder in which case it is known as *idiopathic* carpal tunnel syndrome.

Treatment may include corticosteroid injections to reduce inflammation in the carpal tunnel, or surgery to relieve the pressure on the nerve.

Can diet help with carpal tunnel syndrome?

This is a very contentious issue. Some researchers in the U.S.A. have claimed that patients with idiopathic carpal tunnel syndrome are actually suffering from a deficiency of pyridoxine (Vitamin B_6) and that their symptoms can be greatly relieved by a supplement of this vitamin. This claim has not been widely accepted in the medical world, despite some reasonably good experimental trials in its favour.

Few other researchers or doctors have chosen to investigate this treatment which means there is little evidence to weigh against the original claims for pyridoxine, but it seems that the vitamin is probably relevant for a minority of people with *idiopathic* carpal tunnel syndrome (see above), and irrelevant where this problem is related to rheumatoid arthritis or another long-standing disease. It is certainly the case that a mild deficiency of Vitamin B_6 is quite common, affecting 10–25% of the population.

If you have idiopathic carpal tunnel syndrome and wish to try vitamin treatment, you must discuss it with your doctor first. The recommended dose is 50 mg per day, substantially more than the recommended daily allowance. This dose is probably safe, but there is a small risk of damage to the nervous system, a risk which rises rapidly with larger doses – hence the need for medical supervision. This vitamin should generally be taken as part of a B-complex supplement, for the reasons given on p.286. It may take 12 weeks for the supplement to have any effect on the symptoms. Patients taking the drug levodopa for Parkinson's disease should not try this supplement as it interferes with the action of levodopa.

If you are overweight and have carpal tunnel syndrome, the excess pounds may be contributing to the problem: there is a definite link with obesity. Consult Chapter 2.6 (p.226) for advice on losing weight.

Water retention can also be a causative factor, and a low-salt diet may be helpful if this is the problem. Talk to your doctor before trying this.

· Diffuse Idiopathic Skeletal Hyperostosis ·

This is a very common condition among people over 50, particularly men. It should not cause serious anxiety since it simply produces stiffness of the back, which does not generally deteriorate badly; there is usually only moderate pain. What happens is that bony spurs grow from the vertebrae (the bony units that make up the spine). When one spur meets another spur from an adjacent vertebra they may fuse and form bridges, which then lock the vertebrae together. If many vertebrae are locked in this way, then the spine becomes less flexible.

Diet is most unlikely to make any difference to diffuse idiopathic skeletal hyperostosis.

· Enteropathic Arthritis ·

Arthritic symptoms may sometimes occur in people suffering from certain bowel diseases, including Crohn's disease, ulcerative colitis and coeliac disease. The frequency of arthritis in these patients is higher than in the population at large. About 12% of those with ulcerative colitis are also affected in the joints, as are about 21% of those with Crohn's disease. The percentage of coeliac patients with affected joints is thought to be much smaller.

All these bowel disorders involve damaging inflammation (see p.64) in the wall of the intestine. The inflammation produces great changes in the gut wall, changes that can be seen if a small sample is taken (a biopsy) and viewed under the microscope.

Some researchers believe that the damage to the gut wall might make it more permeable than usual, and so allow through a greater number of food molecules and bacterial antigens (from the bacteria living in the gut, the gut flora – see p.37). These food molecules and bacterial products could thus reach the bloodstream and provoke an immune reaction there. This could produce circulating immune complexes (see p.416), which would then be carried around the body by the bloodstream and deposited in the tiny blood vessels (capillaries) of the joint. The deposited immune complexes might then lead to inflammation and pain in the joint. As yet, there is no firm evidence for any of this.

Surgery for ulcerative colitis will usually get rid of all the joint symptoms, but this is not the case with Crohn's disease. In coeliac disease, a gluten-free diet will generally put an end to the arthritis.

Can diet help with enteropathic arthritis?

Doctors interested in the phenomenon of food intolerance have looked closely at both ulcerative colitis and Crohn's disease. The verdict, after decades of research, is that diet does not influence ulcerative colitis, but that food sensitivity may be a source of symptoms for Crohn's disease. If a change of diet can help the Crohn's disease, it seems logical to assume that it may also help any arthritic symptoms that accompany Crohn's disease.

Pioneering work with **Crohn's disease** has been carried out by Dr John Hunter of Addenbrooke's Hospital in Cambridge, and his results have now been corroborated by independent research which shows that at least 50% of patients with Crohn's disease can recover by using an elimination diet to identify culprit foods, and then avoiding those foods. When patients were closely supervised by Dr Hunter's medical team, who have a great deal of experience with elimination diets, the success rate was higher, with 80% of patients recovering and remaining well after two years.

The form of elimination diet used by Dr Hunter relies on a type of synthetic food known as an elemental diet (p.21) for the first phase, rather than on eating uncommon foods (as described in Chapter 2.4). This approach is used because patients with Crohn's disease tend to be thin at the outset, and further weight loss is not a good idea. With an elemental diet, the number of calories consumed can be as high as usual. As an extra bonus, there is no chance of having a reaction to something that is eaten during the elimination phase – a rare but significant problem with the sort of elimination diet we describe.

No one with Crohn's disease should consider trying an elimination diet without the full agreement and cooperation of their doctor. (If necessary a patient can ask to be referred to a gastroenterology specialist who uses elimination diets for Crohn's disease.) Apart from the potential risk of weight loss, there may be dramatic and unpleasant reactions when offending foods are tested. Unless testing is managed carefully these reactions may produce a severe and lasting deterioration of the Crohn's disease. Indeed, anyone with severe Crohn's disease should only reintroduce certain foods – those most likely to provoke a reaction – under medical supervision in a hospital.

One form of enteropathic arthritis has long been treated with a diet: **coeliac disease**. Patients with this condition must avoid all foods containing the proteins that are collectively called 'gluten'. These are present abundantly in wheat, and in lesser amounts in rye, barley and oats. If the gluten-free diet is maintained religiously, all bowel symptoms, and any arthritic pain, should disappear. Unfortunately, some coeliac patients do not keep to the diet, and thereby expose themselves to the risk of other diseases, including cancer of the digestive tract.

Sometimes coeliacs have persistent symptoms, even though they avoid gluten. This may be the result of a more serious disease and should be investigated by a doctor. For those patients whose continuing symptoms have no obvious cause, the answer may lie in foods other than gluten. Recent research has shown that these patients may have sensitivities to other foods, as a result of the gluten-induced damage to the gut wall – this can make it more permeable to other food molecules which in turn may lead to food intolerance (see pp.190–191). Quite often the offending food is soya (which is a frequent ingredient of gluten-free bread and other products) but it could be any food. Milk, rice, fish and chicken are among those that have been found to affect some coeliac patients. As with other forms of food intolerance, everyone is different, so an elimination diet is the only way to identify the culprit food. Since coeliac disease is a serious condition it is essential that your doctor gives wholehearted consent to trying an elimination diet.

For those with **ulcerative colitis**, an elimination diet is not recommended as it rarely, if ever, produces benefits. Antioxidants notably Vitamin E and Vitamin C, may reduce the damage done by inflammation in the bowel. The mineral selenium, which forms part of another antioxidant molecule, may also be valuable. Advice on boosting your intake of antioxidant nutrients is given on p.000. In theory antioxidants may help with the inflammation in the joints as well as that in the bowel, although there have been no scientific trials that would provide evidence to support this.

· *Enteropathic Spondylitis* ·

Two of the inflammatory bowel diseases – ulcerative colitis and Crohn's disease – can sometimes be accompanied by symptoms that resemble those of ankylosing spondylitis (see p.85). These include stiffness and pain in the lower back and hips. However, there may be arthritis in other joints as well, particularly those of the leg, and this can lead to confusion with enteropathic arthritis (see p.98).

In fact, enteropathic arthritis and enteropathic spondylitis seem to be fundamentally different. In enteropathic spondylitis, the inflammation is more severe and erosion of the small joints can occur. The joint symptoms do not flare up when the bowel symptoms flare up, and wane when the bowel symptoms wane. Nor does surgery for ulcerative colitis cure the joints, as it does with enteropathic arthritis. In short, the spondylitis is not a consequence of the bowel disease but a separate phenomenon: they are thought to appear in the same patient because that person has some underlying abnormality of the immune system which produces susceptibility to both. This abnormality may well be inherited.

About 17% of patients with inflammatory bowel disease develop enteropathic spondylitis. Some people suffer from the spondylitis before they experience any diarrhoea or abdominal pain, but there may already be inflammation of the bowel which has not yet produced any symptoms. If the doctor treating the spondylitis suspects this, a biopsy (see p.414) of the gut will be taken. This will reveal any inflammation and damage in the gut wall.

Can diet help with enteropathic spondylitis?

In the case of Crohn's disease, food intolerance is a possibility, as described on pp.99–100. Only by carrying out an elimination diet can the culprit food or foods be identified, and such a diet requires full medical supervision. Whether avoiding culprit foods will help with the spondylitis, as well as the bowel symptoms, is unknown.

· *Enthesopathy* ·

Inflammation of the points where tendons are joined to bones – see Tendonitis (p.141) for more details.

· *Extrinsic Allergic Alveolitis and Arthritis* ·

The diseases known as bird fancier's lung and farmer's lung (collectively called extrinsic allergic alveolitis) are due to allergens accummulating in the lungs. Arthritis is sometimes among the symptoms, although the main problems are breathlessness, cough and feverishness. Although this is a reaction by the immune system, it is entirely different from the allergic reaction that produces hayfever or asthma.

The arthritic symptoms should clear up if the recommended medical treatment is followed. This usually involves getting away from the source of the allergen. Diet is unlikely to be of any help here, with one rare exception: some patients with bird fancier's lung are sensitive to food containing eggs, due to a cross-reaction. Eliminating eggs for a few weeks, to see if there is any improvement in the joints, might be worthwhile.

· *Feet, Painful* ·

There are a variety of reasons why pain may develop in the feet. Diet is unlikely to be of any help, except in someone who has unexplained pain in other joints as well (see Arthralgia, p.89) or definite signs of food intolerance (see pp.44–5).

There is one condition that causes a sharp pain in the foot, just behind the third and fourth toes, when pressure is applied. Known as Morton's neuroma, it is often mis-diagnosed, which is unfortunate since it can be cured very simply by a small operation.

· *Felty's Syndrome* ·

Patients with this unusual disease suffer from severe rheumatoid arthritis plus a number of other problems, including an enlarged spleen, enlarged lymph nodes, anaemia and reductions in the numbers of immune cells (which makes them more susceptible to infections).

Can diet help with Felty's syndrome?

Elimination diets have never been tried out for patients with Felty's syndrome, and there are good reasons to think that they would not help. The basic problem in this disease seems to be a malfunctioning immune system.

Antioxidants (see p.339) such as Vitamin E and carotenoids are thought to be important in reducing the damaging effects of inflammation. Intake of these antioxidant nutrients can be boosted by eating more of certain foods, and such dietary changes – described on pp.257-9 – will have more general health benefits as well.

· *Gout* ·

Gout often begins unexpectedly with a devastating attack of pain. The joint at the base of the big toe is most often affected (such an attack is called podagra), but gout can also strike at other joints in the foot, or in the knee, wrist or fingers, or indeed almost any joint. The pain intensifies and takes several days or even weeks to subside, but once the attack is over the sufferer usually returns to normal. For some people this gout attack is a one-off event, whereas others have further attacks, sometimes weeks, months or even years later.

Occasionally the first attack of gout is much milder than this, and does not begin so dramatically. In a few people, more than one joint is affected simultaneously. There may also be fatigue and morning stiffness, and in a few patients it is difficult to distinguish gout from rheumatoid arthritis at first, so the doctor will need to make certain tests. Sometimes osteoarthritis is also mistaken for gout.

If gout is left untreated it can attack other joints. With modern treatment, gout rarely develops into a crippling disease as it once did, so joint damage and deformities are now very unusual. Gout is the main form of **crystal arthritis**, in which tiny crystals are found in the joint. These crystals produce severe inflammation.

To understand the process of crystal formation in gout, imagine using warm water to dissolve a crystalline substance such as sugar or salt. After a while all the crystals will disappear, because the sugar has become dissolved in the water. More sugar could be added, and at first it would dissolve, but there would come a point when no more sugar would dissolve. At this point the solution is said to be 'saturated'. Now if you were to pour this solution off from the remaining crystals, so that there was just clear fluid, and then leave it standing in a cool place, after an hour or so you would see the sparkle of tiny crystals that had formed in the liquid. As it cools down, the water can no longer 'hold' all the sugar, and some 'crystallises out'.

This is a very rough-and-ready model for what happens in gout. In the case of someone with gout, the liquid is either blood or one of the body fluids derived from blood, such as that within the joint (synovial fluid). The crystals are a substance called **urate**. When urate dissolves in a liquid, it becomes **uric acid**, and when the uric acid crystallises it becomes urate again. (Urate is said to be a 'salt' of uric acid.)

In fact most healthy people never produce any urate crystals, they simply have a little uric acid in the blood, which is flushed out by the kidneys into the urine. But someone with gout usually has too much uric acid in the blood – so much that their blood is almost 'saturated' (see above) with uric acid. The synovial fluid is partially derived from blood, so it too is saturated with uric acid. A small change in the chemistry of the synovial fluid, such as an increase in acidity, will have the same effect as cooling has on the sugar solution – tiny crystals of urate will form.

These crystals tend to be deposited in the cartilage of the joints where they may provoke inflammation (see p.64). There may also be crystals in various other parts of the body, including the lobes of the ear – they can accumulate in these places without causing any unpleasant symptoms immediately, even though there are enough crystals clustered together to form noticeable whitish lumps in the ear lobe. (These clusters of crystals are called tophi.)

Trouble begins in the joints when the crystals attract the attention of certain immune cells (see p.416) called neutrophils. Their job is to clear up debris wherever they may find it in the body, and they may swallow up the urate crystals in the joints. Once inside these neutrophils, the crystals rupture the external and internal membranes of the cells. Unfortunately, neutrophils contain some very destructive enzymes (see p.415), powerful chemicals whose function is to attack and break down bacteria. Neutrophils store these enzymes for use against any infectious bacteria that they may encounter. When urate crystals rupture the membranes of the neutrophils, a flood of destructive enzymes is released and this sets up the inflammation in the joint.

To make matters worse, aroused neutrophils release a little lactic acid which makes the synovial fluid more acidic and so causes more crystals to form. Damaged neutrophils also emit chemicals that act as panic alarms and attract other neutrophils to the joint. So more crystals are formed and more neutrophils arive to engulf them, setting off another round of enzyme release. In short, the crystals inadvertently provoke the immune system into a damaging over-reaction.

Once it has begun, the inflammation process tends to escalate rapidly, which is why attacks of gout can begin so suddenly and progress to agonizing pain within an hour or so. (It is also the reason why attacks should be treated in their early stages, at the first hint of warning signs. Nothing is gained by being brave and ignoring these initial symptoms, because delay makes the attack much more severe and difficult to treat.)

How do patients with gout acquire so much uric acid in the first place? The answer to this is not entirely known, but it is clear that the underlying cause varies from one patient to another.

Everyone makes uric acid all the time by breaking down chemicals called **purines**. Purines are widely found in all parts of our body, especially our DNA (the hereditary material). Some of the purines that are turned into uric acid come from our own DNA – from dead body cells for example. Other purines come from the food we eat. Turning the purines into uric acid is part of the process of clearing them from the body.

Anyone who is greatly overweight will automatically be producing more waste purines from their own body cells than someone of normal weight. If they are eating food with a high purine content, such as pâté or liver, this will add to the problem. Alcohol makes matters worse, firstly by increasing the rate at which purines are produced, and secondly by making the blood slightly acidic which triggers off crystal formation.

This is why gout has always been associated with a rich diet (although it can also occur in abstemious people – see p.106). In earlier centuries it was thought of as an upper-class disease, which required a stay at a fashionable and expensive spa town for its treatment. Modern-day affluence, at least in food and drink, means that it can now affect many more people.

However, not everyone who overeats and drinks alcohol gets gout. Indeed, not everyone with too much uric acid in their blood gets gout. Some people have very high levels of uric acid but fend off crystal production thanks to the chemistry of their blood. An inability to do this is one of the critical factors leading to crystal formation in the joint. There are various non-dietary inherited factors at work in producing gout.

About 10–15% of gout patients suffer for reasons that are nothing whatever to do with their lifestyle. They are suffering from an 'error of metabolism' – a basic fault in the body's chemistry. The body has to make purines when it needs them, for example to build DNA. Chemical processes which produce purines are normally kept under control, so that they stop when enough have been made. For some unfortunate people, the 'off switch' does not work, so the body simply produces too much purine, which is turned into uric acid. Alternatively, there may be a fault in the normal recycling system which takes some waste purines and reuses them – again this leads to an excessive number of waste purines in the blood. Faults such as these (which are probably there from birth) account for the slim, abstemious person who nevertheless suffers from gout. Uric acid levels are generally low in children, so these gout patients rarely get symptoms until they reach puberty, despite the fact that the underlying fault is there from birth.

For hormonal reasons, men tend to have more uric acid in the blood than women, and the disease is ten times more common in men. Just before the menopause, the uric acid level rises in women, and they are then at risk from gout.

Some drugs prevent the kidneys from taking uric acid out of the blood efficiently, and these can increase the risk of gout. Aspirin can do this, but it is diuretics that are most commonly at fault. These drugs encourage water loss from the body and may be used to combat high blood pressure. About a quarter of new cases of gout are now caused by diuretics. When women suffer from gout there is a good chance that diuretics are to blame, and the early symptoms may be unusual in these cases: the gout often comes on slowly, rather than in a sudden devastating attack, and it tends to affect the hands more than the feet.

Because urate crystals may also be deposited in the kidneys, some people with gout may suffer from kidney stones or other symptoms related to disturbance of normal kidney function.

Can diet help with gout?

At one time, the only treatment for gout was a dietary one. Doctors realised long ago that rich, meaty meals, washed down with plenty of wine and spirits, were often the cause of gout, and they tried to persuade their wealthy patients to reform (rarely with much success!)

Today, someone who has had a single attack of gout may still be treated in this way (but may also receive drugs to help reduce pain and inflammation in the acute phase of gout – usually non-steroidal anti-inflammatory drugs, see p.418). They will be told to lose weight and to reduce their alcohol intake, which will sometimes be enough to banish the gout for ever. If approached in the wrong way, however, loss of weight can actually trigger a fresh attack of gout. For the correct approach to losing weight, and some advice about giving up alcohol, turn to Chapter 2.7 (p.242).

Anyone with recurrent attacks of gout will probably be treated with allopurinol, which tackles the problem so effectively, and (in most people) produces so few side-effects, that patients can continue taking it safely for the rest of their lives.

In rare cases, such as when allopurinol, or other drugs used for gout, have caused problems, it may be valuable to try a diet which is low in purines. This does not have any dramatic effect on the level of uric acid in the blood, because the body still produces its own waste purines. However, a low-purine diet can reduce the purine level in the blood by about 10%, which may be enough to tip the balance and prevent gouty attacks. A low-purine diet should only be tried if other strategies – such as losing weight and reducing alcohol – have failed. It is unlikely to help where the gout is due to a basic error of metabolism. Details of the low-purine diet are given on pp.245–6.

The treatments described so far are relevant if you have experienced attacks of gout in the past, but are not suffering an attack at the present time. Should you be currently suffering an attack of joint pain due to gout, no change in diet can help at this point. See the doctor who will prescribe drugs to ease the pain and calm the inflammation.

· *Hydroarthrosis* ·

This term, taken literally, means 'water in the joint' ('hydro' – water, 'arthro' – joint). The liquid that accumulates and causes the joint to swell up is not actually water but synovial fluid. This is the normal lubricant of all synovial joints (see pp. 420–421), but instead of being present in tiny amounts as it is in a healthy joint, the synovial fluid can become far more abundant in diseases such as rheumatoid arthritis. The overproduction of synovial fluid is part of the disease process, following on from inflammation (see p.64) of the synovial membrane.

'Hydroarthrosis' is a term that is not often used by doctors today. It is not a distinct disease in itself, but a feature of many arthritic diseases.

For appropriate dietary advice, you need first to obtain a more accurate diagnosis.

· *Hypermobility Syndrome* ·

This is a feature of various inherited disorders. The joints are more flexible than in other people allowing some fairly unusual movements. For example, someone with hypermobility syndrome may be able to bend down and place the palms of their hands flat on the floor while keeping their knees perfectly straight.

Because of this unusual flexibility, the joints are more vulnerable to injury, or even to dislocation. This can lead to osteoarthritis at a relatively early age, or to low back pain. There may be swelling, especially of the knee joints. Sometimes there is both pain and swelling of various joints, and this may be mistaken for the early signs of rheumatoid arthritis. On the other hand, while most people become stiff as they reach their later years, hypermobile patients retain normal mobility, so the condition does have some advantages!

Can diet help with hypermobility syndrome?

It is most unlikely that diet would make any difference in this condition.

· *Infective Arthritis* ·

This is an attack of arthritis caused by a bacterium (or, more rarely, another type of microbe) finding its way into a joint and overcoming the immune defences there. The microbe multiplies within the joint, leading to inflammation (see p.64) and painful swelling. Another name that may be used is 'septic arthritis'.

A great variety of different bacteria can infect the joints, including those that cause tuberculosis, bacterial meningitis, gonorrhoea, salmonella poisoning and certain forms of pneumonia. Luckily, it is very rare indeed for any of these bacteria to overcome the immune defences in a joint and set up an infection there. This usually occurs only when the infection is already established in the body generally, so there will often be other symptoms, usually including pronounced fever.

With bacterial infections, the problem is usually confined to just one joint, often a large joint such as the hip, knee, shoulder or wrist. In order to be sure that the arthritic symptoms are really due to an infection, the doctor will take a sample of the fluid from within the joint (the synovial fluid). Sometimes it is necessary to take a small sample of the synovial membrane itself and examine this.

The biggest problem for a doctor, in diagnosing infective arthritis, is when it occurs in someone who already has rheumatoid arthritis. Unfortunately, patients with rheumatoid arthritis are slightly more susceptible, probably because damage to the small blood vessels in the synovial membrane (the membrane which lines the joint) makes it easier for microbes in the blood to pass out of the blood vessels and enter the joint space. From the doctor's point of view, the fact that the joints are already inflamed and swollen makes it hard to recognise the symptoms of infective arthritis.

If you have rheumatoid arthritis and if, during an infection, one joint becomes unusually painful, hot and swollen, be sure to report this to your doctor promptly. You are at somewhat greater risk if you have been taking corticosteroid drugs (see p.414) or if you have had a corticosteroid injection into that joint.

Prompt treatment with antibiotics is vital for anyone with bacterial infective arthritis as the infection can damage the joint permanently and very rapidly, if not brought under control.

Apart from bacteria, other microbes – viruses, multicellular parasites and fungi – can occasionally cause infective arthritis. In the case of fungi, this is very rare indeed and generally affects the joints of the jaw. Multicellular parasites quite commonly cause arthritis but such parasites are uncommon in the temperate regions; only someone who has been in the tropics is likely to be infected.

Among viruses, the only one to actually infect joints is the virus that causes German measles (rubella). Several joints are usually affected, in contrast to bacterial infections which are usually confined to one joint. Rubella virus tends to strike the joints of the hands, wrists, elbows and knees. There is no risk of damage in rubella infection, and the problem usually clears up naturally after a week or so, although it sometimes continues for a few months. No specific treatment is given in most cases.

Doctors make an important distinction between infective arthritis and reactive arthritis (see p.126).

Can diet help with infective arthritis ?

No – antibiotics are urgently required in this form of arthritis and dietary therapy plays no part in treatment.

· *Inflammatory Arthritis* ·

A collective term for several different types of arthritis (see p.65).

· *Inflammatory Polyarthropathy* ·

This term simply means that there is an inflammatory disorder which affects many joints. It may also be called inflammatory polyarthritis. These terms are used to describe patients who, despite having multiple inflamed joints, do not fulfil the diagnostic criteria for rheumatoid arthritis. They are usually seronegative for rheumatoid factor (see p.419) and do not have sufficient symptoms to fulfil the criteria for rheumatoid arthritis set by the American Rheumatism Association – criteria used by rheumatologists worldwide.

Such patients may well be suffering from mild rheumatoid arthritis, or the early stages of the disease. On the other hand, they could be a mixed group which includes patients with a range of different conditions, either in mild form or in the very early stages.

A recent survey in Manchester, England, showed that there were ethnic differences in the occurrence of this disease. While the white population were more likely to have rheumatoid arthritis than the black population (of Caribbean origin), there were far more cases of inflammatory polyarthropathy among the black population. These cases had not generally been diagnosed by the family doctor.

Can diet help with inflammatory polyarthropathy?

Given the possible relationship between inflammatory polyarthropathy and rheumatoid arthritis, an elimination diet might be worth trying. The details of the diet are given in Chapter 2.4 (p.170). Be sure to ask your doctor's advice before trying the diet.

Antioxidants (see p.339) such as Vitamin E and carotenoids are thought to be important in reducing the damaging effects of inflammation. Intake of these antioxidant nutrients can be boosted by eating more of certain foods, and such dietary changes – described on pp.257–9 – will have more general health benefits as well.

· *Juvenile Chronic Arthritis* ·

This is a collection of similar and overlapping diseases, rather than a single disease. Doctors hope eventually to separate them into a number of distinct disorders because this will help in making treatment more precise. At present, they generally recognise certain subgroups within juvenile chronic arthritis, as follows:

Systemic juvenile chronic arthritis, also called **Still's disease** after Dr George Still who described it in the 1890s. It produces a high fever in the afternoons or evenings, and sometimes a rash, often with swelling of the lymph nodes ('swollen glands'). There may be little or no arthritis at the beginning.

Pauciarticular juvenile chronic arthritis involves fewer than four joints, most often the knee, elbow and ankle. Sometimes just a single toe or finger may be affected. It can begin when the child is too young to say that the joints hurt, and parents need to notice if a baby or toddler is avoiding certain actions or having difficulty in walking.

Polyarticular juvenile chronic arthritis involves five or more joints. Some fever may occur occasionally. A few children in this group have rheumatoid factor (see p.419) in their blood, and some of these go on to develop rheumatoid arthritis as adults.

It is natural for parents to worry, but the important thing to remember is that most children make a very good recovery. One survey, which looked at young adults who had once had juvenile arthritis, found that more than 90% of them were largely unaffected by their former illness. Their choice of career was not restricted and many were married and had children.

Compared with adults, young children often do not describe much pain from arthritis, either because there is less pain, or because they do not experience it in the same way, pain having been part of their lives since such an early age. It may be necessary to look for outward signs of joint inflammation because the child will not necessarily report any discomfort. Signs to watch for include swelling of a joint, a slight limp, difficulty in turning taps or using cutlery, or a pattern of movement which suggests that the child is protecting some joints.

Some forms of juvenile chronic arthritis, notably the pauciarticular form, are associated with inflammation of the eyes. Known as **uveitis**, this is usually painless and may easily go unnoticed until it is quite well advanced. Damage to the eyes, and even blindness, can occur. It is therefore vital that the child has regular eye check-ups, and the doctor should organise these.

Physiotherapy is a vital aspect of treatment. Following the advice of the physiotherapist, and keeping to any exercise programmes that are prescribed, is of crucial importance in preventing permanent deformity of the affected joints.

Can diet help with juvenile chronic arthritis ?

Food avoidance may help in rare cases – see p.191–2. Antioxidants (see p.339) such as Vitamin E and carotenoids are thought to be important in reducing the damaging effects of inflammation. Intake of these antioxidant nutrients can be boosted by eating more of certain foods, and such dietary changes, as described on pp.257–9, will have more general health benefits as well.

· *Juvenile Rheumatoid Arthritis* ·

This term is sometimes used instead of juvenile chronic arthritis (see p.111), particularly in the U.S.A. It is not appropriate for all forms of juvenile chronic arthritis, but certain types, such as the pauciarticular kind, can resemble adult rheumatoid arthritis.

· *Lumbago* ·

A term used for pain in the lower back – see Back Pain (p.91).

· *Lyme Disease* ·

This disease is named after the town of Lyme in Connecticut, U.S.A, where it was recognised in 1975. Although particularly common in the eastern United States, it does also occur elsewhere, including Britain, several other European countries and Australia. Cases of Lyme disease were undoubtedly mistaken for other arthritic diseases in the past, including juvenile chronic arthritis and rheumatic fever.

Lyme disease is caused by a bacterium which lives in the blood of certain ticks. These parasites normally infest deer, voles and other wild animals but they can also bite horses, dogs and humans. People are generally bitten by the ticks in woodland areas during the summer.

High-risk woodlands in the U.S.A. now have warning notices about suitable clothing.

The way the skin reacts to the bite of the Lyme-disease tick is highly unusual. It begins with a round red mark which steadily grows in size. As it does so, the skin at the centre recovers its normal hue so that a large red circle remains. There may be some other symptoms at this stage, including fever, headache, stiff neck, tingling in the limbs, flu-like symptoms and swollen lymph nodes ('swollen glands'). If Lyme disease can be recognised and treated with antibiotics at this stage then the arthritis can often be averted.

If left untreated, the heart and nervous system are generally affected by the disease some weeks or months after the initial bite. Arthritis may begin at the same time or may come on later still. The arthritis can die down and then flare up again intermittently over a period of years, which is why the disease was readily mistaken for rheumatoid arthritis. Once Lyme disease has reached this stage it is more difficult to treat and the response is slower. Drugs may help to calm the inflammation in the joints.

Lyme disease could be a form of infective arthritis (see p.108) with the bacterium invading the joints, or a reactive arthritis (p.126). It is even possible that it is hybrid of the two, becoming a reactive arthritis in the more advanced cases.

Can diet help with Lyme disease ?

Diet is obviously irrelevant to this form of arthritis in the early stages, since it is caused by a bacterial infection. Treatment with antibiotics is very effective at this stage and should not be delayed.

No scientific trials of dietary therapy have been carried out in patients with Lyme disease where persistent arthritis has developed.

· *Occupational Arthritis* ·

There are two distinct ways in which a job can increase the likelihood of arthritis developing. The first is a purely mechanical effect which occurs through undue pressure on joints, or overuse of joints; this tends to produce either osteoarthritis (see p.115) or bursitis (see p.95). The second is through substances that are inhaled or absorbed through the skin, and which cause a generalised reaction, probably involving the immune system. This can have a variety of effects on the body, including arthritis.

It has long been known that coalminers are susceptible to osteoarthritis of the spine and knees in later life, while those operating pneumatic drills (jackhammers) may suffer osteoarthritis of the elbows and wrists.

A survey of elderly men, carried out in the U.S.A. in the mid-1980s, extended this observation to manual labourers in general. It showed that men in their 70s and 80s were more likely to suffer from general osteoarthritis if they had done physically demanding jobs, and more likely to suffer from osteoarthritis of the knee if the job had involved a great deal of bending.

Professional sportsmen and sportswomen may also be at a slightly greater risk of osteoarthritis, but this depends very much on the sport. Repeated minor shocks to the joint can lead to osteoarthritis, as in 'wicket-keeper's hands'. In footballers, the knees and ankles are susceptible to osteoarthritis in later life. Among long-distance runners, osteoarthritis of the hip joints is a hazard.

Bursitis is a more immediate reaction to joint misuse, and one which can be treated more effectively than osteoarthritis. It is a specific hazard with particular occupations such as carpet-laying, which may provoke bursitis of the knee (see p.95). Students sometimes develop bursitis of the elbow through long hours studying with their elbows on a desk.

The inhaled substances which can increase the risk of arthritis are mainly rock dusts. Granite workers, who breathe in silica dust while at work, have an increased risk of developing rheumatoid arthritis later in life. There is a considerable time-lag, with the average interval between first exposure to silica dust and the development of rheumatoid arthritis being 25 years.

There may also be some increased risk of rheumatoid arthritis among sandblasters and asbestos workers, as both have a higher level of rheumatoid factor (see p.419) in the blood. Coalminers have a slightly greater risk of developing systemic sclerosis (see p.140), which may include arthritis as one of its symptoms.

Can diet help in occupational arthritis?

In general, it is unlikely to help, but you should refer to the section that concerns your particular diagnosis (eg. osteoarthritis, rheumatoid arthritis, systemic sclerosis).

· *Osteoarthritis* ·

This is the most common form of arthritis and affects elderly people in particular. However, occasionally it can begin in much younger people, even those in their 20s, when it is usually a result of an earlier injury, or unusual use of the joints.

The central event in osteoarthritis is a gradual breakdown of the smooth layer of cartilage (see p.421) that covers the ends of the bones – this is the material that reduces friction between the bones and makes the joint operate smoothly.

The changes in the joint, particularly the erosion of cartilage, mean that there is less to separate the two bones making up the joint. On an X-ray this can be seen as a narrowing of the joint space (the gap between the two bones). The narrowing creates further problems, because the ligaments around the joint – the joint capsule (see p.414) – are looser, like a pair of trousers on someone who has lost weight. This is known as **capsular laxity**, and it makes the ligaments less effective at keeping the joint stable and its movements controlled. The joint is then more vulnerable to damage during movement, which adds to the process of cartilage loss.

Another distinctive feature of osteoarthritis is that the bone at the edges of the joint grows outwards, producing bony knobs or ridges known as **osteophytes**. Exactly why this happens is unknown. In the finger joints, there can also be small lumps beneath the skin near the joint, called Heberden's nodes (if at the fingertip joint) or Bouchard's nodes (if at the mid-finger joint). Again, no one knows why these develop.

Because of the erosion occuring in the osteoarthritic joint, there may be fragments of cartilage and bone floating in the synovial fluid. These may be absorbed by the synovial membrane (see p.421) which then becomes inflamed and swells up a little. Externally the joint will seem swollen, and may be tender and even slightly warm when touched. (In this sense, osteoarthritis does have a little in common with rheumatoid arthritis (see p.129), because there is some inflammation (see p.64) in the joint, but the inflammation is mild in osteoarthritis, and there is no significant overgrowth of the synovial membrane. Moreover the inflammation is a *result* of the disease, not the underlying *cause* as it is in rheumatoid arthritis.)

Once the erosion of cartilage exposes the lattice-like bone underneath, synovial fluid (see p.421) may seep into the small spaces in its lattice. The synovial fluid then erodes the bone from within, creating a larger, fluid-filled cavity, called a subchondral cyst. Later still, this cyst may so thoroughly undermine the bone that part of the joint surface collapses into the cavity. This usually happens only in advanced cases of osteoarthritis, ones which have been in progress for a long time. By this stage, the joint surface is very uneven, and there may be a grating sensation (called crepitus) when the joint is moved.

The primary event in osteoarthritis is the breakdown of cartilage, and this is understood, at least in part. Cartilage is broken down throughout our lives, both by pressure when the joint is used a great deal, and by the body's own cells, which continuously destroy and rebuild the cartilage in the joints for the purposes of maintenance and repair.

What happens in osteoarthritis, is that the 'repair and rebuild' processes fail to keep pace with the rate of breakdown. This may be because the joint has to work very hard and there are repeated small injuries. In this case the condition is known as **secondary osteoarthritis**. Sometimes this is due to a particular type of work or sporting activity (see Occupational arthritis – p.113). Babies born with a dislocated hip may develop osteoarthritis in that hip as adults, because the hip joint works imperfectly and causes unusual stress on the cartilage.

If there is no underlying injury then the condition is known as **primary osteoarthritis**. This shows a characteristic pattern of joint involvement. Joints commonly affected are the hips and knees, and some joints of the spine – those in the neck and lower back. In the hands, it is the joints at the tips of the fingers, and those midway along the fingers, plus the joint at the very base of the thumb just above the wrist. In the foot, the joint at the base of the big toe (the 'bunion joint') may become arthritic. The shoulders, elbows, wrists, knuckle joints and ankles are not usually affected in primary osteoarthritis, and any pain in these will lead the doctor to ask again about earlier damage – if you have osteoarthritis of the ankle, for example, did you play a lot of football when younger?

Primary osteoarthritis tends to run in families, and in some of these families an inherited defect in the chemical constituents of the cartilage has been detected.

The majority of people over the age of 70 have osteoarthritis, as shown by X-rays, although there may be no pain or other symptoms for many of those affected. It is thought that everyone would develop osteoarthritis eventually if they lived to a ripe old age: this seems to be one of the inevitable ills of mankind. Archaeology shows that osteoarthritis affected the Neanderthals, and it has been known throughout history.

On a more optimistic note, most cases of osteoarthritis do not progress rapidly – there may be little change for many years. There are even cases where osteoarthritis of the hip clears up of its own accord. The body's natural repair processes re-establish themselves, and the hip joint recovers its normal structure and function. According to one estimate, this spontaneous healing may occur for as many as 5% of patients with osteoarthritis of the hip.

Treatment of osteoarthritis consists mainly of drugs such as paracetamol and codeine to reduce the pain. Non-steroidal anti-inflammatory drugs (see p.418) may also be prescribed. There is now some concern that certain NSAIDs tend to hasten the destruction of cartilage, although others may protect cartilage. Clearly, the latter are preferable in osteoarthritis, where cartilage breakdown is the central problem. The drug misoprostol, which is often prescribed with NSAIDs to counteract their side-effects on the stomach, may also have a protective action on the cartilage.

Some studies suggest that there are no clear advantages in taking NSAIDs rather than simple pain-killers. Given the side-effects of NSAIDs, pain-killers such as paracetamol may be a better option.

Apart from misoprostol, there are various other drugs believed to have a protective effect on cartilage, known as **chondroprotective agents**. These substances have only been studied to a limited extent, and the results so far are inconclusive. Despite this, chondroprotective drugs are already widely used for osteoarthritis in certain countries including Germany and Switzerland. In time, if their usefulness is proven, they may become more generally available in other parts of the world.

Can diet help in osteoarthritis?

The simplest and most effective dietary measure in osteoarthritis is to lose weight, especially if your hips, knees, ankles or fingers are affected. If you are at all overweight, shedding a few pounds may well produce a marked improvement. The closer you can get to the normal weight for your height the better you will be. Recommendations for losing weight are given in Chapter 2.6 (p.226).

Because osteoarthritis is not primarily an inflammatory disease, it is unlikely that the elimination diet or other dietary treatments, such as oils, will be of much help to most patients. However, there is an element of inflammation of the synovial membrane in some cases of osteoarthritis (see p.115). It is just possible that this inflammation can be alleviated by dietary change, but the benefits are likely to be small.

It might be worth trying an elimination diet if you have other symptoms typical of food intolerance, such as migraine, recurrent headaches, diarrhoea or irritable bowel syndrome, asthma or eczema. The other indication that an elimination diet could help is if you have close relatives suffering from rheumatoid arthritis (suggesting that there is a genetic predisposition to inflammation which may be playing a part in your osteoarthritis) or if osteoarthritis is present in several joints, including the knuckle joints but excluding the finger-tip joints – this too indicates a possible link with inflammatory arthritis. Finally, the elimination diet might be worth trying by younger people (under the age of 50) whose osteoarthritis is puzzling because it cannot be explained by injury. Doctors working with elimination diets have found that such patients somemetimes respond well.

A research team at St George's Hospital in London has tried a pilot study of omega-3 fish oil in patients with osteoarthritis and found a beneficial effect (see p.62). This has not been fully tested, so we cannot categorically recommend it, but there is probably no harm in trying this treatment. If you have red, warm, swollen joints that are tender to the touch – indicating a degree of inflammation – then omega-3 oil is more likely to be of value. Details about the sources of omega-3s are given in Chapter 2.2 (p.143).

Cod-liver oil (which is distinct from omega-3 fish oil) has been tested for usefulness in osteoarthritis in a full-scale scientific trial. It does not seem to be effective (see pp.61–2), although the researchers suggest that this may only be true for patients taking non-steroidal anti-inflammatory drugs (NSAIDs) – see p.418. (If you are not sure whether the drugs you are taking are NSAIDs, ask your pharmacist.)

If you are already taking cod-liver oil and believe it to be helpful, then by all means continue with this, but do not exceed the maximum daily dose because there is a risk of toxicity from Vitamins A and D (see p.285 and p.300). Ensure that you eat enough Vitamin E to cover for the polyunsaturates in the cod-liver oil (follow the guidelines on p.150, but halve the quantities). For those who are considering cod-liver oil, we would suggest you think about omega-3 fish oil instead.

Anyone who has signs of an inflammatory component to their osteoarthritis – see above – might also benefit from a diet that is rich in Vitamin E (see p.305), or from taking a Vitamin E supplement.

Long-term use of aspirin, other salicylates, or NSAID drugs in general, can have adverse effects on nutritional status, and a high dietary intake, or supplements, of certain vitamins may be needed (see p.280).

If you are about to undergo a hip replacement or similar operation, it is a good idea to take some extra vitamins which will ensure that you have all the nutrients you need for rapid healing. Surgery increases the need for nutrients, so even if you eat a good healthy diet a supplement may still be valuable (see p.265 for further details).

· *Osteoarthrosis* ·

This is a newer term for Osteoarthritis (see p.115). It reflects the fact that inflammation ('-itis') is only a small part of the disease in most patients, and that osteoarthritis is therefore an inappropriate name.

· *Osteochondritis* ·

This is a form of arthritis that usually affects knee joints, but can also occur in the ankle, elbow, hip or other joints. It generally follows the separation of a fragment of bone close to the joint.

Can diet help with osteochondritis?

Diet is of no relevance to this disease.

· *Osteomalacia* ·

This is not a form of arthritis, but a disease of the bones themselves, in which the mineral component – calcium phosphate – is gradually lost. The symptoms (see p.299) include muscle weakness, aches and pains, and tenderness around the joints. Osteomalacia is related to problems with Vitamin D which controls the absorption and use of calcium by the body. It is usually a consequence of diseases of the intestine, liver or kidney (which may create a problem with Vitamin D absorption) or a result of over-rapid breakdown of this vitamin.

Can diet help with osteomalacia?

Supplements of Vitamin D, calcium and sometimes phosphate are required to treat osteomalacia, but they must be given with close medical supervision and monitoring. The doctor may offer additional advice about diet, which should be followed carefully.

· *Osteoporosis* ·

This is not a form of arthritis, but a disease of the bones themselves, in which the total density of the bones that give the bones their structure is reduced with loss of both the proteins and mineral component that make bones hard.

As a result, the bones are more brittle and fracture readily. The most vulnerable parts of the skeleton are those where the bone has an open lattice-like structure, known as trabecular bone. The thinning of the bony filaments that make up this lattice leaves a very weak, emaciated, fragile structure which can collapse under pressure.

The topmost part of the thigh bone, close to the hip joint, is made of trabecular bone, and one common result of osteoporosis is a fracture here following a fall, often referred to as a 'broken hip'. The end of the forearm bones, just above the wrist, are also made of trabecular bone and can break easily if the bone is weakend by osteoporosis. Such a fracture, known as a Colles' fracture, often occurs when someone falls and puts out an arm to break the fall: young people rarely suffer a Colles' fracture when they do this, but people over 40, especially women, may well do so. Colles' fractures are often the early warning sign of osteoporosis, appearing a decade earlier than hip fractures – they are a sign that the bones need urgent treatment if things are not to get worse. When osteoporosis becomes severe, the vertebrae (which make up the spinal column) may be crushed spontaneously by the weight of the body, or by a small accident. This produces pain, but it may be disregarded by patients as 'backache'.

Some degree of osteoporosis is a natural part of the ageing process, but thinning of the bones can become very severe in certain individuals, leading to repeated fractures. It is the risk of breaking bones – especially the top of the thigh bone – every time they fall over, that curtails the independence of many old people and forces them into retirement homes prematurely.

Severe osteoporosis tends to affect elderly women far more often than men, and the disruption of the female hormonal balance which occurs at the menopause is partly to blame: oestrogen, the hormone that maintains and controls fertility in women, protects the bones from mineral loss. When it declines with the menopause, women's bones suffer the consequences. Inactivity makes matters worse, because exercise stimulates bones to repair and renew themselves.

Patients with rheumatoid arthritis and other forms of inflammatory arthritis are more vulnerable to osteoporosis than ordinary people, and need to protect themselves against it. Treatment with corticosteroid drugs increases the risk of osteoporosis. So do smoking and drinking alcohol.

Once the symptoms of osteoporosis are evident, a drug treatment may be prescribed. There are some new drugs available and you should consult your doctor if you are concerned – if you have suffered a Colles' fracture for example.

Prevention is much better than cure in osteoporosis, and needs to begin long before there are any symptoms. All preventive measures should be started well before the menopause if possible, to avoid painful and debilitating problems in old age. (But if you have already gone through the menopause, it is not too late to do something about preventing osteoporosis.)

Hormone Replacement Therapy (HRT), used to treat the symptoms of the menopause, is also very useful in preventing osteoporosis. Women who go through the menopause early (before age 45) are more susceptible to osteoporosis and should always consider asking their doctor about HRT. The sooner HRT starts, the better it is at preventing osteoporosis.

Women who have had a hysterectomy (without loss of their ovaries) may not know when they enter the menopause because they do not have periods anyway. If you fall into this category and would like to consider the option of HRT, talk the matter over with your doctor. A blood test can show when the menopause has begun. Women who have had their ovaries removed are at similar risk of osteoporosis as post-menopausal women, and will probably be offered HRT as a matter of course.

Can diet help with osteoporosis?

Diet has an important role to play in preventing osteoporosis, and this is described in Chapter 2.3 (p.161). Exercise is also absolutely essential: this and other self-help measures are dealt with in the same chapter.

· Paget's Disease ·

This is a disease in which certain areas of bone are broken down by the body in an abnormal way. They may later be repaired by the body's natural repair mechanisms but the healthy structure of the bones is not always successfully recreated. Paget's disease may exist for a long time without producing any noticeable symptoms. Once established, it may affect some of the joints, notably the hip and knee joints.

Can diet help with Paget's disease?

Diet is irrelevant to this disease, but drugs may be of considerable benefit.

· *Palindromic Rheumatism* ·

Palindromic rheumatism, also known as **episodic arthritis** (a newer and more accurate medical term), is a disease in which there are recurrent but short-lived bouts of joint pain, with swelling, tenderness and stiffness. It appears to be an inflammatory arthritis (see p.65) like rheumatoid arthritis. The changes in the joint are very similar to those of early rheumatoid arthritis, with swelling and inflammation of the synovial membrane (see p.421), and the over-production of synovial fluid. But the process stops there, and the synovium does not proliferate and attack the articular cartilage or bone as it does in rheumatoid arthritis. The case described on p.17 is a good example.

About one third of people with palindromic rheumatism go on to develop full-blown rheumatoid arthritis later, and at this point the inflammation in the joint begins to progress beyond the initial stage.

Can diet help with palindromic rheumatism?

Diet is often relevant to this disease, which may clear up if certain foods are avoided. Trying an elimination diet (see Chapter 2.4–p.170) is very worthwhile, although you should consult your doctor first. The diet should obviously begin during an attack of the arthritis, but if your attacks are normally short-lived you need to plan ahead and be ready to start the diet promptly, so read Chapter 2.4 which describes the procedure, and work out how you will fit the diet in with your normal cooking and eating routine.

If the exclusion phase of the diet produces an improvement in the arthritis this would be expected to happen within 7–10 days. Any improvement after that time is probably due to the attack burning itself out in the usual way.

Before carrying out an elimination diet, it might be worth simply keeping a detailed food diary while eating your ordinary diet. This may help you relate your attacks of arthritis to intake of a particular food, and could save you the time and effort of an elimination diet. You might want to test the food to prove or disprove your suspicions, especially if it is a food that will be hard to avoid such as wheat or milk. Avoid it for at least two weeks before testing.

· *Pauciarticular Arthritis* ·

A term meaning 'inflammation in only a few joints'. It is often used for one form of Juvenile Chronic Arthritis (see p.123).

· *Polyarthritis* ·

A term meaning 'inflammation in many joints'. It is often used for one form of Juvenile Chronic Arthritis (see p.123), or as another name for Inflammatory Polyarthropathy (see p.110).

· *Pseudogout* ·

This disease has attracted a wealth of alternative names, including pyrophosphate arthropathy, chondrocalcinosis, and calcium pyrophosphate dihydrate deposition disease. It was only identified in 1961, having previously been confused with gout. Both are caused by crystals being deposited in the joint, so they are both forms of **crystal synovitis**.

In pseudogout the crystals are made of calcium pyrophosphate a close relation of the chemical that makes bones hard and strong. Indeed, the calcium pyrophosphate seems to originate from the bone near the affected joint, although what makes it change chemically and migrate towards the joint is unknown. The calcium pyrophosphate crystals form in the cartilage close to the joint initially, and do not cause symptoms although they may be visible on an X-ray. An attack of pseudogout occurs when the crystals are shed from the cartilage into the joint cavity. Severe inflammation follows, similar to that seen in gout, as the crystals are swallowed up by immune cells (see pp.104–5).

Pseudogout can be distinguished from gout by extracting a sample of the fluid within the joint (the synovial fluid) using a syringe. The crystals are viewed under polarised light – those formed in pseudogout scatter the light in a different way from those formed in gout.

The best treatment for pseudogout is with corticosteroid injections into the affected joints. Non-steroidal anti-inflammatory drugs (see p.418) may also be prescribed, or, more rarely, colchicine. These treatments can be very helpful in quelling the inflammation but there is no drug treatment for the underlying disorder, as there is with gout.

Can diet help with pseudogout ?

Diets have never been tried for pseudogout and it seems most unlikely that they would help with this condition.

· *Psoriatic Arthritis* ·

Psoriasis is a disease in which too much new skin is being produced. Layers of skin cells accumulate, forming thickened patches, above which the dead skin flakes off in dry silvery scales. The exact cause of psoriasis is unknown, but the immune system is involved to some extent, producing inflammation (see p.64). Anti-inflammatory drugs are often used to damp down this response.

A minority of those with psoriasis develop painful swollen joints, a condition known as psoriatic arthritis. The synovial membrane within the joint (see p.421) becomes enlarged and begins to cause damaging changes to the cartilage, as happens in rheumatoid arthritis. However, the joints that are typically involved differ from those of rheumatoid arthritis to some extent: the joints at the tips of the fingers are often affected.

Can diet help with psoriatic arthritis?

Psoriasis is very rare among Greenland Eskimos who eat a great deal of oily fish – this may not be a cause-and-effect link, but it prompted medical researchers to try out fish oil as a treatment for psoriasis. The results of these studies are mixed (see p.61) but it seems that fish oil rich in omega-3 fatty acids might give some benefits to patients with psoriasitic arthritis, the good effects becoming apparent within approximately two months. You should discuss this treatment with your doctor .

One of the drugs used to treat psoriasis, etretinate, tends to raise the levels of fats in the blood, and it has been suggested that taking fish oil might be beneficial in reducing them, cancelling out this side effect of the drug, as well as perhaps helping treat the psoriasis itself. If you are interested in the possibility of taking fish oil in combination with etretinate you need to seek the opinion of the doctor who prescribed the drug for you, and who is monitoring its effects: do not try it without his or her agreement. (The same goes for eating regular helpings of oily fish, which will have the same effect.) If you have suffered nosebleeds as a side-effect of etretinate you should not try fish oil (or eating oily fish) as this could aggravate the problem.

For those who dislike fishy tastes, another oil, such as evening primrose oil or borage ('starflower') oil (see p.54) could possibly have a similar effect, but this has not been tested for psoriasis or psoriatic arthritis, only for rheumatoid arthritis.

We have occasionally tried elimination diets (see p.25) for patients with psoriatic arthritis at Epsom General Hospital, but the results have been disappointing. In our experience, this form of treatment is probably not relevant in this condition, although other workers have had more promising results.

A medical team working in Israel has tried out a milk-free, dairy-free, beef-free diet for psoriatic arthritis with slightly more success. Of four patients, one responded very well, with less joint pain and swelling and a reduction of over 50% in the dosage of drugs required. (It is possible that this patient actually had both psoriasis and rheumatoid arthritis, a combination that sometimes occurs and can be mistaken for psoriatic arthritis.)

Zinc supplements have been tried for patients with psoriatic arthritis, and there have been some encouraging results (see p.325).

Antioxidants (see p.339) such as Vitamin E and carotenoids are thought to be important in reducing the damaging effects of inflammation. Intake of these antioxidant nutrients can be boosted by eating more of certain foods, and such dietary changes, described on pp.257–9, will have more general health benefits as well.

· *Raynaud's Phenomenon* ·

This is often referred to as **Raynaud's syndrome**, or simply 'Raynaud's'. It is a circulatory problem that can accompany various diseases including systemic sclerosis. The blood supply to the fingers (and/or toes) is sharply reduced for a while because the muscles in the walls of the small blood vessels go into spasm. This produces numb white fingers and toes temporarily. Cold weather provokes more frequent attacks.

Can diet help with Raynaud's phenomenon?

It may be of some help – see under Systemic Sclerosis, p.140.

· *Reactive Arthritis* ·

In reactive arthritis, bacteria, viruses or other microbes are responsible for arthritis but they are not infecting the joint itself. The infection has occured elsewhere in the body, such as the digestive tract, and the joint symptoms are a response to something carried in the bloodstream, from the site of infection to the joint.

That 'something' may be fragments of bacterial cell walls or other material from the microbes themselves. Alternatively, it may be immune complexes (see p.416). A third possibility is that the joint symptoms are due to immune cells that have engulfed the infecting microbes elsewhere in the body and have then carried them into the joint. Such immune cells might provoke inflammation in the joint.

It is also possible that reactive arthritis involves an **auto-immune reaction** in which the immune system (see p.416) is provoked into attacking the joints. This could happen if the infecting microbe produces antigens (characteristic chemical markers) which are similar to antigens in the joints. The antibodies made to attack the organism might then attack the joints as well.

In reactive arthritis, the infection itself may have cleared up yet the arthritic pains continue for many months or years. In the case of one bacterium which can cause reactive arthritis, *Yersinia*, the bacterial antigens are still found inside the joints many years after the onset of reactive arthritis.

Reactive arthritis is one aspect of Reiter's syndrome (see p.127), in which there may also be inflammation of the eye and the urinary tract. Some of the bacteria that produce Reiter's syndrome, including *Salmonella* and *Yersinia*, can also lead to simple reactive arthritis with no other symptoms.

Rheumatic fever (see p.128) is also a type of reactive arthritis since the bacteria involved do not infect the joints. Most types of viral arthritis (see p.142) are also reactive. The exception is German measles, or rubella, where there is evidence of joint infection.

Several parasitic infections which are endemic in tropical countries can also cause reactive arthritis. The joint symptoms tend to disappear when the parasite infestation is effectively treated by drugs.

See also Infective Arthritis (p.108).

Can diet help with reactive arthritis ?

Little or no research has been done on this. Because the problem begins with an infection, not with any adverse reaction to food, it seems at first glance that diet is most unlikely to help. On the other hand, where a gut infection (such as Salmonella) started the reactive arthritis, it is just possible that a permanent disturbance occurred in the gut flora (see p.37) and that this is responsible for the continuing inflammation in the joints. If so, then a diet which altered the composition in the gut flora might – just possibly – be beneficial. At present, there is no established dietary treatment which can reliably alter the gut flora in a beneficial way (see p.399), but several lines of research are showing that some of the diets that work for other forms of arthritis (such as rheumatoid arthritis) do influence the gut flora. Whether this effect on the gut flora is responsible for the benefits of some diets to some rheumatoid arthritis patients is another matter. In time, this research might throw up results that are relevant to reactive arthritis, but at present there is no dietary treatment that we can recommend. However, antioxidants might be of some help in limiting the damage done by inflammation (see p.339).

· *Reiter's Syndrome* ·

There are three sites of inflammation in classic Reiter's syndrome: the joints, the eye and the urinary tract. Not everyone with the syndrome will show all three, however.

In women, the urinary tract inflammation (urethritis) may be present but not noticeable. Some patients also suffer mouth ulcers, and there may be ulcers on the penis. Sometimes the skin is affected, particularly on the palms of the hands and the soles of the feet.

Reiter's syndrome follows on from an infection, usually beginning within about a month. The infection may be either in the urinary tract or in the bowel. Urinary tract infections are usually acquired sexually, and include the commonplace infection called non-specific urethritis (NSU). The bowel infections responsible include bacterial dysentery, some types of salmonella poisoning and a form of painful diarrhoea caused by the bacterium *Yersinia enterocolitica*.

Once the original infection is over, Reiter's syndrome itself is not infectious.

Most patients with Reiter's syndrome recover from their arthritis after a few weeks or months, but there may be residual aches and pains for years afterwards. In some cases the arthritis is more severe and there is permanent damage to the joints. Quite often the disease dies down completely but then recurs, as much as 10 years later.

There is clearly an inherited factor that makes people susceptible to

Reiter's syndrome. Only one person in 400 who has dysentery goes on to develop Reiter's syndrome, and less than one person in 100 among those who have non-specific urethritis. Of those that do develop Reiter's syndrome, between 60% and 90% carry the genetic marker HLA-B27 (this is the same marker that characterises patients with ankylosing spondylitis (see p.85). Some people with Reiter's syndrome go on to develop ankylosing spondylitis, while a few with skin symptoms as well as arthritis progress to psoriatic arthritis (see p.124).

For persistent arthritis, non-steroidal anti-inflammatory drugs (see p.418) are usually prescribed. If these are unhelpful, second-line anti-rheumatic drugs such as azathioprine and methotrexate may be tried.

Can diet help with Reiter's syndrome ?

See under Reactive Arthritis (p.126).

· *Rheumatic Fever* ·

This was once a common illness of childhood, linked with overcrowded living conditions. Poor nutrition and inadequate medical care were also factors. The disease began to decline following slum clearance programmes in the late 19th Century. It has now virtually disappeared in affluent countries, but it still affects many children in the developing nations.

Rheumatic fever begins with a sore throat or tonsillitis caused by bacteria belonging to the 'beta-haemolytic group A streptococci' group. The sore throat may be so slight that it is scarcely noticed. Only in poor living conditions, or in someone who has previously suffered from rheumatic fever, is the sore throat likely to lead on to rheumatic fever.

In rheumatic fever, symptoms develop in the heart and the joints about 1–5 weeks after the throat infection. Other symptoms include fever and vomiting, small nodules under the skin, and (sometimes) a distinctive type of rash.

There is a danger of permanent damage to the heart valves unless prompt treatment is given, but the joints generally recover in time. Anyone who has suffered one bout of rheumatic fever is susceptible to it again, and penicillin is usually given for throat infections to avert this possibility.

Damage to the heart is probably due to an **auto-immune reaction**, in which the immune system attacks the heart itself. This occurs because the antigens of the streptococci bacteria are similar to certain antigens in the heart. Whether something similar happens in the joints is not known at present. It may do, or there may be other immune reactions involved, similar to those described for reactive arthritis (see p.126).

Can diet help with rheumatic fever?

Good nutrition is probably important in building up resistance to infections and so *preventing the development* of rheumatic fever. There is no other specific dietary treatment.

· 'Rheumatism' ·

There is really no such thing as 'rheumatism': it is an old-fashioned term that covered a wide range of different diseases. You should ask your doctor for a proper diagnosis of your condition.

· Rheumatoid Arthritis ·

This is one of the more common forms of arthritis. It is an inflammatory arthritis, with the main site of inflammation (see p.64) occurring in the synovial membrane or synovium (see p.421) which becomes inflamed and enlarged.

The inflammation in the joint may make it very warm, and the overlying skin can appear red as well as feeling hot. Often the synovium over-produces the lubricating fluid (called synovial fluid) which causes the joint to swell. It becomes uncomfortably distended with fluid and may also be stiff and difficult to move.

The severity of rheumatoid arthritis varies widely. Some people have a very mild form of the disease, while in others it is more severe and the joints may be irreversibly altered by the rampant growth of the synovium, which damages the cartilage and bone. There may be more general symptoms affecting the whole body, such as fever, tiredness and lack of stamina, weight loss and general malaise. 'Swollen glands' are sometimes among the symptoms: these are enlarged lymph nodes (see p.418). All these symptoms are a result of the constant overactivity of the immune system (see p.416).

Sometimes people with the first signs of rheumatoid arthritis (or what looks like rheumatoid arthritis – it is often difficult to diagnose initially) seem to recover spontaneously within a few months of the disease appearing. Exactly what happens is unclear, but this spontaneous recovery is probably aided by complete rest in the early stages.

The joints affected first by rheumatoid arthritis are usually those in the fingers, knuckles and wrist, but not the finger-tip joints. The knees and feet may also be affected early. At a later stage, the disease may spread to the elbows, shoulders, hips and ankles. Sometimes the jaw is affected, where it is hinged to the skull.

Exactly what causes rheumatoid arthritis is unknown, and still hotly debated. The immune system is clearly attacking something. There is some antigen (see p.413) which it perceives as 'the enemy' and against which it battles without victory or respite.

Rheumatoid arthritis was once regarded as a straightforward auto-immune disease (see p.413), but medical opinion is now changing on this because the main auto-antibody involved, rheumatoid factor (see p.419), does not appear in the early stages of the disorder. Some patients with quite severe rheumatoid arthritis continue for several years without developing rheumatoid factor. It seems to be a secondary development, a result of other aspects of the disease, not an underlying cause.

This does not rule out the possibility of some other auto-immune event, rather than rheumatoid factor, being at the root of rheumatoid arthritis. But this other auto-immune event has not been identified. There are certainly antibodies to collagen (see p.414) in some patients but these too are a late development, a result of the destruction of the cartilage, which exposes parts of the collagen molecule that are normally hidden away. Encountering an unfamiliar chemical pattern in these exposed collagen fragments, the immune system mistakes them for alien invaders and mounts an attack.

All that can be said with certainty about rheumatoid arthritis is that the immune system is *overactive*, with the cause of that overactivity being a mystery. Many features suggest that an infectious microbe might be involved. But if this **infective hypothesis** is correct, the microbe concerned is extraordinarily shy. After a century of dedicated searching, the most that researchers have achieved is to rule out active infection by *streptococci*, mycoplasmas, *Listeria*, the German measles virus, the herpes virus, and a number of other one-time suspects.

Thousands of doctors and medical researchers have been intensively looking for this microbe during the past century, using every research tool they could think of, but with virtually no success. More human effort has been expended looking for the cause of rheumatoid arthritis than ever went into the search for the philosopher's stone or the Holy Grail, and yet the search has been equally fruitless.

There are various infective theories which are still regarded as possibilities, but little agreement about these hypotheses. There is some reasonably good evidence for a general disturbance to the gut flora (see p.37), with no specific details about the exact types of bacteria involved. Some studies seem to show that the gut flora is changed by diets which have beneficial effects on rheumatoid arthritis symptoms (see pp.39–40), suggesting that the gut flora might indeed be playing a part.

The auto-immune hypothesis and the infective hypothesis are not mutually exclusive. Some infectious microbes may have antigens which are very similar to certain antigens in the body (**self antigens**), so similar that the immune system might get the two confused. The immune cells may make antibodies to the microbial antigen which then bind to self antigens as well, provoking attack on the body's own tissues. This is a possible cause of some forms of reactive arthritis (see p.126) but there is no firm evidence that it is relevant to rheumatoid arthritis.

Treatment for rheumatoid arthritis relies mainly on drugs that quell the inflammation. An important aim of treatment is to prevent the inflammation in the joint from attacking the cartilage and bone before irreversible and disabling changes have occurred. For this reason it is important to comply fully with the drug regime prescribed.

Can diet help with rheumatoid arthritis?

More research has been done regarding the effects of diet on rheumatoid arthritis than for any other arthritic disease. Despite this it remains a controversial topic. The controversies are described in Section 1 of this book, particularly in Chapter 1.1 (p.15). What follows here is our advice, based on a thorough study of the medical literature, and on the experience of using diet in the treatment of rheumatoid arthritis at Epsom General Hospital over the past fifteen years.

Our first recommendation would be to try an elimination diet as described in Chapter 2.4 (p.170) of this book. Such a diet is designed to diagnose food intolerance or food sensitivity (see pp.415–61 for an explanation of these terms). We have found that a majority of patients show some improvement as a result of trying this diet and avoiding those foods found to aggravate their symptoms. For about 36% of patients the improvement has been dramatic and many are able to give up taking all drugs, at least for prolonged periods of time, and some permanently (see p.33).

Before trying such a diet you should consult your doctor and get his or her agreement because it is not an easy diet to carry out, and you are likely to lose some weight in the first few weeks. If you are already underweight the diet is probably not advisable unless carefully monitored by a doctor. But even if you are not underweight you may well encounter opposition and find your doctor unenthusiastic about the diet – many doctors have not had any experience of using diet to treat rheumatoid arthritis and are sceptical as a result. Also the use of diet in the treatment of rheumatoid arthritis has only been investigated scientifically quite recently and not all doctors know of the good results which may be obtained.

Ideally you should read Chapter 1.1 (p.15) and Chapter 2.4 (p.170) before discussing the diet with your doctor, so that you are ready with all the information you need. The argument in favour of trying an elimination diet can, however, be summarised quite easily, as follows:

A proportion of patients with rheumatoid arthritis improve remarkably when a particular food or foods are removed from their diet (see pp.18–20) – no doctor or rheumatologist who is familiar with the research literature would disagree with this. What is debated is the number of patients affected. In our experience at Epsom General Hospital, the number who benefit substantially is quite high, about 36%, and this makes it worthwhile looking systematically for food-related symptoms in those of our patients who are interested in this type of treatment. Even if the proportion were only 5%, as the more conservative estimates suggest, it would still be worth looking for food reactions if patients themselves were willing to accept the odds involved: in return for a few weeks of effort and doing without some familiar foods you have a one-in-twenty chance of substantial improvement in rheumatoid symptoms to the point where you may no longer need any drugs, or far fewer than you would otherwise have needed. Such odds should seem very favourable to anyone with the pain, disability and anxiety that rheumatoid arthritis brings, particularly since there are no serious side effects from the diet, and you can always return to drugs in a few weeks if the diet does not help you.

Bearing in mind that rheumatoid arthritis can progress rapidly, and that serious joint damage may be incurred, it is important that treatments which can affect the disease process should begin as early as possible. If an elimination diet is to be tried, it makes sense to try it now rather than in six months' or a year's time. But if such a diet is tried and is clearly not working, then the sensible reaction is to abandon the elimination diet promptly and to continue tackling the inflammation with the appropriate drugs. Do not be tempted to go on experimenting with more and more diets while ignoring conventional medical treatments, and do remain under medical supervision.

If the elimination diet does work well for you, you are unlikely to need other types of dietary treatment. For those who are not helped by the elimination diet, however, there are other possibilities. The most promising are fish oil, olive oil and the GLA oils (evening primrose oil, borage or 'starflower' oil, and blackcurrant seed oil), all of which can be helpful in reducing inflammation. The doses and likely effects of these are described in Chapter 2.2 (p.143), while the story of how they became accepted by the medical profession is told in Chapter 1.2 (p.46). Other changes to fats in the diet, such as reducing the quantity of saturated fat eaten, might also be beneficial – see Chapter 2.2. If you suffer from easy or spontaneous bruising, as some people with rheumatoid arthritis do, fish oil is not advisable. Before taking fish oil, check Table 4 on p.152 for other conditions in which it may be damaging.

Several different vitamins have potential benefits for those with rheumatoid arthritis, including Vitamin B_5 or pantothenate (see p.291) and Vitamin C if the symptoms suffered include spontaneous or easy bruising. Antioxidants (see p.339) such as Vitamin E and carotenoids are thought to be important in reducing the damaging effects of inflammation. Intake of these antioxidant nutrients can be boosted by eating more of certain foods, and such dietary changes, described on pp.257–9, will have more general health benefits as well.

Several of the drugs prescribed for rheumatoid arthritis can affect absorption or loss of vitamins and minerals, producing nutrient shortages in the long term (see p.280). High-dose Vitamin C can make rheumatoid arthritis worse (see p.295), and so can iron supplements on rare occasions (see p.321).

Anyone with rheumatoid arthritis is at a higher risk than normal of developing osteoporosis. Dietary measures to protect against this problem are described in Chapter 2.3 (p.161).

Finally, an inadequate diet can cause a disease that is not rheumatoid arthritis but resembles it very closely (secondary hyperparathyroidism). The deficiency concerned is a shortage of calcium, which may occur for anyone who has avoided all dairy products for some time (see p.313).

· *Rheumatoid-like Arthritis* ·

An umbrella term that covers rheumatoid arthritis and palindromic rheumatism (episodic arthritis) – see p.17.

· *Rickets* ·

This disease is caused by a lack of Vitamin D in a child's diet, and a lack of sunlight (see p.298). Rickets can be mistaken for arthritis because one symptom is swelling of the wrists or ankles.

Can diet help with rickets?

Vitamin D supplements are needed to treat rickets once it has become established: follow your doctor's advice carefully.

Calcium supplements may also be needed to treat rickets (see p.229). If the condition does not respond to Vitamin D and calcium, this may indicate a need for magnesium supplements as well (see p.326); this is known as 'refractory rickets'.

Whenever Vitamin D is taken at high doses for a long period of time (as for refractory rickets) there is a risk of calcification of soft tissues: careful monitoring of calcium levels in the blood and close medical supervision are necessary to prevent this damaging side-effect.

Preventing rickets involves encouraging children to spend more time out in the sun and making certain changes to the family's diet (see pp.297–9).

Mothers who are breast-feeding should note that their breast milk alone does not contain enough Vitamin D (see p.299), but breast-feeding is still preferable to bottle-feeding.

· *Sarcoidosis* ·

This rare disease produces inflammation (see p.64) in many parts of the body, particularly the skin, eyes, lungs and liver. It can also produce arthritis. Fortunately most patients recover completely within two years and many do so without any treatment. However corticosteroids may be prescribed to quell the inflammation if there is a risk of blindness or lung damage.

Can diet help with sarcoidosis?

If you would like to feel that you are doing something to aid your recovery, you could perhaps try olive oil or evening primrose oil, as described in Chapter 2.2 (p.143). Before doing this you must obtain your doctor's agreement. Note that these oils have not been tested at all in sarcoidosis, and it is only extrapolation from other inflammatory diseases that suggests they might be helpful.

Fish oil supplements are not advisable in sarcoidosis unless the product concerned is guaranteed to contain little or no Vitamin D as large doses of Vitamin D can be very damaging to people with sarcoidosis (see pp.300–301), and you should not take multi-vitamin supplements, or cod-liver oil, without medical supervision. Eating too much of foods that are reinforced with Vitamin D, such as margarine, should also be avoided.

Antioxidants (see p.339) such as Vitamin E and carotenoids are thought to be important in reducing the damaging effects of inflammation. Intake of these antioxidant nutrients can be boosted by eating more of certain foods, and such dietary changes – described on pp.257-9 – will have more general health benefits as well.

· *Seronegative Arthritis* ·

Rheumatoid arthritis in which tests for rheumatoid factor (see p.419) are negative.

Can diet help with seronegative arthritis?

They may well be able to help. In particular, those with rheumatoid arthritis who respond to an elimination diet are more frequently seronegative. See Rheumatoid arthritis (p.129).

· *Seronegative Spondarthritis* ·

An umbrella term that covers ankylosing spondylitis, Reiter's syndrome, psoriatic arthritis, spondylitis associated with inflammatory bowel disease and certain other disorders. Ask for a more precise diagnosis and then refer to the entry concerned.

· *Sexually Acquired Reactive Arthritis* ·

Sometimes abbreviated to SARA, this term refers to cases of Reiter's syndrome (see p.127) which follow on from a sexually transmitted infection, such as non-specific urethritis (NSU). (Note that Reiter's syndrome can also follow dysentery.)

Gonorrhoea and (more rarely) syphilis can also produce arthritis, but this is due to direct infection of a joint, so it is an infective arthritis (see p.108).

Can diet help with SARA?

The simple answer to this question is that diet is most unlikely to help – clearly the problem begins with an infection, not with any adverse reaction to food.

However, antioxidants (see p.339) such as Vitamin E and carotenoids are thought to be important in reducing the damaging effects of inflammation. Intake of these antioxidant nutrients can be boosted by eating more of certain foods, and such dietary changes, described on pp.257–9 will have more general health benefits as well.

· *Sicca Complex, Sicca Syndrome* ·

A name sometimes used for the dry eyes and dry mouth that are part of Sjögrens syndrome.

Can diet help with sicca complex?

It may be of some help – see Sjögrens syndrome.

· *Sjögrens Syndrome* ·

A distressing condition in which the flow of both tears and saliva is greatly reduced because the body's immune system (se p.416) is attacking the glands that produce these secretions. The nose, throat and vagina may also suffer dryness. Accompanying these symptoms there may be rheumatoid arthritis, or another disorder such as systemic lupus erythematosus, systemic sclerosis or polymyositis.

Anti-inflammatory drugs may be prescribed to treat the underlying condition. Artificial tears, that are put into the eye with a dropper when needed, help to ease the irritation of dry eyes and reduce the risk of infection or damage. Lozenges that stimulate the flow of saliva and artificial saliva sprays may also be provided.

Can diet help with Sjögrens syndrome?

There is no really good research on this subject, but one trial looked at the effect of evening primrose oil and found no benefit.

Another trial found that patients with Sjögrens syndrome may react badly to Vitamin B_3 or niacin (see p.291).

Sjögrens syndrome affects all the body's moist surfaces and it is likely to make the gut more permeable to food molecules. This is known to predispose to food sensitivity, because more intact food molecules reach the bloodstream. Although no research has been done to check this, if sensitivity to food does occur more often in people with Sjögrens syndrome then this could be a factor in their arthritis (where rheumatoid arthritis accompanies the other symptoms). An elimination diet might be worth trying, if your doctor agrees. See Chapter 2.4 (p.170) for details.

If you have difficulty chewing and swallowing refer to p.226 for advice on this problem.

Antioxidants (see p.339) such as Vitamin E and carotenoids are thought to be important in reducing the damaging effects of inflammation. Intake of these antioxidant nutrients can be boosted by eating more of certain foods, and such dietary changes, described on pp.257–9, will have more general health benefits as well.

A study of patients with Sjögren's syndrome in Japan showed that their antioxidant levels in the blood were unusually low, a common reaction to generalised inflammation. Supplements of Vitamin E seemed to reduce the inflammation, in so far as they produced improvements in several laboratory tests, such as C-reactive protein. Rather than just taking Vitamin E, it would seem sensible to increase consumption of all the major antioxidants. Boosting antioxidant levels is something that can be done in combination with other dietary treatments.

· Still's Disease ·

Old name for one form of juvenile chronic arthritis (see p.111).

· *Synovitis* ·

This is inflammation of the synovial membrane (see p.421) within the joint. This occurs in rheumatoid arthritis and several other forms of inflammatory arthritis. It is not a diagnosis in its own right.

· *Systemic Lupus Erythematosus* ·

This is an auto-immune disease in which the body's natural defences are turned against certain body parts, (see p.64) causing inflammation. The most commonly affected organs are the joints, the skin and the kidneys. The over-active immune system often produces more general symptoms as well, notably tiredness, fever, loss of appetite and malaise. Hair loss sometimes occurs.

If the disease is not treated adequately it can progress and become more serious. Damage to the kidneys by the ongoing attacks of the immune system can, in the worst instances, lead to kidney failure. Treatment is much more effective now than it was 20 years ago, and deaths from kidney failure are now much less common: out-of-date medical books which refer to systemic lupus erythematosus as 'usually fatal' are inaccurate and cause much unnecessary worry. Many cases are now known to be mild and easily managed.

Treatment includes the use of anti-inflammatory drugs or immunosuppressive drugs to damp down the auto-immune response. Patients whose symptoms get worse when they are exposed to sunshine can improve matters by wearing sun-block cream, but should ensure that they are getting enough Vitamin D from their diet (see p.297).

Can diet help with systemic lupus erythematosus?

There is one way in which diet, or a commonly sold 'food supplement', can actually make systemic lupus erythematosus worse, and everyone with the disease should be aware of this danger. Alfalfa seeds and alfalfa sprouts contain a substance called L-canavanine which is toxic to mammals, including human beings, if eaten in sufficient quantity. When fed to macaque monkeys in slightly smaller, sub-lethal doses it eventually, after several months, produces a disease that closely resembles systemic lupus erythematosus. The possibility that alfalfa might have the same effect on humans is impossible to test scientifically without putting people at serious risk, but the experiment has been inadvertently carried out by patients with systemic lupus erythematosus taking alfalfa tablets bought at a healthfood shop. Two cases are described in the medical literature, both women with a long history of systemic lupus erythematosus who were being successfully treated with drugs and whose disease had become inactive, with normal blood tests. Each began taking alfalfa tablets without the knowledge of their doctors, and their lupus became active again within 6–12 months, with severe symptoms and rising levels of anti-nuclear antibodies (the hallmark of lupus) in the blood. Although there is no absolute proof that the alfalfa tablets caused this deterioration, given the effects of alfalfa on monkeys it seems plausible that the alfalfa may indeed have been responsible. No one with a history of lupus, or with lupus in the family, should take these tablets. It might also be advisable to avoid alfalfa sprouts.

Supplements of omega-3 fish oil should also be avoided by patients with lupus as they make the condition worse.

One other trial is of interest, although we cannot recommend the diet it studied because this was only a pilot study and further experiments are needed to confirm its benefits – or show them to be illusory, as often happens when treatments are tested more fully. Patients were asked to stop using vegetable oil, margarine and other sources of polyunsaturated fatty acids, but to continue using saturated fats. This experimental diet – which of course is contrary to all current recommendations for healthy eating – was based on results with a breed of laboratory mouse which spontaneously develops a disease similar to systemic lupus erythematosus. Feeding the mice a diet containing saturated fats but no unsaturated fats delayed the development of the disease considerably. People are not necessarily like mice, yet the saturated fat diet did seem to have benefits for over half the patients tested in this study. However this was an open trial (not a double-blind placebo-controlled trial – see p.27) so the results have to be interpreted cautiously. Because the diet could increase the risk of heart disease and be damaging to general health, it should not be tried out until its effects on lupus sufferers have been assessed more fully.

Antioxidants (see p.339) such as Vitamin E and carotenoids are thought to be important in reducing the damaging effects of inflammation. Intake of these antioxidant nutrients can be boosted by eating more of certain foods, and such dietary changes, described on pp.257–9, will have more general health benefits as well.

Those whose kidneys are affected by lupus may have to restrict their intake of potassium (see pp.330–331) and possibly protein (see p.348). You should follow your doctor's advice about this. Do not make major changes to your diet without medical approval.

· *Systemic Sclerosis* ·

This is a disease in which the skin and other connective tissues (those tissues that surround, cushion and support various organs) become thicker and harder than normal. This affects the skin of the fingers and face most severely, and it often causes problems in many other parts of the body, notably in the blood vessels, the oesophagus and other parts of the digestive tract, the heart, lungs and kidneys.

Arthritis is, therefore, just one symptom among many. Only about one third of patients with systemic sclerosis develop joint pain.

Alternative names for this condition are **scleroderma** (meaning 'hardened skin' and used when the skin alone is affected) and **progressive systemic sclerosis**, used when the disease is more generalised. The immune system (see p.416) seems to be involved in causing the disease, but exactly what goes wrong is far from clear. In some cases, the disease seems to be precipitated by exposure to dust or a synthetic chemical: silica dust may produce the disease in miners, while vinyl chloride, toluene, benzene, trichloroethylene and epoxy resins have all been linked to the disease in chemical workers. The 'toxic oil syndrome' which resulted from the sale of adulterated olive oil in parts of Spain in the early 1980s, was similar to systemic sclerosis.

There is, at present, no proven treatment for the underlying disease, although various drugs are being tried. Medicines may be prescribed to help alleviate some of the symptoms. Those affected by Raynaud's phenomenon (see p.125) can help minimise this problem by keeping warm, wearing thick gloves or mittens when out in cold weather, and, if they smoke, giving up tobacco which aggravates the circulatory problems.

Can diet help in systemic sclerosis ?

Various studies have been carried out to see whether taking omega-3 fish oil or evening primrose oil could help with the symptoms of Raynaud's phenomenon that often accompany systemic sclerosis. It seems that a high dose of evening primrose oil may be helpful, but that fish oil might be damaging (see p.61).

One odd 'side effect' was noticed in the trial of evening primrose oil. Almost all those taking this oil felt less depressed at the end of the trial than before.

The question of whether diet could beneficially influence the underlying disease process in systemic sclerosis has been little investigated, but it seems unlikely that it could. One rather bizarre dietary experiment with systemic sclerosis and rheumatoid arthritis took place in Japan about forty years ago (see p.352).

Antioxidants (see p.339) such as Vitamin E and carotenoids are thought to be important in reducing the damaging effects of inflammation. Intake of these antioxidant nutrients can be boosted by eating more of certain foods, and such dietary changes, described on pp.257–9, will have more general health benefits as well.

· *Tendonitis, Tenosynovitis* ·

Tendonitis is an inflammation (see p.64) of the tendons, the fibrous 'cords' that connect muscles to bones so that they can pull against them.

The tendons have a sheath around them and the inner lining of these resembles the synovial membrane found in the joints. If this lining becomes inflamed the condition is known as tenosynovitis.

If the inflammation occurs at the point where the tendon is joined to the bone, this is called enthesopathy. It is a feature of the seronegative spondarthritides (see p.135), but can also occur independently of these diseases.

Can diet help with tendonitis?

The real answer to this is that no one knows. However, there is some limited evidence that an elimination diet may be worth trying (assuming your doctor agrees). See Chapter 2.4 (p.170).

· *Vaccination and Arthritis* ·

Occasionally, vaccination for German measles (rubella) can produce a brief attack of arthritis which begins 2–4 weeks after the vaccination. This should clear up within a few days, although some people are unfortunate enough to suffer the symptoms for several weeks or months or occasionally even longer. No treatment is required as recovery occurs spontaneously.

Can diet help with vaccination-induced arthritis?

Diet is irrelevant to this form of arthritis.

· *Viral Diseases Causing Arthritis* ·

One virus, the one which causes German measles or rubella, can actually infect the joints; see infective arthritis (p.108).

Most viral infections seem to cause arthritis indirectly, because there is no trace of the virus in the affected joints: they are forms of reactive arthritis (see p.126).

The viral infections linked with arthritis include mumps, infectious hepatitis, infectious mononucleosis ('glandular fever'), chickenpox and HIV (see AIDS, p.81). Occasionally a bout of arthritis occurs during a recurrence of herpes in people infected with this persistent virus. In certain parts of Australia, the Ross River virus can cause epidemics of arthritis.

Arthritis associated with viral infections clears up naturally within a few days or weeks in most cases. No specific treatment for the arthritis is needed.

Can diet help with virally caused arthritis?

Diet is irrelevant in these forms of arthritis.

· *Whipple's Disease* ·

A rare condition in which joint pains are only part of the wide spectrum of symptoms. Important features of the disease include diarrhoea, abdominal pain and weight loss, caused by failure to absorb nutrients from food. There may also be fever, anaemia, changes in the skin pigments and swollen lymph nodes.

The disease is thought to be caused by a bacterial infection in the digestive tract, but the bacterium responsible has not been identified. A long course of antibiotics – usually taken for a year – seems to be effective in treating the disease.

Can diet help with Whipple's disease?

Dietary supplements are given to help compensate for the shortfall in nutrient absorption: follow the doctor's instructions carefully. Apart from that, it would be sensible to eat a good balanced diet with plenty of fruit and vegetables, whole grains, nuts, eggs, cheese, lean meat and fish. Avoid drinking tea with meals as this interferes with the absorption of some nutrients. So do wheat bran, oat bran and various other foods (see pp.309–310).

Chapter 2.2

USING OILS IN THE DIET TO REDUCE INFLAMMATION

Changing the types of oil and fat that you eat can produce improvements in rheumatoid arthritis and certain other inflammatory diseases. This idea, which would have seemed highly implausible to most doctors twenty years ago, is now widely accepted on the basis of a wealth of recent scientific evidence. That evidence is described in Chapter 1.2 (p.46), here we are just concerned with practical advice for anyone wanting to try out oils for themselves.

Firstly, as with all diets, ensure that this one is appropriate for your particular form of arthritis. *The main part of this chapter deals with rheumatoid arthritis only*. Other forms of arthritis are dealt with at the end of the chapter on p.159. If you do not have a firm diagnosis yet, it is probably best to be cautious about oil treatments until you do: it is certainly not advisable to take high doses of omega-3 fish oil at this stage, since it may have some non-beneficial effects in certain disorders, such as systemic lupus erythematosus (see p.152). The very early stages of systemic lupus erythematosus are often not distinctly different from the early stages of rheumatoid arthritis, so you should steer clear of fish oil until you have a firm diagnosis of rheumatoid arthritis.

· Oils for Rheumatoid Arthritis ·

All the oil-based dietary treatments have certain things in common. Firstly, their effects build up very gradually: they generally take at least three months to achieve their full benefit, although olive oil may be a little quicker than this when taken at a high dose. Secondly, if you stop taking the oil, after taking it regularly for three months or more, the benefits continue for many weeks, or even months, thereafter. This is because the human body accumulates stores of the useful fatty acids.

Thirdly, the positive effects of these oils are modest but worthwhile. Most people get some benefit, and the degree of improvement does not vary hugely from one person to another – there is no distinct group of 'good responders' who have a very marked improvement as there is with the elimination diet (see p.29).

All these factors combine to make it very difficult to assess the effects of an oil, and to distinguish these effects from the normal ups-and-downs of a fluctuating disease. When the oils are tried out in research studies, large numbers of patients are included, to overcome such problems, and they are compared with a control group taking a placebo (see p.27). Even then it is quite hard to accurately assess the benefits of the oils.

For the individual trying out an oil at home, it is far more difficult: there will be no sudden improvement when you begin, and nothing much will change if you stop taking the oil – not for many weeks anyway. In these circumstances, how can you be sure this treatment is helping you? The answer is that you cannot be entirely certain, but you can have confidence in the oils because so many research studies have now been carried out showing that these oils do indeed help the majority of patients. These studies should reassure you: if you stick with the oil treatment for 6–12 months, and if you feel better than you did at the outset, you can be reasonably confident that the oil has contributed to this improvement, and that it is therefore worthwhile to continue.

Because this is a long-term diet, not a 'quick fix', you need to be sure that the dietary programme you have devised for yourself is both practicable and appetising enough to be maintained indefinitely. Fortunately, you can lapse occasionally – that is one of the advantages of the beneficial fatty acids being stored in the body. A few days off the diet will not do any damage, and once you have been taking the oil for a year or more, you can safely lapse for a few weeks without ill-effects.

· *Olive Oil* ·

The simplest and cheapest change you can make is to add olive oil to your daily diet. Several lines of evidence show that, for many patients, olive oil has a significant effect in easing the syptoms of rheumatoid arthritis (see p.54).

The amount that has given the greatest benefit when used as a supplement in research studies is 22 ml (1 1/2 tablespoons) per day. This has been shown to help with pain, joint tenderness and morning stiffness for most patients, although it may not be effective for patients taking corticosteroids.

A smaller daily dose of olive oil, 7.5 ml (1½ teaspoons), also has some limited benefit in reducing pain and joint tenderness, but does not seem to improve morning stiffness. The larger dose may produce effects more promptly, sometimes in less than three months.

There are several different approaches that you might take to introducing olive oil into your diet. The simplest is to take it in addition to your ordinary diet, which is how it was given in most of the scientific trials that found beneficial effects. However, you may not get maximum effect from the olive oil in this way: bearing in mind the findings from Greece, described on pp.47–8, it seems that rheumatoid arthritis patients may reap more benefit by a general shift in their eating habits, away from meat, eggs and dairy products, and towards olive oil and more fruits and vegetables. (You might also want to add more oily fish and shellfish to this diet, given the Greek findings, but we deal with fish later, on pp.148–150.)

The health benefits of this type of 'Mediterranean diet' are now thought to be substantial. Heart disease is much less common in Mediterranean countries, probably due to the combination of olive oil, the low levels of saturated fat, and the high levels of antioxidants (see p.339), notably carotenoids, from fresh vegetables such as red peppers. Olive oil is also thought to protect against heart disease, because it is very rich in monounsaturated fatty acids, which are now considered to be better for health than either saturated or polyunsaturated fats (see p.357). A Mediterranean-style diet may also protect against some forms of cancer.

For some people, such a radical shift in eating habits is not possible, because other family members do not wish to change their menu, or because most meals are eaten away from home. If you fall into this category, then you should simply add olive oil to your present diet, and cut down a little on butter, margarine, cream or cooking oil, so that your overall intake of fat and oil stays about the same.

If you can face taking olive oil straight from the spoon then by all means do so, but few people can manage this on a daily basis. The easiest alternative is to incorporate olive oil into your main evening meal, by adding a bowl of salad, and dressing this with plain olive oil, or olive oil mixed with a little lemon juice or wine vinegar. Make sure you do not lose too much of the oil at the bottom of the bowl – you can wipe the bowl clean with a piece of bread, Greek-style, to ensure none of the olive oil is wasted.

Another option is to consume your olive oil at breakfast, since this is the most flexible meal of the day for most families. A traditional Mediterranean breakfast is fresh crusty white bread dipped into a bowl of olive oil, and eaten with some fresh fruit or salad. This is delicious, and an excellent start to the day. When eating olive oil in this way, it is important to find one that you really like: the flavours vary enormously, with some more peppery than others, some more bitter or astringent. For breakfast eating, a mild and fruity olive oil is best. Large supermarkets and delicatessans have a good range, and the labels often give a guide to the flavour; you can also try specialist Italian or Greek shops.

Traditionalists might prefer to make toast in the ordinary way and then spread it with solidified olive oil: you can make this by putting your ration of olive oil into a small plastic container in the freezer the night before. (You can also pour liquid olive oil onto toast from a spoon, although it takes a little practice to get it evenly spread.)

For those who cannot learn to love the taste of olive oil, the following recipe is well worth trying for a quick and filling breakfast.

1. Chop two large bananas.
2. Put into a blender with 22 ml ($1^{1}/_{2}$ tablespoons) of olive oil, 142 ml ($^{1}/_{4}$ pint) water and a dash of vanilla essence or some grated nutmeg.
3. Blend for 2 minutes, then pour into a large glass.

The blended mixture tastes like a banana milk-shake: the olive oil is virtually undetectable. This meal-in-a-glass gives a breakfast of 335 calories.

Anyone who cooks their own main meal of the day can incorporate olive oil into this, simply by substituting it for ordinary cooking oil. If you do this, make sure that you are getting the full dose of olive oil, and not leaving much of it stuck to the plate or cooking pan. Use olive oil in your salad dressings as well.

If you decide to make a substantial change in your eating habits, along the lines of the Greek Lenten diet (see p.47), then you should incorporate more fresh vegetables into your meals, and substitute some beans, chickpeas and fish for the usual servings of meat, eggs and dairy produce.

You can do this perfectly well with some traditional favourites such as baked beans on toast or sardines on toast (miss out the butter and spread your toast with olive oil instead), adding a salad to boost the vegetable content, and some fresh fruit to round off the meal.

Alternatively you can introduce some Mediterranean recipes such as hummous (see p.212), taramasalata (see p.223), or sweet red peppers stuffed with herbs and rice and cooked in olive oil. Ratatouille is a prime example of good Mediterranean cooking and is easily made.

1. Combine 454 gm (1 lb) each of chopped tomatoes, aubergine and courgettes, with 222 gm ($\frac{1}{2}$ lb) each of chopped onions and green peppers.
2. Add 4 tablespoons of olive oil, salt, pepper and a clove of crushed garlic.
3. Put into a casserole dish with a lid and cook at 180°C (350°F, Gas Mark 4) for about an hour or until the vegetables are all cooked (but not soft and disintegrating).
4. Add a generous handful of chopped parsley just before serving.

This feeds three or four people as a main meal: serve with bread, rice, new potatoes or baked potatoes. Some sardines grilled with herbs make a good addition to the meal.

There are many other excellent Mediterranean recipes using olive oil. Some useful recipe books are listed on p.429.

Nutritionally, olive oil is a balanced food: it has slightly more Vitamin E than required to offset all the polyunsaturated fatty acids it contains. If you are watching your weight, the suggested olive oil supplement of 22 ml (1$\frac{1}{2}$ tablespoons) supplies 166 calories, which you can compensate for by cutting out an equivalent amount of oil or butter.

There are various brands of margarine, with attractive pictures of olives and olive leaves on the package, that may seem like a good alternative to olive oil. In fact they only consist of about 20–21% olive oil – the rest is other fats and oils. As usual, it pays to read labels carefully!

· Fish Oil ·

Note that high doses of omega-3 fish oil (whether from capsules or from whole fish) can have adverse effects on some diseases. Consult Table 4 (p.152) to check that this form of dietary treatment is safe for you.

There are two ways to get a therapeutic dose of fish oil: either by eating oily fish or by taking omega-3 fish oil in capsules. In principle, we would always advocate real food rather than a supplement, but there are pros and cons to both options here.

The three main concerns are cost, calories and convenience. Cost and calories both relate to the amount of fish oil needed, and we would recommend taking 1.8 gm of EPA per day if possible (equivalent to 3 gm of total omega-3s in most supplements, but not in whole fish, where a larger intake of total omega-3s would be required to give 1.8 gm of EPA). If you cannot achieve this intake, a smaller amount of EPA may have some lesser benefits, but there is probably no point in taking less than 0.8 gm per day. (The rationale for the dose of 1.8 gm of EPA is given on p.58.)

The problem with this dose is that most of the moderately priced fish oil supplements sold in healthfood shops, if taken in the amount recommended by the manufacturer, will not supply nearly enough. These recommended doses have been decided with heart disease in mind, and a much lesser quantity of omega-3 is required to prevent heart disease. To the best of our knowledge there are no toxic constituents in these inexpensive fish oils that would prevent a larger dose being taken, but we cannot recommend this unless you obtain a written assurance directly from the manufacturer that the daily dose you wish to take is safe.

One product, made by Solgar and sold in healthfood shops, is based on hydrolysed Norwegian salmon oil and does provide enough EPA omega-3 fatty acids if taken at the recommended dose (4 capsules per day). The daily cost would be about £1.11.

The other product that can supply enough EPA is the original omega-3 supplement called MaxEPA, which is only available from chemists' shops. The daily dose would be 10 capsules, and the cost about £2.50 per day. One advantage of this supplement is that it has been used in all the major trials of fish oil conducted to date, so it has scientific credentials that other supplements cannot really match. However, other supplements should, in theory, be as good as MaxEPA if they supply enough EPA.

Obtaining the same dose of omega-3 fatty acids from fish itself is a slightly uncertain business, because the amounts of omega-3 present in oily fish vary enormously from one catch to another. You may have seen claims that 100 gm ($3\frac{1}{2}$ oz) of smoked mackerel will give 3.5 gm of omega-3s per day: this was based on an unusually high concentration of omega-3s found in one particular batch of mackerel. Using more realistic average figures, you would need to eat about 200gm (7 oz) of mackerel, herring or sardines per day to be sure of getting enough EPA. This is about the weight of two large smoked mackerel fillets, or two tins of sardines. A smaller quanitity of pilchards, or a much larger quantity of salmon, would give the same dose of EPA (see Table 3 p.150).

Only wild, sea-living fish have omega-3 naturally – it is derived from their food. Wild salmon, as used for canning, contain reasonable levels of omega-3, but farmed salmon only have omega-3s if fish oil is added to their feed. This is now common practice on fish farms in Scotland and Norway, where most of the fresh salmon and smoked salmon sold in the U.K. originates. The situation may not be the same in other countries, and you should make enquiries of the producers if you intend to rely on salmon for some of your omega-3s. (Note also that farmed fish may contain some arachidonic acid, unlike wild sea fish – see p.155.)

White fish such as cod, being low in all oils, has low levels of EPA as well. The richest source is halibut, but 600 gm (1 lb 5 oz) per day would be required to get an average daily dose of 1.8 gm of EPA (and this would supply rather a high level of mercury – see p.152). Most catches of shellfish have about the same content of EPA as halibut, although the levels in crab and lobster are occasionally higher. Thus, white fish and shellfish can make some small addition to your intake of omega-3s, but are unsuitable as the main source.

Fresh tuna fish supplies some omega-3s, but again levels are low and if tuna was your only source you would need to eat 600 gm (1lb 5 oz) a day to give 1.8 gm of EPA. (Like halibut, tuna can be high in mercury, and large daily portions are not advisable – see p.152.) The particular canning process used for tuna removes the natural oil, so most tinned tuna contains little or none. (The exception is a variety of canned tuna sold only in France at present and called *'tuna au naturel'*.)

Other tinned fish, such as sardines, pilchards and mackerel fillets, are just as good a source of omega-3s as their fresh counterparts. Go for fish canned in brine, water or tomato sauce, rather than vegetable oil, since your intake of oil from the fish itself will be high, and it is better not to boost it with added vegetable oil. If you can only buy fish canned in oil, drain the fish well and pat dry with kitchen towel to remove as much vegetable oil as possible.

Smoking does not destroy omega-3s, so kippers and smoked mackerel can be useful, but they should not be eaten too often as the smoking process creates some substances that are very weak carcinogens – harmless if eaten occasionally but not recommended in large amounts every day.

The cost of 200 gm (7 oz) of mackerel or herring is less than 60 pence per day. For this money you are getting a nutritious high-protein meal, as well as your omega-3s, which is one substantial advantage over capsules. You are also getting over 400 calories, which is fine if you are underweight, but not a good idea if you are trying to slim. By comparison, the daily dose of oil in capsules would supply only 48–90 calories. These figures are summarised in Table 3.

Table 3: Sources of EPA

Sources of 1.8 gm of EPA	Cost	Calories
170 gm (6 oz) pilchards	£0.40	214 calories
200 gm (7 oz) herring	£0.55	467 calories
200 gm(7 oz) mackerel	£0.55	446 calories
200 gm (7 oz) sardines (tinned in brine, drained)	£0.60	400 calories
320 gm (11 oz) salmon	£2.75 (fresh) £1.60 (tinned)	410 calories
10 capsules of MaxEPA	£2.50	90 calories
4 capsules of hydrolysed Norwegian salmon oil	£1.30	48 calories
57 gm (2 oz) of *Omega spread margarine (see p.000)	£0.13	362 calories

Other fish:
Bloaters are as rich in EPA as pilchards.
Sprats may contain as much EPA as salmon, but they are highly variable and some catches contain none at all

---

*Check that the margarine contains at least 5.2 gm of omega-3s per 100 gm.

The best option for many people will be to eat fresh or tinned fish on some days, and take capsules on others.

Some cooking methods reduce the omega-3 content of fish, including baking and grilling, although the losses are not huge. Steaming and poaching affect the omega-3 content the least.

The need for Vitamin E

The polyunsaturated fats in oily fish are potentially damaging unless you protect yourself with Vitamin E (see p.342). If you are eating whole fish rather than taking capsules, be sure to maintain a high intake of this vitamin. For example, 200 gm (7 oz) of an oily fish such as mackerel contains about 6.6 gm of polyunsaturates. This requires an additional 2.6 mg of alpha-tocopherol (the most potent form of Vitamin E – see p.302) per day which could be obtained from:

10 gm (1 level tablespoon) sunflower seeds
14 gm (1/2 oz) almonds or hazelnuts
16 gm (1 heaped tablespoon) wheatgerm
86 gm (3 oz) sweet potato or peanuts
140 gm (5 oz) avocado (half of one very large avocado)

15 ml (1 tablespoon) sunflower oil
30 ml (2 tablespoons) safflower oil
18 gm (²/₃ oz) sunflower margarine

Sunflower seeds are much tastier if toasted, but this will reduce their Vitamin E content a little, so use a *heaped* tablespoon to compensate for this.

There is no need to take a Vitamin E supplement, since the vitamin is so easily obtained from common foods. If you are trying to minimise your fat consumption, note that sweet potato and sunflower seeds are the least fatty sources of this vitamin.

Capsules of fish oil have added Vitamin E, but one study (see p.303) suggests that the polyunsaturates in the fish oil 'use up' all of this Vitamin E, leaving no safety margin. Since polyunsaturates can be damaging if not fully covered by Vitamin E, and since a little surplus Vitamin E is likely to be useful in rheumatoid arthritis anyway (see p.304), it might be wise to err on the generous side and consume more of this beneficial vitamin. This can easily be done by adjusting your food intake (see above) rather than taking supplements.

Side-effects of fish oil

Nausea and indigestion do affect some people when taking fish oil in capsules. These side-effects usually pass after a while, so do not give up too soon.

If you are feeling nauseous, halve the number of capsules taken, wait until the side-effects have subsided, then gradually increase the dose again over a period of 2–3 weeks.

Hazards of fish oil and oily fish

Never take excessive amounts of omega-3 fish oil capsules because the omega-3s affect the ability of the blood to clot. On the dose recommended above this effect will scarcely be noticeable, unless you are prone to nosebleeds, in which case you may find that they last longer and recur more easily. Very high doses of fish oil have more serious and potentially dangerous effects on blood clotting, at least for Europeans. (It seems that Eskimos, who eat massive amounts of omega-3 fatty acids, have a different type of metabolism, having adapted to such a diet over thousands of years, and do not suffer as much with this problem.)

Because of the effect on clotting, people with certain diseases affecting the blood, such as haemophilia, should not take omega-3

Table 4: Diseases and drugs incompatible with fish oil supplements

---

Who should avoid high doses of omega-3 fish oil?
Asthmatics, if sensitive to aspirin
Epileptics
Haemophiliacs
Those with Raynaud's syndrome
Those with spontaneous or easy bruising
Anyone with a family history of haemmorhagic stroke
Non-insulin dependent diabetics
Those with systemic lupus erythematosus
Those with multiple sclerosis
Anyone taking Warfarin or other anti-coagulant drugs

Who should avoid a diet rich in oily fish?
All those listed above
Gout sufferers (fish oil supplements are safe, as they are not rich in purines, unlike the fish themselves)

---

supplements. Nor should those taking anti-coagulant drugs such as Warfarin – these too reduce the blood's ability to clot. Fish oil may make some conditions worse, including Raynaud's syndrome, where the fingers or toes go white and numb temporarily, especially in cold weather. A comprehensive list of diseases and drugs with which fish oil is incompatible is given in Table 4.

You may notice that you bruise a little more easily after some months of taking omega-3 oils. This again is a result of changes in the blood's capacity to clot. It is a harmless side-effect, but those who already suffer spontaneous or easy bruising, as part of their rheumatoid arthritis symptoms, would be best advised not to try fish oils.

Fish and pollutants

If you take an interest in environmental issues, you may be aware that some years ago the Swedish government warned people not to eat fish more than twice a week, because of concerns about mercury poisoning. This is no longer a cause for concern. Mercury pollution of the seas has been declining over the past 20 years, thanks to more stringent environmental laws. This is true for all the developed countries, although there may still be fairly high mercury levels in fish caught along parts of the Italian coast, and in certain types of large fish elsewhere in the world, notably tuna, halibut, shark, marlin and swordfish. Because it is the cumulative effects of mercury that cause problems, eating the occasional meal of fish with a higher mercury content does not matter at all, but large helpings of fish such as tuna or halibut should not be eaten every day. With other fish, levels of mercury are now so low that it is safe for adults to eat 250–500 gm (9–17$\frac{1}{2}$ oz) per day. Pregnant women should be a little more cautious, and not eat more than 250 gm (9 oz) per day.

What of other pollutants? In some parts of the world, such as the Great Lakes of North America, or the Baltic Sea, there is a potential problem with pollutants from factories such as dioxins and furans, which may act as carcinogens. No actual effects on health have been observed, even among those with a high intake of fish caught in these waters, but researchers believe that people should be cautious and not eat too much fish from such sources.

In general, then, there is no cause for concern about pollutants, even if you are eating large daily helpings of fish.

Fish oil supplements (as opposed to whole fish) have a very low content of mercury and other pollutants.

Omegas in everything

The surge of interest in omega-3 fatty acids has spawned a number of new products, such as bread and margarine, fortified with omega-3s and claiming to supply the consumer with useful quantities of these fatty acids. The buyer should beware, however, because the claims for these products relate to the prevention of heart disease, which involves a far lower dose than that required by people with rheumatoid arthritis. So you should ignore statements on the pack about the amount needed each day to fulfil recommended allowances. Over ten times as much would be needed to have any effect on rheumatoid arthritis.

One brand of margarine currently available, 'Omega spread', could fulfil your daily dose of omega-3s without requiring you to eat margarine in huge quantities. It supplies 5.2 gm of omega-3s per 100 gm (3$\frac{1}{2}$ oz) of margarine, so you could obtain the daily dose that we recommend – 3 gm of total omega-3s – by eating 57 gm (2 oz). This means margarine on everything, and not too thinly spread, but it is possible. Check that the brand you buy does contain 5.2 gm of omega-3s per 100 gm (3$\frac{1}{2}$ oz) – other brands contain much less, notably Pact which only contains 1.4 gm per 100 gm (3$\frac{1}{2}$ oz). Make sure that you are eating a full 57 gm (2 oz) per day.

The omega-3 enriched bread currently on sale does not contain anything like enough omega-3s to be useful to someone with rheumatoid arthritis. Half a loaf would be needed simply to give the low dose that can help prevent heart disease.

Cod-liver oil and rheumatoid arthritis

Many people with rheumatoid arthritis take cod-liver oil and are convinced that it helps them, but the dose of EPA – the useful ingredient in omega-3 fish oil – that can be obtained from a teaspoonful of cod liver oil is only 0.4 gm, which is probably far too little to have an effect on rheumatoid arthritis in the space of a few months (see p.58). Whether it might help if taken consistently for several years, owing to the build-up of EPA in the body, is an interesting question, but not the sort of question that scientific trials can easily answer.

Cod-liver oil contains large amounts of Vitamins A and D, which are toxic if taken in excess. They, too, accummulate in the body, and it is very important to be careful about the amount consumed. Vitamins A and D from other sources (such as margarine) will add to the daily dose. It is therefore vital not to take more than a teaspoonful of cod-liver oil each day.

In general, we would advise against taking cod-liver oil for rheumatoid arthritis because omega-3 fish oils are much more likely to be helpful. If you have been taking cod-liver oil and you do decide to continue taking it, note that unlike omega-3 oils it does not generally contain Vitamin E, so you need a good source of Vitamin E in your diet – follow the guidelines on p.150, but halve the quantities.

These comments also apply to other fish-liver oils, such as halibut-liver oil.

Linseed (flax-seed) oil

Despite the claims that are sometimes made for it as a substitute for omega-3 fish oil, linseed oil is unlikely to produce any benefits (see pp.59–60).

· Changing Other Fats in your Diet ·

There is some limited evidence that saturated animal fats might aggravate the symptoms of rheumatoid arthritis (see pp.52–3), and further evidence that arachidonic acid in the diet might also have an adverse effect (see p.55).

Table 5: Arachidonic acid in food

Very high	*Moderate to high*	*Low*
Kidney	Turkey	Milk
Calf liver	Heart	Milk products
Eggs		*Farmed salmon
	Moderate	Trout
High	Lamb	
Venison	Pork	*Little or none*
Veal	Chicken	Rabbit
Lamb's liver	Beef	Duck
	Trout	Grouse
		Pheasant
		*Wild salmon

(* Most fresh salmon and smoked salmon sold in the U.K. is farmed, whereas tinned salmon tends to come from wild fish).

It is easy enough to cut down on saturated animal fats, if you would like to, and this undoubtedly has other health benefits (see pp.260–262) even if your joints do not improve. The Mediterranean type of diet described on p.145, with the addition of some oily fish, would simultaneously decrease saturated fat while increasing your intake of olive oil and omega-3s.

By reducing the amount of meat eaten, this diet will also reduce the quanitity of arachidonic acid consumed. You could even choose to go one step further and cut out arachidonic acid completely: this can be done by choosing certain meats and avoiding others, as well as avoiding eggs and freshwater fish such as trout. The meats that are virtually free from arachidonic acid are, unfortunately, all rather expensive meats (see Table 5).

An alternative tactic is to avoid completely those meats that are high in arachidonic acid (namely kidney, liver, veal, venison, heart and turkey) while eating only small amounts of meats with moderate levels of arachidonic acid (pork, lamb, chicken and beef). This will reduce your intake of arachidonic acid to very low levels.

· *GLA Oils* ·

The GLA oils are evening primrose oil, borage oil ('starflower oil') and blackcurrant seed oil. The main active ingredient in all of them is a fatty acid called gamma-linolenic acid or GLA (see p.51).

We are including these oils in this chapter because their effects have something in common with those of fish oil. However, they are not foods – they are sold only as supplements, in capsules. The active ingredient, GLA, would never be eaten in significant quantities on any normal diet.

The amount of GLA shown to be effective against rheumatoid arthritis in experiments is 540 mg per day, which tends to produce a small but steady easing of symptoms, sufficient to allow many patients to reduce their dose of NSAIDs (see p.418). The benefits take at least three months to materialise, and it may be nine months before the maximum effect is achieved.

None of the supplements sold in shops at present has a recommended dose giving 540 mg per day of GLA, but some can be taken at 300 mg per day. Look for a brand that contains 90–100 mg of GLA per capsule, and suggests a maximum dose of three capsules per day. The cost will be substantially less than omega-3 fish oil, at about 35 pence per day. Although 300 mg per day will not have as much effect as 540 mg per day, it should be of some benefit. (There are 'high strength' brands sold by post that can be taken at a dose of 500–660 mg per day – see p.433 for the address of the supplier. The cost would be about 60 pence per day.)

Blackcurrant seed oil contains two additional ingredients, called alpha-linolenic acid (ALA) and stearidonic acid. Both are omega-3 fatty acids and can, in theory, be converted to EPA, the active ingredient of fish oils. In practice, it seems that very little alpha-linolenic acid is converted (see pp.59–60). These two additional ingredients do not seem to give blackcurrant seed oil any great advantages over evening primrose oil or borage ('starflower') oil.

Capsules of evening primrose oil should be swallowed whole, never chewed, because the oil is irritating to the throat and can cause a persistent, hacking cough. For this reason, the oil sold 'loose' in bottles is not recommended.

Reasons for choosing GLA oils

GLA oils are a good choice for strict vegetarians who do not wish to take fish oil. They are also useful for anyone who is allergic to fish, and for those who dislike the taste of fish, since even when fish oil is taken in capsules it tends to produce fishy burps later. If you have suffered persistent side-effects from fish oil, you may find that a GLA oil is less problematic (but the reverse could also be true – people vary greatly in their ability to tolerate these oils).

Cost may also be an incentive, since GLA oils are cheaper than omega-3 fish oils. On the other hand, the highest recommended dose of GLA (300 mg per day) from the supplements currently sold in shops is only 55% of that used in experiments with rheumatoid arthritis. You will have to buy through mail order to obtain a GLA oil whose recommended dose matches that used in experiments.

Combining GLA oils with other oils

There are good grounds for combining olive oil with fish oil (see p.47), but could it be valuable to combine GLA oils with olive oil, or with fish oil?

On purely theoretical grounds, the different oils should complement each other's effects, as they are all thought to work in different ways. Scientists are reasonably certain about how omega-3 fish oils work (see pp.50–51), and the same is true for GLA oils (see pp.51–2) – these two modes of action are certainly not the same. How olive oil works is a mystery, but it lacks the active ingredients of the other two so, in theory, it could complement the action of either fish oil or GLA oil.

Only one research group has looked at the effects of combining fish oil with evening primrose oil, and they used a lesser dose of evening primrose oil plus very small amounts of fish oil, only 13% of our recommended dose. At these levels, fish oil and evening primrose oil produced the same sort of benefits as evening primrose oil (at the full dose) alone. It is possible that a larger dose of both would, when combined, be of more substantial benefit.

If you want to try combining a GLA oil with either olive oil or an oily-fish diet, or with omega-3 fish oils, there is no obvious reason not to. (You could even combine all three as long as you suffer no undue side-effects, such as nausea or indigestion.) Combining different types of oils may be of additional help, and is unlikely to do you any harm as long as you are careful to restrict other fats and oils in your diet, so that your total intake of fats and oils is not too high. According to current guidelines, the oil and fat intake should be no more than 30% of total calories. Assuming you eat about 2000 calories per day, this is equivalent to 67 gm (2 1/3 oz) of fat per day.

Use Table 6 to assess the fat intake of your chosen therapeutic diet. Keep the intake of other fats down as much as possible.

Table 6: Amount of fat in various oil supplements and therapeutic diets

Supplement/oil	Recommended daily amount	Fat content
Olive oil	22 ml (1¹/₂ tbspns)	18 gm
EPA sources		
Pilchards	170 gm (6 oz)	10 gm
Herring	200 gm (7 oz)	37 gm
Mackerel	200 gm (7 oz)	33 gm
Sardines	200 gm (7 oz)	23 gm
Salmon, canned	320 gm (11 oz)	26 gm
MaxEPA	10 capsules	10 gm
Hydrolysed Norwegian salmon oil	4 capsules	5 gm
*Omega spread margarine	57 gm (2 oz)	40 gm
GLA sources		
**Evening primrose oil	3 gm (=300 mg GLA)	3 gm
**Blackcurrant seed oil	1.5 gm (=285 mg GLA)	1.5 gm
**'High strength' evening primrose oil (see p.156)	5 gm (=500 mg GLA)	5 gm
**'High strength' starflower oil	6 gm (=660 mg GLA)	6 gm

*Check label for omega-3 content – see note to Table 3.
**Brands vary – check label for actual GLA content of brand. Some may be less concentrated, so you would need to take more oil to achieve the same intake of GLA.

Side-effects of GLA oils

There may be nausea or indigestion from evening primrose oil or other GLA oils. This problem may be alleviated by taking the capsules during the course of a meal. Some people also suffer with diarrhoea as a side-effect.

Hazards of evening primrose oil

Those with a history of epilepsy should not take evening primrose oil, as it can precipitate attacks. Other GLA oils may well have the same effect and should therefore be avoided.

. *Using Oils for Other Forms* .
of Arthritis

Systemic lupus erythematosus

If you have systemic lupus erythematosus, it is inadvisable to take omega-3 fish oil, or to eat large amounts of oily fish, as there are no long-term benefits, and your condition may deteriorate if you later stop taking the oil (see p.60). (For anyone with lupus already taking this oil, the best course is probably to continue if you have been taking it regularly for more than three months.)

Raynaud's phenomenon

Fish oil supplements or an oily fish diet are not advisable for anyone with Raynaud's phenomenon (also called Raynaud's syndrome – see p.125). Evening primrose oil may be helpful (see p.61), and you should take the maximum dose available from capsules (see p.156). Olive oil might also be beneficial, although this has not been so thoroughly tested – follow the guidelines on pp.144–7.

Psoriatic arthritis

There is at present some limited evidence that omega-3 fish oils might help with psoriasis and psoriatic arthritis (see p.61). This is a fast-moving field of research, and we would suggest that you ask your doctor about the latest recommendations regarding omega-3 fish oil and psoriasis.

Osteoarthritis

There is no guarantee that omega-3 fish oil will help with osteoarthritis, but it might be of some benefit (see p.62), especially for those who have red, swollen, tender joints – indicating a degree of inflammation. You can either take fish oil in capsules, or eat oily fish – follow the guidelines on pp.147–154.

Cod-liver oil is probably not beneficial, at least for those taking NSAIDs (non-steroidal anti-inflammatory drugs). The research study that demonstrated this is described on pp.61–62. We would suggest that you choose omega-3 fish oil capsules or eat oily fish instead.

Table 7: Quick guide to the ingredients in oil supplements

Ingredient	Abbreviated to	Found in	Usefulness
Eicosapentaenoic acid	EPA	omega-3 fish oil; (also in cod-liver oil, but not in useful amounts)	Valuable for rheumatoid arthritis but only if dose is adequate (see p.148). Might be useful for psoriatic arthritis (see p.159) and possibly for osteoarthritis if there is significant inflammation (see p.62). (Also valuable in prevention of heart disease.)
Docosahexaenoic acid	DHA	omega-3 fish oil (also in cod-liver oil in small amounts)	May be valuable in rheumatoid arthritis but this is uncertain. Valuable for prevention of heart disease, and for health of brain and nervous system. An essential fatty acid – which may be lacking among vegetarians and those who rarely eat fish – see p.355.
Linoleic acid	LA	All vegetable oils, and almost all other fats, both plant and animal	Not effective against rheumatoid arthritis. An essential fatty acid but so ubiquitous in food that shortages are virtually unknown (see p.354).
Gammalinolenic acid	GLA	Evening primrose oil; Blackcurrant seed oil; Borage oil ('starflower' oil)	Valuable for rheumatoid arthritis (see p.156). May also be helpful for Raynaud's syndrome (see p.61).
Alpha-linolenic acid	ALA	Linseed/flaxseed oil; Soya bean oil; Blackcurrant seed oil	Not thought to be effective against rheumatoid arthritis (see pp.59–60).
Stearidonic acid	—	Blackcurrant seed oil	Might, in theory, be converted to EPA, but no evidence that it is. Of no proven value against rheumatoid arthritis (see p.60).

Chapter 2.3

DIETS TO PREVENT OSTEOPOROSIS

Osteoporosis is a growing problem in industrialised countries, and the number of fractured hips among the elderly is rising steadily. It is a particularly insidious disease because there is usually no outward sign of thinning bones until a fracture occurs – often a type of broken wrist known as a Colles' fracture, or the spontaneous collapse of a vertebra producing back pain, loss of height and sometimes a stooping posture or 'dowager's hump', as the front part of each vertebra gives way while the back does not.

It is not too late to do something about osteoporosis at this stage, but prevention should ideally begin much earlier.

Most of us, especially women, need to be concerned about osteoporosis, which can bring a heavy toll of pain, suffering and loss of independence during old age. It should be of particular concern to anyone with rheumatoid arthritis, ankylosing spondylitis or any other inflammatory arthritic condition, all of which increase the risk of osteoporosis. This applies to men as well as women. Although the bones close to inflamed joints are the most badly affected, there is also a general loss of bone density throughout the body.

Inactivity, which is often forced on arthritics by their painful or stiff joints, also increases the risk, for people of all ages and both sexes.

Among those with healthy joints, or with a mainly non-inflammatory disease such as osteoarthritis, it is principally older women who are most at risk of osteoporosis because the menopause ('the change of life' when monthly periods stop) causes a more rapid loss of bone density. The greater the bone density before the menopause, the less damaging this loss will be: building a sound healthy skeleton in early life is thought to be important in preventing osteoporosis later. For this reason, younger people – women in their twenties and thirties – should also concern themselves with selecting a diet that benefits their bones.

For more background information on osteoporosis see p.120. Should you be concerned about osteoporosis, and would like to know if you have the early signs of the disease, your bone density can be measured. Ask your doctor about this test.

· *Diet and Osteoporosis* ·

As explained on pp.314–5, calcium intake is important in preventing osteoporosis, but there are many other nutrients that also matter. A diet which encourages the loss of calcium from the body in the urine (because of high protein and cereal intake, combined with few fruits and vegetables) cannot necessarily be remedied by taking extra calcium.

Shortages of other crucial nutrients such as Vitamin D and Vitamin K also need to be considered. The diet outlined here is designed to correct all the deficiencies in the modern diet that might be contributing to the rising levels of osteoporosis. The important elements of the diet are dealt with in turn.

What to eat and what to avoid

First and foremost, you need a reliable source of absorbable calcium. Ideally, we would recommend a calcium intake of 800–1,000 mg/day, to be combined with a magnesium intake of *at least* 400–500 mg/day so that the ratio is 2:1.

For anyone who eats dairy products, this calcium intake is quite easily achieved. For example, almost 700 mg of calcium could be obtained by eating the following:

250 ml ($1/2$ pint) milk, whole or skimmed – 300 mg calcium
100 mg ($3^1/2$ oz) plain yoghurt – 200 mg calcium
28 gm (1 oz) cheddar or other hard cheese – 187 mg calcium

(Note that we would not advocate eating larger portions of cheese, for the reasons given on p.164.) The rest of the daily allowance would come from other foods, such as bread and vegetables.

If you wish to calculate exactly how much calcium your typical daily diet contains, refer to the figures on pp.315–7.

Vegans will probably find it difficult to achieve a calcium intake of 1000 mg per day unless they eat a calcium-enriched product such as fortified soya milk. If fortified products are not eaten, then a supplement is advisable.

Achieving an intake of 500 mg of magnesium per day is difficult on a typical diet, because the kinds of foods that are rich in magnesium, such as nuts, and lentils, are not generally eaten in the quantities required. By choosing only magnesium-rich foods, using the list on p.328, it is possible to devise a balanced and nutritious diet of less than 2000 calories per day which also yields 500 mg of magnesium per day, but it would be tough sticking to such a diet because the number of suitable foods is limited. For this reason, a modest supplement of magnesium may be advisable. Check first that you are not already taking laxatives or indigestion remedies that contain magnesium (see p.329).

Avoid foods that bind calcium and magnesium and block their absorption, such as wheat bran, oat bran, unleavened bread and spinach (see pp.309–311). Do not drink tea with meals. The lower your calcium and magnesium intake, the more careful you need to be about these foods and drinks that block mineral absorption. If you eat at least 1000 mg of calcium per day you can afford to be a little more relaxed about eating some 'mineral blockers'.

Ensure that you are getting enough Vitamin D, either from sunshine or from your food (see p.297). If you are entirely housebound, there is a risk of Vitamin D deficiency, because foods contain relatively small amounts. You should eat some margarine or eggs, or take cod-liver oil, or another form of supplement.

Include some rich source of Vitamin B_6 (pyridoxine) in your diet several times a week. If you are a meat-eater, this could be chicken, turkey, pork or fish. Vegetarians can choose from eggs, soyabeans, brown rice, oats, walnuts or peanuts. Note that freezing food reduces the content of this vitamin, as does keeping cooked food warm for long periods of time.

Meat and eggs will also supply manganese, as will milk. Some vegans, or those on macrobiotic diets may be short of this mineral (see p.332) and should consider taking a multi-mineral supplement to boost their supply. Taking calcium, iron or magnesium supplements increases the need for manganese.

Eat some dark green leafy vegetables every day, and make your portions large. At least some should be uncooked, such as parsley, watercress or the dark green forms of lettuce, such as cos or sweet romaine. These will give you a good supply of folic acid or folate (one of the B vitamins) which is destroyed by boiling. It will also boost your magnesium intake.

These green salads, along with other green vegetables such as broccoli and cabbage, will also supply Vitamin K. This too is believed to be valuable in preventing osteoporosis, and may be particularly important for anyone with ankylosing spondylitis.

Eat generous helpings of other vegetables as well, and plenty of fruit. The special value of fruit and vegetables, apart from their vitamin content, is in counteracting the acidifying effect that some foods have on the urine. This reduces the amount of calcium and magnesium lost from the body by this route (see p.407). Foods that contribute to acidity of the urine are cheese, eggs, meat, fish, cereal grains (wheat, rice etc.), pulses and some nuts.

Weight-for-weight, hard cheeses such as cheddar are by far the most serious offenders in this respect. You should eat only small amounts of such cheeses and aim to match the cheese with 6–7 times its weight in fruit and/or vegetables – so 28 gm (1 oz) of cheese should be accompanied by at least 170 gm (6 oz) of salad, fruit or fruit juice. A small glass of apple juice or 3 large sticks of celery would fit the bill.

Avoid processed cheese, reduced-fat cheeses and Parmesan as these are exceptionally high in acid-producing substances.

Meat, fish, eggs, rice, oats and pasta should be matched with three times the weight of vegetables. Potatoes count as vegetables in this context, since they have the same effect in counteracting acid.

Bread, beans, lentils and cream cheese should be matched by an equal weight of fruit or vegetables.

Milk, yoghurt, ice cream, cream, butter, margarine, oil, jam, honey and alcoholic drinks do not need to be matched.

Peanuts, walnuts and most other nuts need to be matched with twice their weight of fruit or vegetables, but hazelnuts do not need matching at all. Sultanas and raisins count as fruit but are worth four times their actual weight in these equations: so you could match 57gm (2 oz) of peanuts with 27 gm (1 oz) of raisins.

These rules, which are summarised in Table 8, may seem cumbersome at first, but after a few days of weighing foods you should have a fair idea of what balances out and be able to judge by eye alone. Notice that substituting potatoes for rice, bread or pasta helps considerably in getting main meals to balance.

Some fruits and vegetables are better than others for neutralising acid foods: carrots, celery, courgettes, potatoes, bananas and blackcurrants are among the best. Do *not* eat cranberries, plums or prunes as they contain a particular type of acid that is not fully broken down (see p.406) and which therefore acidifies the urine. Avoid dried apricots unless they are the unsulphured kind (sold in health food shops). Other dried fruit that is heavily treated with sulphur dioxide should also be avoided, since the sulphur will be acid-forming.

Very large doses of Vitamin C – more than 1 gm per day – could also acidify the urine, and should be avoided. Such doses are not likely to be obtained from food, but only from Vitamin C supplements, which are unnecessary on a diet rich in fruit and vegetables, such as the one outlined here.

Table 8: Matching foods to avoid calcium losses

Acid-forming foods	*Amount of fruit, vegetables or potatoes needed to match*
Reduced fat cheese, Parmesan, processed cheese	9–10 times weight
Cheddar cheese Other hard cheeses	6–7 times weight
Meat Fish Eggs Cottage cheese Rice Oats Wheat-based breakfast cereals Pasta	3 times weight
Peanuts Walnuts All other nuts, except hazelnuts Cornflakes	twice weight
Bread Cake, biscuits Beans, lentils Cream cheese Chocolate	equivalent weight

Choosing fruit and vegetables:
Avoid cranberries, plums, prunes and dried apricots (unless unsulphured).
Favour carrots, celery, courgettes, potatoes, bananas and blackcurrants.
Raisins and sultanas count for four times their weight.

Organic fruits and vegetables are now available in most supermarkets, and while they may cost more, it is worth buying them when you can. They are likely to contain more boron, a trace mineral that is thought to play a part in preventing osteoporosis. Honey is also a good source of boron, and could be used in place of sugar. Avocados are also quite rich in boron.

The diet outlined above should provide you with an adequate intake of zinc, another mineral which may have some relevance to osteoporosis. Meat is the main source of this mineral, so if you are vegetarian you should check that you are eating enough zinc-rich foods, using the figures on p.324.

Check also that you are eating some foods which supply copper, such as beans, lentils, shellfish, liver or nuts. Consider taking a multi-mineral supplement if none of these items feature on your menu regularly.

Cut down on salt which increases losses of calcium in the urine. It would also be wise to avoid phosphate food additives as high intakes of phosphate may contribute to osteoporosis. These additives are found most often in cooked meat products such as sliced ham or turkey sold packeted, 'meat loaf', some sausages (eg. pastrami) and some types of pâté. Check on the label for mono-, di- or tri-phosphates.

Coca-cola, pepsi and other cola drinks also contain phosphorous: when checking unfamiliar soft drinks look on the label for 'phosphoric acid'. Occasionally, phosphates may be identified on food labels by their E numbers, which are E338–341, E450–452 and E1410–E1414.

The caffeine in coffee and tea can be bad for the bones unless your calcium intake is adequate. Anyone eating less than 800 mg of calcium per day should restrict themselves to 1–2 cups of fresh-brewed coffee daily. (The same amount of caffeine is found in 4 cups of instant coffee, 4 cups of strong tea, 5 cans of cola or 5 chocolate bars.) For those with an intake above 800 mg, there is probably no need to restrict caffeine intake.

Heavy, or even moderate, drinkers should be aware that alcohol also increases bone loss (see p.168).

· *Active Bones Stay Hard* ·

Diet is only part of the battle against osteoporosis. Staying as active as possible is of vital importance. For those who have good mobility, exercise should include running, walking or sports such as tennis, which exercise the limbs against the pull of gravity – this is the best way to stimulate regeneration of the bone. If you cannot take this kind of exercise because of disability, swimming will probably be beneficial because the muscles have to work against the resistance of the water. While at the pool, try walking for five or ten minutes at the shallow end – the water should be just below your waist. This is marvellous exercise for the thigh muscles which lose their tone if you cannot walk very far normally. Thanks to the water resistance, every step in the water is as good as six on dry land. The muscular force against your thigh bone will benefit the uppermost end of the bone: the part that breaks in a 'hip' fracture. It is one of the areas of the skeleton that is especially vulnerable to osteoporosis.

For those who cannot manage any such exercise, there is still some hope: regular stretching of the arms and legs, and clenching and unclenching the fists can be done, even in bed or in an armchair, and will give the bones some stimulus to regenerate their mass. The muscles of the thighs and buttocks can be clenched and unclenched too, as can most muscle blocks, the opposing muscles being tightened at the same time so that they pull against each other. Practise doing this with the buttock and thigh muscles, then experiment with other muscle pairs.

Even in bed the feet can be moved in circular patterns, the back arched, the head and neck rotated – and so on. All such movement will help prevent osteoporosis, as well as improving your general well-being and promoting the healthy circulation of the blood. Devise new movements for yourself and aim to exercise as much of the body as possible. Obviously you should not do anything that might result in a fall because there is always the risk of breaking a bone when osteoporosis has set in.

Many sports aids are now available that can be of use to those who are relatively immobile but still want to stay fit. There are small dumb-bell weights, or, if you cannot grip easily, weights that strap around the wrist or ankle with a velcro fastening. 'Thigh toners', where you work your muscles against a spring, can also be valuable. Take care when using such aids and consult a physiotherapist if you are in any doubt about what you should attempt to do. Your doctor should be able to refer you to a physiotherapist if you request this.

· *Other Changes in Lifestyle* ·

Cigarette smoking makes osteoporosis more likely, so you can help protect yourself by giving up smoking. The other health benefits of doing this include drastic reductions in the risks of heart disease, lung cancer, chronic bronchitis and emphysema. Hints to help with quitting cigarettes are given on p.176.

Drinking heavily also adds to the risk of osteoporosis in later life. Again, there are many other health-related reasons for reducing alcohol consumption. Advice about changing your drinking habits can be found on p.243. A magnesium supplement may be particularly useful if you have been a heavy drinker, as alcohol encourages loss of magnesium from the body, which may contribute to the osteoporosis associated with alcohol abuse.

· *Hormone Replacement Therapy (HRT)* ·

With the menopause or 'change of life', comes a sudden drop in the levels of the female hormone oestrogen. This decline has an unfortunate effect on the bones, which begin to lose their mass at an unprecedented rate.

This phase, during which 1–2% of the bone mass is lost each year, lasts for 5–10 years. Then the bone mass stabilises to some extent and the annual rate of loss is not as rapid.

Replacing oestrogen during the years immediately after the menopause is the single most effective treatment in the prevention of osteoporosis among older women. This treatment is called Hormone Replacement Therapy (HRT). The HRT pills are taken daily and contain progesterone, another hormone, as well as oestrogen. The cycle of monthly bleeding may be re-established by the treatment, according to the type of HRT prescribed. Some HRT does not induce monthly periods.

Questions are often raised about the safety of HRT. When first introduced, oestrogen alone was given, and this involved an increased risk of cancer of the endometrium (the lining of the womb). The addition of progesterone eliminates this risk entirely. If used for more than ten years, HRT does increase the risk of breast cancer slightly, but few women actually take HRT for this length of time. On the positive side, HRT reduces the chance of dying from a heart attack by 40–50%. Overall, the protective effects greatly outweigh the risks, and HRT increases life expectancy by about 2 years. These facts are based on HRT using oestrogen alone. It is believed that the combined oestrogen/progesterone pill now used will give similar results. Given its considerable benefits in preventing osteoporosis, HRT is a treatment that every woman should at least consider.

· *Osteoporosis before the Menopause* ·

One word of caution about exercise: you can have too much of a good thing. Young women who go overboard on exercise – usually runners – sometimes stress their bodies so much that oestrogen levels fall. Their periods stop, and the low oestrogen levels in the blood produce changes in the bone just like those seen in post-menopausal women. If they continue with their punishing exercise regimes, such women are at risk of osteoporosis.

Any young woman whose periods have stopped spontaneously should be seen by a doctor and treated to reduce the risk of osteoporosis. Loss of bone mass can begin to be seen after just six months without menstruation. This also applies to women with anorexia nervosa whose periods stop.

Chapter 2.4

THE ELIMINATION DIET

An elimination diet is not a dogmatic diet of the kind that says 'Everyone with arthritis must cut out meat, red wine and citrus fruits'. All the good, objective research shows that different foods affect different patients (see Chapter 1.1, p.15). Citrus fruits might well provoke joint symptoms in one person with rheumatoid arthritis, but for another person they are harmless, whereas cheese and milk are the culprits. For many others, food is irrelevant to their disease.

The elimination diet, then, is a form of diagnosis – a way of testing your own body to see if any foods provoke symptoms in the joints. At the end of the diet you may come to the conclusion that foods are not a factor in your arthritic symptoms. Or you may discover that a certain food, or two or more foods, make your joints much worse.

What you do after that is up to you. Most people who have found that foods make a difference then try to avoid the culprit foods as far as possible, because the benefits easily make up for the inconvenience of a restricted diet. Sometimes people find they can go back to eating the culprit food occasionally, or in small amounts, after they have stayed away from it for a year or so. However, if the food is eaten regularly again, symptoms tend to recur.

One advantage of the elimination diet is that you get an answer very quickly. Within three weeks you should have a 'yes' or a 'no' response to the question 'Do foods affect my joints?' If the answer is no, you can abandon the special diet straightaway. If the answer is yes, you then begin the process of testing foods to see which ones are the culprits.

The testing process might take a couple of months, but your diet is becoming less restricted all the time, so it is not as arduous as the initial stage.

An elimination diet is only worth trying for certain types of joint disease. The main ones to respond are arthralgia (simple joint pain), episodic arthritis (also called palindromic rheumatism) and rheumatoid arthritis (particularly seronegative rheumatoid arthritis). Some of the rarer forms of arthritis may also be worth investigating with an elimination diet and you should consult Chapter 2.1 (p.79) to see if this diet is at all relevant to your condition.

Arthritis accompanying Crohn's disease is also a good candidate, and the bowel symptoms may improve as well. However, this is a serious disease and cannot be self-treated. You may need a special form of diet and you *must* have close medical supervision.

In some people there may be other symptoms, as well as arthritis, in response to the culprit food – symptoms such as headaches, fatigue, diarrhoea or aching muscles. The umbrella-term **food intolerance** is used to describe all these reactions and to distinguish them from food allergy (see pp.43–5). To be honest, food intolerance is one of those medical terms which means 'Well, we don't entirely understand it, and we are not sure what causes it, but we know how to treat it'. (There are more of these terms used in medicine than most doctors would like to admit!) Certainly the basic causes for food intolerance are not yet understood.

· *Keeping a Symptom Diary* ·

As soon as you begin thinking about going on an elimination diet, start a 'symptoms diary'. Note how painful your joints are, for example, how long your joints remain stiff in the morning, and how long you can keep active before becoming fatigued. Also note down any other unpleasant symptoms, such as headaches. The purpose of the symptom diary is to have something which you can refer to later, when you are testing foods. It should give you some idea of how ill you were at the outset. Equally important, it can give an idea of how variable your symptoms are from day to day, which is useful in evaluating your response to the diet.

· *Seeing your Doctor* ·

Before trying an elimination diet you need to see your doctor and check that there is no medical reason why it might be risky for you. If you are already seriously underweight this might rule out the diet because it can cause some weight loss in the initial stages. Whatever advice the doctor gives about the safety of the diet in your particular case, *you must follow it*.

Be prepared for your doctor to perhaps be a little sceptical, or even hostile, when you raise the question of diet and arthritis. The reasons for such reactions by the medical profession are explained on pp.22–3, and you will find it helpful to have read this section before the appointment. Be calm and patient, and be prepared to listen – the doctor has good reasons for these opinions.

Please also read this chapter *in full* before the appointment, so that you understand exactly what the elimination diet entails. Take the book with you in case your doctor wants to know more about the details of the diet. If the doctor is firmly set against the elimination diet, try to establish whether this is simply because he or she believes it is useless, or because the diet poses a real threat to your health.

· *Understanding Elimination Diets* ·

Many years of experience with food intolerance have established certain key facts:

1. There is quite often more than one food at fault.
2. Commonly eaten foods such as wheat and milk are most often the culprits, although there may be foods that you eat more rarely which are also causing problems.
3. The reaction to the food is fairly slow, usually taking at least an hour to begin and up to 48 hours for certain foods. The symptoms produced may continue for several hours, or even days in the case of joint symptoms.
4. Because the problem often lies with foods eaten at least once a day (perhaps at almost every meal), and because the reactions are slow, on a normal diet the effects of one meal tend to run together with reactions from the next. For this reason, it is not at all obvious, in an everyday setting, which particular food is causing the symptoms. So the simple test of eating a large amount of a suspect food and watching for symptoms will rarely work.
5. Unless all the problem foods are cut out at the same time, there may be no significant improvement. So simply cutting out milk for a few weeks, then wheat for a few weeks, then another food, and so on, is unlikely to reveal anything. (Doctors who are unfamiliar with food intolerance may well suggest such an approach.)

The basic design of the elimination diet takes these five factors into account. It begins with an **exclusion phas**e, in which you cut out most foods and only eat a very limited range of foods which are unlikely to provoke symptoms. If foods really are at fault in your case, you should improve considerably during the exclusion phase. The improvement will begin quite quickly – in one to three weeks, depending on how severe your arthritis is and how long it has been established.

If you do not experience any improvement after three weeks, then you should abandon the diet altogether. You may want to try another dietary approach, and you should turn to Chapter 2.1 for guidance, consulting the relevant section for your particular form of arthritis.

If you do improve, you then proceed to the **reintroduction phase**. This is a systematic testing of single foods, one-by-one, to see if they provoke symptoms. Because you have not eaten the foods for over a week, the reaction to them should be fairly prompt and clear-cut. The 'running-together' of symptoms from one meal to the next, as described above, will no longer be there to obscure your reactions to individual foods.

The outline of the elimination diet given above may sound so simple that you are inclined to start immediately, but this would be a mistake. Thoughtful planning is needed, especially in relation to the timing of the diet. Please read the whole chapter carefully before you begin.

· *Preparing for the Diet* ·

An elimination diet is not like a slimming diet or a health-fad diet, where you can cheat for one meal, or for a whole day, then go back to the diet. To get a clear result using the elimination diet, you must eat *absolutely nothing* but the allowed foods. Even a single sip of coffee or a nibble of some prohibited food could confuse the result, so you need iron discipline during the diet. (Be assured that, if you get well, it will all seem entirely worthwhile in six months' time.)

The best advice for an elimination diet is: 'Do it once and do it well.' Trying the diet for a second time may be difficult and you might not get such good results, so plan ahead to ensure that your first attempt goes smoothly.

Since you need to be sure of what you are eating, it is best not to have any ready-made foods or restaurant meals until the diet is over. (Towards the end of the testing phase, a simple meal out, such as steak and salad with a baked potato, may be possible, assuming you have already tested all the foods in the meal.) If you need to eat in a canteen at work, check with the cook whether anything has extra ingredients, or whether some foods come from a tin (vegetables, for example). Tinned foods are excluded at first.

If possible, make all your own food – that way you know exactly what you have eaten. Lunches can be prepared and taken in a picnic box. During the winter months, if you prefer to have hot food, a wide-necked vacuum flask is ideal, and is inexpensive to buy.

Invitations to lunch or dinner can be a problem, especially in the early stages of the diet. With good friends, explain exactly which foods you are allowed and make it clear that there must be nothing added – no sauce, gravy, butter, herbs, spices or other flavourings for example. Alternatively, you can accept the invitation but say that you will bring your own food. This can be pre-cooked, and arranged on a plate to be warmed up in an oven or microwave, so that you do not inconvenience the host or hostess. For a buffet party or reception, you can always eat beforehand so that you do not need food once you are there.

Christmas, weddings and big family gatherings may be more difficult and in making your plans you should try to ensure that these do not fall in the first two or three months of the diet. (On the other hand, if you have a progressive disease such as rheumatoid arthritis, and if you are indeed reacting to food, the sooner you detect and avoid the culprit food the better. So do not delay the diet for too long.) Mark the expected phases of the diet in a diary or calendar, so that you can plan social engagements accordingly.

The first week of the diet is always the worst. During this phase it is best to avoid meals out altogether. You will be on a very restricted diet, and you may feel more unwell than usual (further details on this later). Try not to let this first week coincide with an especially demanding time at work, or at home. Take some time off if you can, or at least plan it so that the second and third day of the exclusion phase are at a weekend. Buy a good novel or rent some videos to take your mind off how you feel.

Once the first week or so is over, everything changes. If you are not improving then you know that you can stop the diet soon (it is not worth continuing beyond three weeks). If you do experience an improvement in your arthritis, this will encourage you so much that it should be easy to keep going.

· *Pitfalls in Elimination Dieting* ·

Some people sail through the elimination diet with no trouble and come out with clear-cut answers. A few people improve on the exclusion phase but then encounter problems and, unless they are guided carefully, will finish up feeling confused and not much better, despite the fact that food really *is* at the root of their problems.

This chapter has been carefully planned to guide you through the elimination diet, overcoming any difficulties if they arise. Pitfalls and problems may seem to loom very large as you read the chapter for the first time, but do not be put off by this. *The chances are that you will not encounter any of them.*

· *Related Foods* ·

When you come to testing foods, you need to understand a little about how related foods can **cross-react** with one another. If two plants, or two animals, are related to one another, the foods obtained from them will be chemically similar. Things do not need to look alike to share chemical constituents. Your DNA only differs from that of a gorilla by 1% – so you should not be surprised if a courgette and a melon, which originate from the same plant family, are sisters under the skin. Despite superficial differences, they are fundamentally alike in terms of their chemical constituents. This similarity may mean that they both provoke symptoms in a food-allergic or food-intolerant person.

The most clear-cut example comes from the cereals, all of which are grasses (members of the family Gramineae or Poaceae). The cereal that causes problems most frequently (particularly in countries where bread is a staple food) is wheat, while maize (corn) runs a close second, particularly in Canada and the U.S.A. where more maize is eaten. Wheat belongs to the subfamily Pooidae, along with rye, barley and oats. Neatly correlated with this is the observation that many people who react to wheat also have problems with rye and barley, and some react to oats as well. Maize is in a separate subfamily, and rice in yet another subfamily. This fits in with the fact that most people who are troubled by wheat or maize can still tolerate rice.

Not all foods behave in quite such an orderly manner, and sometimes in true allergy there are cross-reactions between items that are unrelated, such as almonds and walnuts, or birch pollen and apples. The reasons for this are not understood, but it seems that certain chemical constituents are shared because they are useful to the plant (as with nuts from different plant families) or by sheer coincidence (as with birch pollen and apples).

Conversely, there are some plant families that rarely show cross-reactions. Many people are allergic or intolerant to peanuts, for example, but surprisingly few of them react to other foods from the family Leguminosae, such as lentils, peas, beans and soyabeans.

Despite these exceptions, there is a tradition of looking at family relationships and watching for cross-reactions. For many foods, it is more a matter of faith than science, but the families are still thought to be a useful guide. The food families, and other relevant relationships, are given in Appendix I (p.422).

In the reintroduction phase of the diet, as described later in this chapter, the tests are planned so that there are at least four days between the testing of related foods. For this reason, you should keep to the order of testing precisely. The only foods that may be rescheduled are those that have no close relatives. These are marked with an asterisk (*), and may be swapped with other asterisked items only. Do not alter the time-spacing of items that have no asterisk.

At the end of the testing phase, if you have experienced some positive reactions, check those foods against the lists in Appendix I. If there are related foods which you might want to eat and which you have not already tested, then you should test them individually. For example, if you have reacted to tomatoes, peppers or potatoes, you may want to test aubergines or cape gooseberries, which belong to the same family. Approach each food with an open mind, however, and do not anticipate a reaction – psychogenic reactions (see p.18) can occur if you convince yourself that you must be sensitive to a food before testing it.

· *Stopping Smoking* ·

If you smoke cigarettes or other forms of tobacco, you should stop, at least while on the diet, and preferably for ever. The adverse health effects of smoking are enormous and are *not* exaggerated, despite the myths put about by inveterate smokers and pro-smoking campaign groups.

Among the serious diseases that are caused or worsened by cigarettes are lung cancer, mouth and throat cancer, chronic bronchitis and disease of the large arteries leading from the heart (which can contribute to heart attacks). Emphysema, an incurable, often disabling and potentially fatal lung disease, is frequently caused by cigarette smoking. Smokers are also at risk of damaging the arteries in the legs to such a degree that, in severe cases, amputation may be required. Pregnant women who smoke may damage their unborn babies, while the children of smokers are more at risk of asthma and other breathing problems.

There is some evidence that tobacco smoke may contribute to rheumatoid arthritis. People who smoke have higher levels of rheumatoid factor (see p.419) and of other autoantibodies – elements of the immune system that are directed against the body itself and which can play a role in several forms of arthritis. Smokers seem to succumb to rheumatoid arthritis rather more frequently than non-smokers. Among people with established rheumatoid arthritis, those who smoke are more susceptible to complications involving the small blood vessels in the skin.

Unfortunately, nicotine is a highly addictive drug. According to former heroin addicts who have also renounced cigarettes, nicotine is in some ways more addictive than heroin. This is worth knowing because it explains why attempts to give up frequently fail unless tackled with gritty determination, and why smokers are prepared to delude themselves endlessly about cigarettes, claiming that they are 'not really dangerous' in the face of damning medical evidence.

Because giving up smoking is so difficult, you would be well advised to do it *before* you embark on the elimination diet, rather than face both hurdles at the same time. There are now a number of aids available, including chewing-gum that contains nicotine, and patches which are applied to the skin and which gradually release nicotine into the bloodstream. These give you an alternative source of nicotine so that initially you simply have to get used to not lighting up and puffing away. Once you are out of the smoking habit, you can then, very gradually, reduce the dose of nicotine from the substitute. Chemists' shops stock these products and you may want to talk to the pharmacist about them and ask what he or she recommends. Ideally you should have weaned yourself off the nicotine substitute, as well as the cigarettes themselves, before beginning the elimination diet, although some people, driven by a powerful wish to get better, do manage to eliminate both cigarettes and foods together. Ideally you should stop abruptly and have a firm resolve never to smoke again. Cutting down on cigarettes gradually is not the best approach to giving up since you remain a smoker for longer and, unless you have great self-discipline and a definite programme of steady reduction, you tend to cheat and not to achieve success. This does not mean that a limited reduction in the number of cigarettes smoked each day is not useful – but even a low consumption of cigarettes can kill you, and the only safe option is to stop completely.

Hypnosis can be valuable in strengthening your determination, and acupuncture is also said to help. There is also one useful technique which you can do alone and which helps considerably in giving up cigarettes. When you have decided that you will give up, sit down and smoke three, four or more cigarettes in quick succession: as many as you can until you feel ill. This is a simple way of telling your addicted body that cigarettes are toxic – you are conveying the message in a simple language the body can understand. Throw away any unsmoked cigarettes but keep the stubs from the last few that you smoked, placing them in a glass jar with a little water. Over the next few weeks, whenever you feel tempted by the thought of a cigarette, have a sniff at the mixture in the jar. The foul smell will remind you of just how unpleasant tobacco is. (A glass jar with a tight lid is ideal as you can carry it about with you.) Avoid friends who smoke, also parties and bars, at least for a while.

If you can give up smoking *and* undertake dietary treatment you have two ways in which you can hope to tackle your rheumatoid arthritis (as well as improving your general health). If you really can't give up smoking completely before your diet, then reduce your cigarette consumption to the lowest possible level.

THE ELIMINATION DIET

· Exclusion Phase ·

This will last for at least seven days, and possibly longer. If there is no improvement after three weeks, then discontinue the diet.

During the exclusion phase, you are only allowed the following:

Trout, salmon and cod
Carrots
Pears
Kiwi fruit
Sweet potatoes
Bottled mineral water (still or sparkling)
Salt

Do not use tinned foods of any kind. All foods may be cooked if preferred, but you should not add anything in the cooking process, so only boiling (in mineral water), grilling or baking is allowed. Pear juice can be made by removing the pear skins and pips, then liquidising the fruit with spring water. Carrots eaten raw are a good snack.

If you normally eat any of these foods *every* day then you should *not* eat them during the exclusion phase. Choose alternative foods that you never eat normally making sure that these foods are not related to foods that you eat regularly (see pp.422–8 for food families).

Nothing else at all must pass your lips, apart from your usual medicines, and the following:

> On the first day, in the morning, take three teaspoons of Epsom Salts dissolved in half a pint of warm water. (Note that this will induce one or more urgent bowel movements about an hour or so later.) The purpose of this 'dose of salts' is to clear out residual foods from the bowel, so that, if you are going to respond to the exclusion phase, you do so more promptly. (Should you suffer from constipation later on in the exclusion phase, you can repeat this treatment.)

Hidden food substances

Before beginning the dietary programme it is important to have discussed with your doctor what medicines you should take.

Many tablets, capsules and liquid medicines contain food substances as 'fillers', mainly lactose (the sugar found in milk) and corn starch, which might interfere with your elimination diet if you have a sensitivity to either milk or corn (maize). The colourings used in some medicines might also create problems if you are sensitive to these. Unfortunately medicines are exempt from the kind of labelling regulations applied to food, and the fillers and colourings do not have to be listed.

When using the elimination diet at Epsom General Hospital, we try to take most patients off their drugs before starting the diet, with the exception of the pain-killer paracetamol, which has no additives. This gives a completely clear interval during the exclusion phase, when no unidentified food substances might be consumed in the guise of medicines. We also believe that patients respond more clearly to food withdrawal and reintroduction if their symptoms are not being damped down by drugs.

If you want to try doing the elimination diet in this way, *you must have your doctor's wholehearted agreement.* The withdrawal of drugs must be medically supervised: in particular, there are some drugs, notably corticosteroids (see p.414), *which it is dangerous to stop taking abruptly.*

An alternative approach is to switch to similar drugs that do not contain food substances. Your doctor can find out about these by contacting a Drug Information Service.

Toothpaste may also contain cornstarch and other hidden ingredients that could interfere with the diet. Ideally, you should avoid using toothpaste and should clean your teeth with sodium bicarbonate dissolved in warm water. Toothpaste should be introduced only in the reintroduction phase (see below) and should be tested just as foods are tested. Avoid licking stamps or envelopes as the gum on these may also contain cornstarch – use a damp sponge or cloth.

Do not eat huge amounts of the foods that are allowed on the exclusion phase as there is a danger of developing new sensitivities to foods eaten in large quantities. Have three meals a day and keep each meal relatively small, rather than starving yourself and then eating one large meal in the evening.

Keep a comprehensive record of all symptoms that you notice on each day. It is not just joint pains and stiffness that are relevant but other symptoms such as headaches, fatigue, dizziness, aching muscles, catarrh or swollen ankles. It is thought that back ache and catarrh, for example, are closely associated with food intolerance so if you develop these symptoms, you should be encouraged to persevere. Headaches, muscle aches and swollen ankles are also commonly reported as withdrawal symptoms (see below) during the early stages of an elimination diet and are an encouraging sign.

What may happen . . .

You feel much worse initially.
This is a good sign, unlikely though it may seem at the time! The reasons for such 'withdrawal symptoms' are not understood but they usually show that food is indeed a factor in your illness. Persevere and the worst should pass after about four days although some withdrawal symptoms may take a week or even a little longer to settle completely.

You feel much worse, then much better
This is excellent. You may now go on to the reintroduction phase.

You are just the same at first then steadily get better
This is another possible pattern of reaction. Younger people, in particular, are more likely to sail through without 'withdrawal symptoms'. You may begin the reintroduction phase any time after day seven.

You feel much worse, then better, then worse again
Occasionally there is a second smaller phase of 'withdrawal symptoms'

at about the end of the first week. Keep going because this should only last for a day or two. Go on to the reintroduction phase when this second set of withdrawal symptoms has settled down.

You feel worse at first and do not improve
There are three possible explanations. One is that you are not food-intolerant and that simply cutting down on food has made you feel unwell, perhaps because you were malnourished at the outset, which can happen, especially in rheumatoid arthritis.

The second possibility, if you stopped taking certain anti-inflammatory drugs before the diet, is that you are not food-intolerant and the down-turn is due to the loss of the effect of these drugs.

The third possibility is that you have food intolerance to some of the items eliminated (so you have experienced 'withdrawal symptoms'), but you are also sensitive to an item that is allowed on the exclusion phase, and eating rather more of this than usual is maintaining your symptoms.

To test for the third possibility, switch to the rare-food diet, which is an alternative exclusion-phase diet, given on p.182. Stay on this for a week and see what happens. If you do not improve on this diet, it seems unlikely that you have food intolerance. Go back to your normal eating pattern and medication.

After feeling worse initially you get much better, but then steadily get worse again
This may indicate that you are food-intolerant and that, although you were not initially intolerant of anything allowed on the exclusion phase, you develop new intolerances to foods quite easily if you eat too much of them. Simply eating them in large amounts, more than once a day, may set off a new sensitivity in some people.

Fortunately this does not happen to many people, but if you are among the unlucky few you should think carefully about what to do next. You need to begin a new 'exclusion phase' with none of the present foods, and without acquiring new sensitivities. You could switch to a rare food diet, as described on p.182, and see if you improve.

After a week, you feel much better but still have some symptoms
Go on to the reintroduction phase on day seven. When you have tested several foods and found six that do not affect you, cut out all the foods that you were eating on the exclusion phase and just eat the six new foods for a few days. If you improve this suggests that something

allowed during the exclusion phase was affecting you a little. Continue with the reintroduction phase, testing foods in the set order. Keep off the foods that you ate in the exclusion phase. At the very end of the reintroduction phase, test each of the foods from the exclusion phase, one per day, to see which of them was the cause of your symptoms.

Alternative exclusion phase diet

This is a rare food diet, and can be used when a replacement is needed for the standard exclusion phase (see p.178). Choose two or more foods from each line of the list below, avoiding any foods that you have been eating regularly. These foods can be found in the larger supermarkets, although some are seasonal.

Turkey, duck, goose or rabbit
Okra, asparagus, swede or chow-chow.
Mangoes, pomegranates, lychees, passion fruit, blueberries, tamarillos
Parsnips, turnips, yam, dasheen.
Spring water, still or sparkling
Salt

If you have never eaten any of the foods listed in the standard exclusion phase (see p.178) – kiwi fruits for example – you can include this food in your exclusion phase as well.

· Reintroduction Phase ·

Only begin this phase when you have improved and have markedly less joint pain, stiffness and swelling. If you have found the exclusion phase very trying, because your diet was so restricted, this next phase should cheer you up considerably because you will be broadening your diet every day.

Stage One of the reintroduction phase

The object now is to obtain a list of about twenty foods to which you are not sensitive. This will give you a reasonably wide range of foods that you can safely eat, so that you have a more varied diet. You should also be aiming to broaden your diet so that you can eat less of each individual food to reduce the risk of developing new sensitivities.

The foods tested in Stage One are unlikely to cause symptoms. Some people will react to one (or possibly more) of these foods, but for most people this testing stage should pass uneventfully, and the improvement in the joints will be maintained.

Keep to the order of reintroduction given here. It starts with the 'safest' foods, which is beneficial since you need to broaden your diet as quickly as possible. The order is also designed to provide a gap of at least four days between related foods (see p.176).

Where two or three foods are shown for a day, you should introduce only one at each meal. It is up to you to choose which one to introduce at breakfast, which at lunch, and which in the evening meal. You should leave a gap of *at least five hours* between meals since otherwise symptoms from a food taken at breakfast may develop after you have eaten lunch, which will confuse you. You can snack on established safe foods in between meals if you feel hungry but try to keep the snacks varied and not to eat one food repeatedly. As before, you must not eat tinned foods, or any form of the food which may have additional ingredients, unless these have already proved safe.

If there is no reaction within five hours you can consider that food blameless. The most common time for a food reaction to begin is about two to three hours after it has been eaten, but the full-blown reaction might take longer to develop. Should you have symptoms first thing in the morning, before breakfast, they are probably related to the food tested at your evening meal on the previous day.

Not everyone is completely symptom free when they begin to test foods. You may have improved considerably during the exclusion phase but still have some joint pains as you enter the reintroduction phase. Some people who are in this situation worry that they will not know whether they have really provoked a reaction when they test a food. In practice, this is not really a problem. You should simply see whether your symptoms have changed after taking a food and ignore any symptoms which were present throughout the test. For example, if you had a painful ankle at breakfast time when you tested the new food and still have the same ankle pain at lunchtime, but without any new symptoms, the breakfast food is safe because nothing has changed. But if, by lunchtime you have a painful swollen knee, in addition to the painful ankle, then your symptoms have changed and the newly painful, swollen knee could well be a reaction to the food tested at breakfast time.

When symptoms do arise, wait until they have subsided before testing any more foods. You may have to eat safe foods only for the next few meals – or even for two or three days if there are persistent symptoms.

When you restart testing foods, begin again where you left off. (This means that, if you had a reaction at the end of Day 5, for example, and then spent two days recovering, you should start again with the tests listed for Day 6 although in fact it is Day 8.)

Reactions vary in both intensity and type – one food might provoke a headache, another will cause joint swelling and pain, while a third will just produce drowsiness and depression. Take note of *all* reactions, not just those that affect the joints, and avoid any food to which you reacted.

A food which has not provoked symptoms is considered to be safe and can be added to your allowed list of foods on the following day. Sometimes you may not be sure whether a food has or has not provoked symptoms. For example, if you tested a food at breakfast, then went shopping, and came back from shopping with painful feet, you may not be sure whether the pain in your feet is the result of the food or of the shopping. Do not guess. Avoid that food for the moment and simply test it again when five days have elapsed.

Throughout this time, keep a diary of everything you eat, and all your symptoms, including the time when they occur.

The foods to test in Stage One are as follows:

Day 1   **Broccoli**, fresh or frozen.
           Avocado pears *.

Day 2   **Green beans**, fresh or frozen.
           Fresh pineapple *. If eating this on an empty stomach, heat it for ten minutes in some mineral water first since it may cause indigestion otherwise.
           Fresh turkey * (or frozen turkey if free from additives).

Day 3   Fresh **tomatoes**.
           Olive oil * or **safflower oil**.
           Pork, either grilled or roasted in its own fat.

Day 4   **Tap water** *; drink two glasses at least.
           Rice
           Lettuce

Day 5   **Bananas** *
           Grapes
           Soyabeans. Even if you do not eat these beans normally it is important to test them because they appear, as soya flour or soya meal, in a variety of prepared foods. You can buy

see p. 176 for explanation

soyabeans from a health food shop. They should be soaked overnight and boiled for 1¹/₂ –2 hours or until soft. If you prefer, drink two large glasses of soya milk, or eat some tofu (soya curd).

Day 6 **Cow's milk**; drink two large glasses. If you have not drunk milk habitually for some months before the elimination diet you should not try this test, as you may react adversely to the milk sugar, lactose (see pp.215–6). Test plain **Cheddar cheese** instead.
Cabbage
Fresh chicken, (or frozen chicken if free from additives).

Day 7 **Tea** *; whatever type of tea you usually drink. You can add milk if you did not react to milk yesterday, but do not add sugar as this needs a separate test.
Apples
Parsnips

Day 8 **Butter**; only test this if you did not react badly to milk.
Leeks
Lamb; either roast lamb or grilled lamb chops.

Day 9 ***Sensodyne* toothpaste** – original flavour, not mint; this brand is used because it does not contain cornstarch.
Plaice
Courgettes or **marrow**

If any of the above foods are unavailable, you could substitute **dates**, or fresh **melon** of any kind.

At the end of Stage One of the reintroduction phase, you should have a fairly wide choice of safe foods. You can now plan a reasonably varied and satisfying menu, remembering, as before, never to over-indulge in one particular food.

Stage Two of the reintroduction phase

Now that you have a less restricted diet you can test the foods that are most likely to be a source of arthritic symptoms. Whatever you do, try not to anticipate a reaction to any of these foods. You must approach each test with an entirely open mind or there is a risk of psychogenic reactions (see p.18).

Two foods are tested on most days, one at breakfast and one at your evening meal. Cereals (wheat, corn, rye and oats) are given two whole days to themselves as they tend to produce very slow reactions.

Day 10
Morning: **Yeast**. Take yeast tablets sold as a vitamin supplement: these are available in chemists' shops or health food shops.
Evening: **Potatoes**; freshly prepared, *not* instant mashed potato.

Day 11   **Eggs** *

Days 12 & 13 **Wheat**. Only test with bread if you did not react badly to yeast. Eat two slices of wholemeal bread *with all three meals* for two days. Be sure to test bread that is made with pure wheat flour. Read the label carefully if buying packaged bread, or check with the baker if you buy from a bakery. Some loaves contain mixtures of flours which will confuse the test result.

If you had a positive reaction when you tested yeast, do the wheat test with a non-yeast – containing pure wheat product such as Shredded Wheat or Puffed Wheat cereal, or wholewheat pasta. In all cases, check labels to ensure the food is 100% wheat with nothing added. You could also try bulgar wheat (crushed wheat, sold in health food shops; cook for about 20 minutes in a little stock and serve like rice). If you did not react to eggs, you can use wholewheat flour to make a pancake-type mixture.

Day 14
Morning: Fresh **coffee** made using coffee beans.
Evening: Ground **black pepper** *.

Day 15
Morning: **Cane sugar**; use West Indian demerara sugar, eg. from Jamaica or Trinidad.
Evening: Any **flavouring** you particularly like, such as chilli powder. Choose something with a single ingredient, not a mixture.

Day 16
Morning: Fresh **oranges**.
Evening: Plain **peanuts** with no additives.

see p. 176 for explanation

Day 17

Morning: **White sugar**. This may be made from pure beet sugar, or a mixture of beet and cane sugar. If you felt well after eating cane sugar but react badly to white sugar, you can deduce that you are sensitive to beet sugar.

Evening: **Bacon**; only test this if pork did not affect you.

Days 18 & 19   **Corn (maize)**; eat this at every meal for two days, as described for wheat. You can eat corn-on-the-cob, or frozen 'sweetcorn', or use two tablespoons (or more) of cornflour to thicken some meat juices, milk (to make a white sauce) or other liquid. Polenta, available from Italian food suppliers, is made from maize. Polenta or maize meal is also available in some health food and wholefood shops. Read the label to check there are no other ingredients in the polenta that you should still be avoiding at this stage.

Day 19

Morning: **Onion**

Evening: **Cheese**, Cheddar or similar; only test this if milk and butter were both negative. Even if you are tolerant of milk you may still react to cheese bcause it contains chemical substances produced by bacteria and moulds during the cheese-making process. If you had a very strong reaction to yeast, you may also react to cheese whch contains traces of yeast.

Day 20

Morning: **Spinach**.

Evening: **Peas**.

Day 21

Morning: **Celery**.

Evening: **Grapefruit**.

Day 22

Morning: **Cucumber**.

Evening: **Cauliflower**.

Day 23

Morning: **Honey** *.

Evening: **Mixed herbs**.

Days 24 & 25   **Rye**: use a pure rye crispbread (check the label). Eat several slices with all three meals for two days.

Day 26

Morning: **Saccharin** * tablets. You need to test these because saccharin is found in many soft drinks and some convenience food.

Evening: **Walnuts**.

Day 27

Morning: **Grapefruit**.

Evening: Green or red **sweet peppers**.

Day 28

Morning: Any **seasonal fruit** eg. strawberries, peaches, rhubarb (test one fruit only)

Evening: **Prawns** or **shrimps**, if liked.

Day 29

Morning: Fresh **lemon**

Evening: **Tinned carrots**. This is a test for sensitivity to the phenolic resin used to line the can.

Day 30

Morning: **Raisins** or **sultanas**.

Evening: **Garlic**, if liked.

Day 31   **Malt extract**. This needs to be tested because malt is a common ingredient in many packaged foods. Malt extract can be bought from most chemists. Spend a whole day on this, taking 2 teaspoonfuls with each meal.

Days 32 & 33 **Oats**: use oatcakes or oatmeal (either eaten raw with milk or fruit juice, or cooked as porridge). Eat some oats three times a day for two days.

Day 34   **Instant coffee**. Test Nescafé Gold Blend which does not contain cornstarch. This is a test for chemical residues derived from the processing of instant coffee.

If you have not tested any foods that you commonly eat, then you can proceed to check these over the coming week, at a rate of two per day.

Many foods are mixtures of those so far tested, and can be eaten when all the ingredients have been tested singly. If you have a bad reaction to such foods, check the ingredients label again. Be aware of the '25% rule' for compound ingredients (see p.193), and look for compound items such as 'sausage' on the label. If this does not seem to explain your reaction, then you may be sensitive to a food additive used in the product. By trial and error you should be able to work out which additives affect you. Monosodium glutamate is one that can be tested singly, as it is sold in large supermarkets and Chinese groceries; sprinkle a little on some meat for the test.

If you reacted positively to bacon or ham, but not to fresh pork, you should consider the possibility that you are sensitive to **nitrates**. These are used as food additives in 'cured meats' including bacon, ham, gammon, salt beef, and some frankfurters. Any meat with the pinkish colour typical of ham or bacon has probably been prepared with nitrates. Nitrates are also applied as fertilisers to farmland, and run off the fields in the rain to end up in our drinking water. Some commercial crops, such as spinach, may have high levels of nitrate in them, due to its use as a fertiliser. To reduce your nitrate intake to a minimum you should cut out bacon and other cured meats (see above), eat organically-grown vegetables or those from your own garden (don't use fertilisers, obviously) and drink a mineral water (but not Perrier as it is as high in nitrates as some tap water). Check the labels for the analysis and look for one that has less than 0.5 mg per litre of nitrates.

The reintroduction phase should take about six weeks. If it takes any longer than this, there is a risk of lost sensitivity: some people become less reactive after avoiding their culprit food for a time, or do not react as promptly, so that the results are unclear. (Note, however, that most people take many months or many years to lose their intolerance. Some are still sensitive to the food after ten years of strict avoidance.)

If you have still not tested all foods seven weeks after starting the exclusion phase, then you should reintroduce all those which have not yet been tested. Eat all of them every day for a week. If, after a week, there is no reaction, then you can consider them all safe. If there *is* a reaction, stop eating them once again, and avoid them for five days, or until your symptoms disappear, if this takes longer. Then retest each of those foods in turn, using the same procedure as before.

Incomplete testing

If something goes wrong during the testing – you might get a bout of 'flu for example – then you may have to stop testing foods. Try not to eat untested foods while you are ill, then go back to testing when you recover. This will be a setback, of course: as explained above, there is no point in trying to test foods beyond seven weeks. If you are unable to test all the excluded foods, then you should go back to your normal diet for about a month. Eat whatever you like, but if there *are* any foods which gave a positive reaction when tested, then you should continue to avoid these.

Keep a record of your symptoms, and review the situation at the end of the month. If you are reasonably well, then continue with this diet, avoiding the suspect foods. If, after a month on this diet, your symptoms have returned, then you should start the exclusion phase again. Any foods that you previously tested and found safe can be eaten in addition to the standard exclusion-phase foods, but if your symptoms have not cleared after a week, then you should exclude these foods as well.

Assuming your symptoms clear up on this new exclusion phase, then you can test the excluded foods as described above.

· *After the Elimination Diet* ·

Assuming that you have successfully identified your culprit foods, the next step is to establish an adequate menu that excludes those foods. Make a list of the foods you cannot eat, and a list of those that you can. Look at pp.194–204, especially the 'Crucial nutrients' section, for those foods you must avoid, and ensure that your diet is nutritionally adequate.

Some forms of food intolerance seem to abate after a year or more of avoiding the culprit food, so that a little of the food can be eaten from time to time. *This does not necessarily happen with rheumatoid arthritis.* We have seen patients who, after years of avoidance, have gone back to eating their culprit food occasionally, have had no ill-effects initially and have therefore assumed the food was safe, only to suffer a serious recurrence of their old symptoms soon afterwards. One patient relapsed in this way after ten years of avoiding the culprit food, while several have relapsed after four years' avoidance. In a few cases, returning to their strict diet did not put things right again, and they bitterly regretted that they had deviated from the original diet. For this reason we would advise you to avoid your culprit food or foods indefinitely.

Once you have established a workable diet, try to keep your food varied. If you find yourself eating one sort of food very regularly, take a week off from it and then eat it only once every three or four days. Continue to eat healthily, with plenty of green vegetables and not too much processed food (see Chapter 2.8–p.252).

Avoid anything that irritates the gut lining and makes it more permeable: see Table 9. The more permeable the gut is, the more intact molecules pass through into the bloodstream, and this is thought to increase the risk of food intolerance.

Table 9: Items that increase the permeability of the gut wall

Strong coffee
Strong tea
Highly spiced food
Raw pineapple
Raw papaya (pawpaw)
Excessive amounts of alcohol

Certain drugs also make the gut more leaky, notably aspirin and other non-steroidal anti-inflammatory drugs (see p.418). You should only take these if you really need them. Paracetamol does not affect the gut wall in this way, and is a useful pain-killer.

· *Knowing When to Give Up* ·

One of the hazards of elimination dieting is not knowing when to give up. Very occasionally, people who have had a small improvement that seems to be related to cutting out food, or have had a rather confusing and variable response to the elimination diet, become obsessed with the idea that food avoidance is the answer to all their problems. They cut out more and more foods until they are on a highly restricted diet, with perhaps only two or three foods allowed. This is a serious mistake, and carries with it the risk of malnutrition. You must therefore be very careful to avoid this pitfall. In the long run, you need an ample and varied diet to maintain your health, and this must be the overriding concern. This is why an elimination diet is best conducted under medical supervision – we would strongly recommend that you seek your doctor's advice and help while on the diet.

· *Food Avoidance and Juvenile Arthritis* ·

The question of whether children should ever be put on restricted diets is a very contentious issue. There are cases of children having malnutrition and stunted growth because of supposedly therapeutic diets imposed on them by their parents. This has, understandably, made many paediatricians very hostile to the whole idea of food intolerance.

In general, food rarely seems to play a part in juvenile chronic arthritis. On the other hand, the case history described on p.7 shows that food can occasionally be a relevant factor and that avoiding the culprit food can produce a very marked improvement. There is also a report in the medical literature of food elimination proving useful in juvenile chronic arthritis. The patient was a 14-year old girl who had suffered from arthritis for six years. When milk was cut out of her diet she recovered and remained well, and when challenged with milk she again developed arthritis. It would be sad if such patients did not receive the substantial benefits that a dietary change can bring.

However, we would certainly not advocate a full elimination diet for children. A more limited diet in which the most likely culprits are avoided during the exclusion phase may be worth trying. The foods to avoid would be milk and milk products, eggs, citrus fruits, peanuts, wheat, corn and other grains. *You must not try this diet without the full consent and close supervision of your child's doctor.* A calcium supplement is essential when milk is avoided, and other vitamins may also be needed, particularly Vitamins A and D.

Do not become 'convinced' that food is at the root of your child's joint symptoms – keep an open mind. A recent study identified certain arthritic children who had clear-cut food intolerance manifesting itself as eczema and diarrhoea, but whose arthritis was unrelated to food.

Chapter 2.5

LIVING HAPPILY WITH A RESTRICTED DIET

If you have completed the elimination diet (see Chapter 2.4) and found that certain foods consistently provoke symptoms, then you will need to avoid those foods scrupulously in future (see p.190). You will need to find replacements for these foods, and to ensure that you are not missing out on any important nutrients in the process. This chapter is designed to help you in this, and to ensure that you do not go hungry despite a restricted diet.

Avoiding some foods is relatively easy, but others, such as wheat, corn, milk, egg and soya are so widely used in ready-made food that you have to be on guard against eating them inadvertently. Look up the ingredient you are avoiding in the first section of the chapter, and familiarise yourself with all the foods where it could be a hidden ingredient. Learn the synonyms used on food labels so that you can detect it in packaged food.

If you have a true allergy to any food, as indicated by symptoms such as tingling or swollen lips, tingling in the mouth, nettle rash (hives) or breathing difficulties after eating, you need to be especially careful about reading labels. Subsequent exposure to the food can provoke a violent reaction known as anaphylactic shock, which is sometimes fatal.

Be aware of the 25% rule on composite ingredients: if a composite ingredient (eg. sausage on a pizza) comprises less than 25% of the product, its individual constituents do not have to be listed, just the item itself. So a label might say 'sausage' and not mention that this contained peanut oil, soya or egg.

When eating in restaurants, be very cautious about hidden ingredients in dishes, and ask to speak to the chef if you are in any doubt – waiters and waitresses are often an unreliable source of information about the food.

Finding substitutes for staple foods can be difficult. In the first half of this chapter you will find a guide to substitutes for the particular food you are avoiding. Any words shown in **bold type** can be looked up in the second part of the chapter (pp.205–225), where there is information on how to cook the more unfamiliar foods, and some useful recipes.

Be alert to the possibility of cross-reactions to related foods (see pp.175–6), and eat these sparingly. However, you should not worry about cross-reactions excessively. They do not occur for many people, and worrying about a food can provoke a psychogenic reaction (see p.18) to it.

Avoiding problem foods

**CORN
(MAIZE)**

Found in:
Corn-on-the-cob, sweetcorn, 'corn niblets'.
Cornflakes, Cheerios, Corn Pops, some other **breakfast cereals** (p.208), some muesli.
Soups, soup mixes.
Cornflour, custard powder.
Gravy and gravy mixes, white sauce, Bechamel sauce, parsley sauce and many other sauces (for substitutes see **thickeners** p.224).
Some packet snacks such as Doritos, Monster-Munches (read all packet labels).
Many ready-made meals and sauces.
Tortilla chips.
Corn bread, polenta.

Hidden ingredient in:
Some **baking powder** (p.205).
Many ready-made foods – read labels with great care.
Gum on stamps and envelopes.
Many tablets (including some prescribed for arthritis).

Substitutes:
(See entries marked in **bold type** above.)

Possible cross-reactions:
Other cereals, such as wheat, rye, barley, oats, rice or millet could start to cause reactions if you eat too much of them.

Label watch:
Look out for: 'cornmeal', 'cornstarch', 'corn syrup', 'dextrose', 'cereal starch', 'edible starch', 'food starch', 'glucose syrup', 'modified starch', 'starch', 'vegetable gum', 'vegetable oil', 'vegetable starch'.

EGGS   *Found in:*
Quiche, soufflé.
Meringues (egg white only).
Batter, pancakes, waffles, Yorkshire pudding.
Rich shortcrust pastry, cheese straws.
Crème caramel (except cheaper versions – check the label), mousses, egg custard, custard tarts, many different desserts.
Crème patissière (found in fruit tarts etc.).
Sponge cake, Madeira cake.
Brioche and some other rich breads; Danish pastries, eclairs, choux buns.
Marzipan.
Egg noodles, egg pasta.
Advocaat.

Hidden ingredient in:
A very wide range of ready-made foods – always read labels.
Egg glazes on pastry.
Some margarine (as lecithin).
Some ice cream.

Substitutes:
Nothing really tastes like eggs themselves, but there are substitutes for baking which reproduce their cooking qualities (see p.214).

Possible cross-reactions:
The eggs of other birds are very likely to cross-react.
People with a true allergy to eggs sometimes react to vaccines if they have been cultivated in eggs.

Label watch:
Look out for: 'ovalbumin', 'lecithin' (but lecithin could be made from soya).

Crucial nutrients:
Ensure you have other sources of B vitamins (see p.287) and Vitamin D (see p.297)

MILK   *Found in:*
Cream, butter.
Cheese, cottage cheese, cream cheese.
Yoghurt, fromage frais, crème fraîche.
White sauce, Béchamel sauce, parsley sauce etc.
Custard, rice pudding, semolina, tapioca and sago
pudding.

Hidden ingredient in:
Most margarines.
A great many packaged foods – always read the labels.
Pastries, buns, cakes, biscuits, scones.
Home-made pastry is often made with butter.
Some medicines contain lactose, or milk sugar, as a
filler. This does not necessarily affect everyone who is
sensitive to milk (since most are reacting to milk
proteins, not lactose) but it may cause problems for
some. Diarrhoea and flatulence are the usual reaction.
In the U.S.A., many white breads contain milk solids,
but this is not the case in the U.K.

Substitutes:
See **milk substitutes** (p.216), **butter substitutes**
(p.209), **cheese substitutes** (p.211).
Look for items labelled 'Dairy free' or 'Suitable for
vegans'.
See **cakes** (p.210) and **biscuits** (p.206) for milk-free
recipes.

Possible cross-reactions:
Some people cross-react to beef but this is highly
unusual. A cross-reaction to goat's milk, or to sheep's
milk is more common.

Label watch:
Look out for: 'whey', 'casein', 'caseinate', 'lactalbumin',
'lactose'.

Crucial nutrients:
If you avoid milk and other dairy products you run a
serious risk of calcium deficiency. It *is* possible to get
enough calcium from fish such as sardines, eaten whole,
but you would need to eat a good portion of such fish
every day. It is also possible to get enough calcium from

purely vegetable sources, and vegans successfully do this, but it requires a high consumption of calcium-containing vegetable foods (see p.317) and a very disciplined approach to eating, which is difficult for most people. A calcium supplement may be the best option or a calcium-fortified food, such fortified soya milk (see p.312). A supplement which also contains magnesium in the correct ratio (about 2:1) is probably a good idea, unless you have a very high intake of green leafy vegetables and other magnesium-rich foods (see p.328).

Apart from calcium, milk also supplies protein, some of the B vitamins and some Vitamin D. You are unlikely to be short of protein, unless you eat very little fish, meat or eggs; if this is the case, check with the figures on pp.350–351. Ensure that you are eating other sources of B vitamins (see p.287) and that you either get enough sunlight to make Vitamin D for yourself, or eat some foods rich in this vitamin (see p.297).

NUTS   *Found in:*
Nougat, marzipan, praline and many other sweets and chocolate products.
See also PEANUTS (p.198)

Hidden ingredient in:
Many bakery products, such as cakes, biscuits and cookies, savoury pastries, and desserts.
Stuffing mixes; special vegetarian foods.
Gluten-free breads may contain ground almonds.
If you are sensitive to peanuts as well as other nuts, the range of food to be cautious about is even wider (see po.198–9).
Should you have any symptoms of true allergy (see p.83) in response to nuts, beware of all unlabelled foods and restaurant food; ask before you taste.

Substitutes:
Seeds are a good substitute nutritionally, and for their value as snacks, and in vegetarian cooking.

Possible cross-reactions:
All nuts are potentially capable of cross-reacting, one

with another, even though they are from unrelated plant families. Those that are related (eg. pecan and walnut) are the most likely to cross-react. Reactions with peanuts (see below) are also likely, even though these are not true nuts.

Label watch:
There are no synonyms for most nuts, but there are some for peanuts (see p.199).

Food manufacturers and supermarkets have suddenly become very 'nut conscious' because of fatal reactions to nuts by people with a true allergy to them. If you have such an allergy, do not be lulled into a sense of false security by this: there will still be many producers and many shops that fail to label nut-containing products carefully. The 25% rule for composite ingredients is of particular concern to those with severe nut allergy (see p.193).

Crucial nutrients:
Almonds and hazelnuts are a good source of Vitamin E, an important nutrient for anyone with rheumatoid arthritis. **Sunflower seeds** (p.221) are an alternative source, as are sunflower spread and sunflower oil. There are also some other sources (see p.301). If not eating plenty of these then a supplement of Vitamin E may be advisable.

Nuts are also a good source of many B vitamins (but not Vitamin B_{12}). Again, seeds can act as a replacement source, as can various other foods (see p.287).

PEANUTS *Found in:*
Peanut butter.
Satay sauce (as in chicken satay); many other Thai dishes.

Hidden ingredient in:
A wide range of foods, especially biscuits, cakes, cookies, savoury snacks and desserts.
Bakery products sold loose, without ingredients' labels, should always be 'suspected' in case they contain peanuts.
Many curry sauces, some Chinese egg rolls.
Some brands of Worcester sauce.

If you have any symptoms of a true allergy to peanuts (eg. tingling or swollen lips, nettle rash, or difficulty in breathing) then you must also be very cautious about eating in restaurants and cafes, and religiously read the labels on packeted food.

There is a new product in America, which could be exported to other countries: it is made from peanuts stripped of their original flavour by chemical treatment, reflavoured as almonds or other more expensive nuts, and moulded to the appropriate shape. The packets declare their ingredients of course, but beware the bowl of nuts on a bar or party table. There are also now available pretzels with a peanut paste filling which is quite unexpected, and therefore potentially dangerous.

Vitamin tablets and drops sometimes contain traces of peanut oil. So do some sweets eg. Jelly Babies.

Substitutes:
As for NUTS (see p.197).

Possible cross-reactions:
All other nuts, even though they belong to different plant families. Nuts seem to share some common constituents that trigger allergy and intolerance.

Cross-reactions to pulses or legumes are also possible, because peanuts belong to the same plant family. The members of this family include: kidney beans (also called haricot beans, navy beans, white beans and 'baked beans'), lima beans, broad beans, butter beans, black-eye peas, chickpeas, lentils and mung beans. Carob is also a legume.

Label watch:
Look out for: 'groundnuts', 'groundnut oil', 'peanut oil'.
Peanut oil can also be described as 'vegetable oil', and as 'arachis oil' (usually in creams, soaps and cosmetics).

Be aware of the 25% rule on composite ingredients (see p.193) if you have a true allergy to peanuts, and see the 'Label watch' section for NUTS (p.198).

Crucial nutrients:
As for NUTS, (see p.198).

POTATOES *Found in:*
Chips, French fries. Crisps and many other savoury snack foods, including Quavers (real all labels).
Many ready-made meals, soups.
Cornish pasties, many vegetarian pasties.

Hidden ingredient in:
Some Indian dishes (eg. Sag aloo – 'aloo' means potato).
Some ready-made foods.

Substitutes:
Barley (p.205), **breadfruit** (p.208), **buckwheat** (p.209), **cassava** (p.211), **chestnuts** (p.212), **cornmeal** (p.213), **dasheen** (p.214), mashed **chickpeas** (p.212), **millet** (p.217), parsnip, **plantains** (p.220), **pumpkin** (p.220), quinoa, rice, **sorghum** (p.221), swede, **sweet potato** (p.222), turnip, **yam** (p.224).

Possible cross-reactions:
Occasionally there are reactions to other vegetable foods from the same plant family; tomatoes, aubergines, sweet peppers, chilli peppers, paprika, cayenne and cape gooseberry (Physalis). Sweet potato belongs to an entirely different family and should not cross-react.

Label watch:
There are no unfamiliar synonyms for this food, but look for 'potato flour'.

RICE   *Hidden ingredient in:*
Many Indian and Japanese sweetmeats, which are made with rice flour.
Spring rolls (the pastry is made with rice flour).
Some noodles (rice noodles are very white, unlike wheat pasta).

Substitutes:
Wild rice (p.224), **sorghum** (p.221), **millet** (p.217), quinoa, **cornmeal** (p.213), **buckwheat** (p.209), **barley** (p.205).

Possible cross-reactions:
Wild rice. Occasionally cross-reacts with other grains such as wheat or corn (maize).

Label watch:
There are no unfamiliar synonyms for this food, but look for 'rice flour'.

SOYA   *Found in:*
Soya beans, soya meal, soya flour.
Soy sauce, miso.
Textured vegetable protein (TVP).
Vegetarian burgers, risotto, 'sausage' rolls and most other meat substitutes.
Soya milk, soy yoghurt, soy cheese.
Many gluten-free breads and other gluten-free products.

Hidden ingredient in:
Many packaged foods: always read the labels.

Substitutes:
Toasted sesame oil makes a reasonable substitute for soy sauce.
For alternatives to soy milk see **milk substitutes** (p.215). For wheat-free, soy-free bread you can bake your own or try one of the substitutes, such as rice cakes, listed under **bread** (p.206).

Possible cross-reactions:
Some people who become sensitive to soya later react to other pulses or legumes (members of the bean family). These include kidney beans (also called haricot beans, navy beans, white beans and 'baked beans'), lima beans, broad beans, butter beans, black-eye peas, chickpeas, lentils and mung beans. Carob is also a legume. Beansprouts could well cross-react. Peanuts are also members of this family and cross-reactions to peanuts are possible.

Label watch:
Look out for: 'lecithin', 'vegetable gum', 'vegetable protein', 'textured vegetable protein' (TVP), 'vegetable starch'.

Crucial nutrients:
Soyabeans are an important source of protein for vegetarians and vegans. Vegetarians can fulfil their protein needs by using eggs or dairy produce, assuming

they can tolerate these. Vegans should ensure that they eat protein-rich vegetable foods (see pp.349–351). (Eat other beans in moderation to reduce the risk of cross-reactions.) **Quorn** (p.221) may be useful.

Soyabeans also supply some B vitamins but there are many other sources for these (see p.287).

WHEAT   *Found in:*

Bread (p.206), pitta bread, nan bread, some poppadoms, chapattis.

Breadcrumb coatings (eg. on fish fingers).

Flour (p.215).

Cakes (p.210), **biscuits** (p.206), buns, scones, teacakes, crumpets, muffins, cookies etc.

Pancakes (p.219) unless made with pure buckwheat flour.

Pastry (p.219) of all kinds, pasties, pies.

Sauces and gravy may contain wheat flour rather than cornflour (see **thickeners**, p.224 for substitutes).

Pasta (p.219): spaghetti, tagliatelle, macaroni, egg noodles, pasta shells and bows, vermicelli.

Wheat Flakes, All-bran, Bran Flakes, Weetabix, Puffed Wheat, Shredded Wheat, Shreddies, Cheerios, Corn Pops, Clusters and many other kinds of **breakfast cereals** (p.208) even if 'wheat' does not appear in the brand name: check all labels.

Many kinds of muesli.

Samosas may contain some wheat flour (check the label).

Cous-cous, bulgar wheat, semolina.

Hidden ingredient in:

Most kinds of rye bread (unless guaranteed 100% rye).

Some rye crispbreads, some oatcakes.

Many ready-made foods: read labels with care.

Sausages.

Taramasalata (often contains breadcrumbs).

Baking powder.

Mustard powder and English mustard. (French mustard is usually wheat-free, but check the label.)

Substitutes:

See entries marked in **bold type** above. And see **millet** (p.217) for a sandwich substitute. Rice, potatoes, and some of the starchy substitutes for POTATO (see p.200) may prove useful in keeping your diet as varied and filling as possible while avoiding wheat and other grains.

Possible cross-reactions:
Rye, barley and oats are closely related to wheat, and could well cause cross-reactions. If you *can* tolerate them you should still be cautious and not eat too much of them to avoid becoming sensitive. Rye is the most likely to cause problems, oats the least.

Corn (maize), rice and millet are also grains, although less likely to cross-react. Again, eat these in moderation.

Label watch:
Look out for: 'flour', 'cereal binder', 'cereal filler', 'cereal protein', 'cereal starch', 'edible starch', 'food starch', 'modified starch', 'starch'.

Bulgar wheat is also true wheat, but buckwheat is not. 'Gluten-free' products are also wheat free (but the reverse is not the case: rye bread, for example, may be wheat free but it still contains gluten).

Crucial nutrients:
In the U.K., all bread except wholemeal is fortified with calcium, and constitutes an important source of this mineral. If you avoid dairy products as well as not eating bread, a calcium supplement is advisable, unless you eat substantial portions of other calcium-containing foods (see p.317). If you are not replacing wheat bread with other whole grains take care to eat other foods that supply B vitamins (see p.287), zinc (see p.324) and iron (see p.322).

YEAST   *Found in:*
Yeast extract (Marmite, Vegemite).

Hidden ingredient in:
Stock cubes (p.222).
Bread (see p.208), including sourdough bread, but excluding soda bread, most brands of pitta bread, chappatis, most nan bread.
Danish pastries, doughnuts, Chelsea buns, American 'coffee cake', teacakes (and any other cake with a bread-like texture).

Pizza.

Rolls, most croissants.

Beer, wine, cider (other alcoholic drinks, such as whisky and gin, also contain some yeast but not as much).

Vinegar (hence in salad dressing, pickles, chutney etc.)

Many vitamin tablets, especially B vitamins.

Many ready-made meals and packet foods – read the labels.

Any food that is fermented or has a long processing time (eg. sour cream, buttermilk, cheeses, sauerkraut, dried fruit, soy sauce, miso, black tea). Test these individually to see if you react.

Very ripe fruit.

Juice or jam that has been opened and kept for a while.

Substitutes:
See entries marked in bold above.

Try spirits instead of beer and wine. Toasted sesame oil is a good substitute for soy sauce.

Possible cross-reactions:
You might react to mushrooms or other edible fungi, either to the items themselves or to moulds and yeasts growing on them. Quorn, a protein-rich food derived from fungi, could also cause problems.

Label watch:
Look out for: 'hydrolysed protein', 'hydrolysed vegetable protein', 'leavening'. 'Citric acid' may be derived from yeast. So may 'monosodium glutamate'. 'Mycoprotein' is another name for Quorn.

Crucial nutrients:
If you eat a lot of bread made without yeast, you may run the risk of certain mineral deficiencies, because it contains substances which block the absorption of calcium, magnesium, iron, zinc, manganese and copper (see p.309). Ensure that you eat plenty of the foods that are rich in these minerals (see Chapter 3.3) or take a multi-mineral supplement.

Yeast is a good source of most B vitamins, and you should consume other foods that are rich in these vitamins (see p.287) or take a yeast-free B-complex tablet.

· *Guide to Individual Foods* ·

The primary purpose of this section is to help those who have successfully completed an elimination diet and know that they have to avoid certain foods in their diet. It offers advice on finding substitutes for common foods such as bread, milk and egg, and information on cooking some of the more unusual foods.

Baking powder

Baking powder usually contains a small amount of wheat flour, and anyone who is very sensitive to wheat should buy a wheat-free brand or make their own. Mix 60 gm (2 oz) of sodium bicarbonate with 130 gm (4½ oz) of cream of tartar. Add 60 gm (2 oz) of potato flour, rice flour or another flour which you are allowed. Sieve four times to ensure thorough mixing and then store in an airtight jar. Cream of tartar can be bought from most groceries or supermarkets. Sodium bicarbonate is sold by chemists, or on the medicine's counter of most supermarkets.

Barley

This grain can act as a substitute for potatoes, rice or bread, although it may cross-react with wheat or rice. You can get barley very cheaply from supermarkets and health food shops. It makes a homely, filling addition to stews, casseroles and soups but it needs to cook for quite a long time (about 1–1½ hours). Try a simple winter stew of barley, carrots and tomatoes with garlic and a hot spice. Add some meat, beans or chickpeas to supply protein.

Beans

Beans are rich in protein, fibre and certain vitamins. They are also cheap and filling, although the amount of fuel needed to cook them does make them slightly more expensive than they seem initially. Tinned beans, whether plain, or in the familiar guise of baked beans in tomato sauce, are a convenient alternative, and contain just as much protein.

Beans must be cooked properly to destroy the natural toxins: never eat half-cooked beans. Pick out discoloured beans and soak the rest overnight, then cook in twice their volume of water until soft (about 1½ hours). Beans may cause problems with flatulence but removing the skins after cooking can diminish this effect.

Note that the protein in beans is not as 'good', nutritionally, as animal protein, and meals need to be planned accordingly (see p.349).

Biscuits

If you must avoid wheat, but can eat oats, flapjacks are a good substitute for biscuits, and easily made. Heat 125 gm (4 oz) of margarine or butter with 4 tablespoons of honey. When melted, add 250 gm (8 oz) rolled oats and 50 gm (2 oz) chopped nuts. Mix well, spoon into a shallow greased tin and bake at 180°C (350°F, Gas Mark 4) for 20–30 minutes. Cut into fingers while still warm, but do not remove from the tin until cold.

Your favourite biscuit recipes can be used with non-wheat flours, such as rye flour, rice flour or carob flour (see **flour**, p.215). If the flour of your choice is a low-protein flour, an egg is a useful addition to the mixture: reduce the quantities of the other added liquids and the butter/margarine a little, to compensate for the extra fluid and fat in the egg.

Gluten-free biscuits can be bought at most health food shops, and these will be wheat free. Milk-free biscuits can easily be made using margarine, and most shop-bought biscuits are milk-free, but check the label. See also **egg substitutes** (p.214).

Bread and bread substitutes

Avoiding wheat:
Assuming you have an *intolerance* of wheat (rather than coeliac disease or a true food allergy) it is worth checking that it is *all* parts of the wheat grain you must avoid. It may be the proteins in the wheatgerm that affect you, or something in the outer coat of the wheat grain. If this is the case, you will be able to eat white bread and white flour, but should avoid wholemeal bread, granary bread, and any products (eg. crackers) containing wheatgerm.

The proteins in wheat flour, which include gluten, are what makes wheat so good for bread-making. Trying to make bread without wheat involves finding a substitute for this protein. Other high-protein flours (see **flour**, p.215) such as rye flour or soya flour, are frequently used. Rye flour unfortunately contains gluten (as do oats and barley) which makes it unsuitable for coeliacs. Non-coeliacs who are sensitive to wheat may also cross-react to rye, barley or oats.

Gluten-free bread is sold in some health food shops and chemists' shops, or you can buy a gluten-free flour and make your own. Those with coeliac disease can get some gluten-free products on prescription. All gluten-free products are free of all wheat, rye, barley and oats.

Mixtures of different flours are used to make gluten-free flours eg. rice flour, rice bran, maize flour, potato flour, soya flour, split pea flour, carob flour, corn starch and ground almonds. You can improvise with simple mixtures of your own – eg. equal quantities of rice flour, soya (or gram) flour and potato flour. Note that the mixture must always include at least one type of high-protein flour (see p.215), such as soya, gram or lentil. Use yeast and make in the ordinary way, but without kneading the bread. It will inevitably have a heavier texture than ordinary bread, and will probably taste better if toasted. Should you have to avoid yeast as well, it is possible to make soda bread using gluten-free flour. The manufacturers of gluten-free flour usually supply recipes for use with their particular flour mix.

Remember that most gluten-free mixes contain soya flour or other bean-derived flours. Make sure you are not eating soya and related foods (see p.201) too regularly, especially if you are vegetarian – they feature in most commercial meat substitutes and 'vegeburgers', and they are found in many packet foods and instant meals, both vegetarian and non-vegetarian.

Rye bread is *not* gluten-free, but it is suitable for some wheat-sensitive people. Good rye bread has a better texture than most gluten-free bread, though it cannot rival wheat. If you buy unlabelled rye bread from a local bakery be sure to check that it is 100% rye and does not have a little wheat flour added – speak to the manager, *and ask to be notified if they change the composition of the bread*. Rye flour often contains some traces of wheat anyway, because wheat grows as a weed in fields of rye.

Similarly, with rye crispbread, check that it is pure rye: some now have wheat bran added.

Oatcakes are not gluten-free, but are useful to many who are sensitive to wheat. They can be found in most good supermarkets, delicatessens and health food shops. Oats are preferable to rye since they are less likely to cross-react with wheat. Check the label, as a few types are made with wheat flour as well as oats.

Rice cakes and rice crackers are gluten-free. Both can be bought from delicatessens and health food shops. The 'cakes' are actually savoury – rather like a crispbread, but made from puffed grains of rice. They may look like polystyrene ceiling tiles, but they actually taste very good, and are well worth trying.

Gram-flour poppadoms are sold in Indian groceries and can be eaten as an accompaniment to a meal. Check that they do not contain wheat flour. Grams are small beans, and you should not eat them too often if you are already sensitive to soya or other beans. Here is a traditional Indian recipe for gram-flour bread:

1. Mix two cups of gram flour with a small, finely chopped onion, 1/2 teaspoon cumin seeds, 1/2 teaspoon salt and a pinch of chilli powder.
2. Rub in 1 tablespoon of butter (see p.000).
3. Add a little water – enough to make a stiff doughy mixture.
4. Take small balls of this and press down lightly with your hand on a floured surface.
5. Fry on a griddle or hot plate, turning once.

Avoiding yeast:
Soda bread is yeast-free. Most pitta bread is made without yeast, but check the label. Chapatis and some other Indian breads (phulkas, parathas and nan bread) are also yeast-free in most cases. Rye crispbreads, oatcakes and rice cakes are both yeast-free and wheat-free.

Breadfruit

This is a truly exotic food, from the islands of the Pacific. It makes an excellent substitute for potatoes or other starchy foods. Breadfruit is only sold in a few specialised Indian and Chinese groceries, but is well worth looking out for. It is a large green spherical fruit with a delicate honeycomb-like pattern on the surface. Pierce the skin to allow steam to escape, then bake it whole at 190°C (375°F, Gas Mark 5) for 1 1/2–2 hours. The white flesh is firm, with a subtle flavour and creamy texture. Meal-sized portions can be frozen after cooking. As it can be sliced and eaten straight from the skin (like a slice of melon) breadfruit is useful for packed lunches.

Breakfast cereals

If you are sensitive to wheat, choose Cornflakes or Rice Krispies. Always check labels before trying a new product: a little wheat is often added to cereals based on oats, corn or rice.

Plain porridge oats or rolled oats can be used raw as a breakfast cereal, and they are far more filling (and cheaper) than most packet cereals. If you allow the milk to soak in for a few minutes before eating they will be more digestible. Raisins and chopped apple make a tasty addition.

If you react to wheat, oats *and* corn, then you could try rice flakes or millet flakes, both available from good health food stores. Serve as for oats (see above). Do not eat too much of any grain as you will run the risk of acquiring a new sensitivity: have something other than cereal for breakfast several times a week.

Packeted breakfast cereals are usually reinforced with several different B vitamins. If you eat a good mixed diet, the loss of the added vitamins in a daily bowl of cornflakes is unlikely to cause any deficiency, but check the natural sources of B vitamins on p.287 and make sure you eat plenty of these.

See also **porridge** (p.220).

Buckwheat

This is a nutritious brown grain with a strong, earthy flavour, available in most health food shops. Despite the name, it is not of the wheat family. Use it in soups or stews with other strong flavourings to dilute its taste. To prepare the grains, wash them well and cook in twice the quantity of salted water. Weaken the taste if you wish by changing the water after the first boil, simmering for 15 minutes until the buckwheat is softened. Season generously with herbs or spices.

Buckwheat flour is useful in baking and pancakes, and buckwheat noodles can replace wheat **pasta** (p.219). However, you should not eat too much of it, as it has a reputation for causing sensitivity reactions.

Butter substitutes

Margarine is the simplest substitute for butter, but some brands (eg. Flora) contain small amounts of milk solids. The brands that do not, eg. Granose, Tomor and Vitasieg, are available from large supermarkets and from health food shops.

For those who dislike the taste of margarine, there are other possibilities. One is **tahini** (p.223), or ground sesame seeds, preferably the light variety. Another is sunflower-seed spread which is very nutritious. Note that sunflower seed spread is especially rich in Vitamin E, whereas tahini does not contain sufficient Vitamin E in relation to the quantity of polyunsaturated fatty acids it contains (see p.301). **Nut butters** (p.218) spread thinly are also good: cashew butter is the smoothest, but almond butter and hazelnut butter are richer in Vitamin E. The flesh of an avocado pear, lightly mashed, is an excellent substitute for butter. It is very rich in oils and spreads well.

In sauces, creamed coconut can sometimes act as a substitute for butter, although it only suits certain foods. Try melting creamed coconut in orange juice over a low heat, adding salt, garlic and finally ground almonds to thicken the mixture – this makes a tasty sauce to accompany chicken or pork. Do not eat this too often, as coconut is very rich in saturated fat.

If you rarely get out in the sun, and are eating neither butter or margarine, make sure you have some other source of Vitamin D in your diet (see p.297).

Cakes

A typical cake includes egg, wheat flour, butter and, frequently, milk. If you are avoiding wheat, you should be able to find gluten-free cakes in a health food shop, or you can make your own substituting an alternative **flour** (p.215), or mixture of flours for wheat. You need some high-protein flour, or the result will be rather heavy. An extra egg can help to give better texture to cakes made from low-protein flour; obviously, you must decrease the milk or other liquid to compensate for the additional liquid. Making a cake without milk is not difficult: use any **milk substitute** (p.215), or just use water, or a mixture of water and a little beaten egg. Replace the butter in your recipe with milk-free margarine (see p.209).

Making a cake without egg is more difficult. The best answer is egg replacer, available by post (see p.432 for addresses) or occasionally found in some health food shops. Recipes are usually supplied with such products. The replacer is designed to reproduce the baking qualities of eggs and give the cake its characteristic lightness and texture – it does not replace the flavour of eggs. To simulate that rich eggy taste try adding some vanilla essence. In fruit cakes and tea breads, where lightness is not essential, a mashed avocado can enrich the mixture. Mashed bananas also give richness: look in any good cookery book for a recipe for banana bread (actually a cake, rather than a bread). See also **egg substitutes** (p.214).

Carob

Carob is a substitute for chocolate. It can be bought from health food shops in several forms, as a flour, in carob drops or as a concentrated syrup for making drinks. The pea-sized carob drops can be eaten in place of sweets and chocolates: you could mix them with a selection of dried fruit and nuts. They can also be melted for use as icing or sauce.

Carob flour is quite adaptable. It can be added directly to baking mixtures in place of cocoa for an alternative 'chocolate' cake. You can also wet it with a little honey to make an icing or a filling for cakes.

Cassava

This is a starchy root with an excellent flavour, texture and colour that makes a good substitute for potato or rice. It is not widely sold, but you may find it in Indian or West Indian stores. Boiling in plenty of water is essential for this root crop, to remove toxic compounds: it should *not* be baked. Peel, dice and boil for about 15 minutes, or until soft. (There is no need to soak before cooking for the types of cassava that are sold in Britain, but this may be necessary for cassava bought elsewhere: some types contain larger amounts of toxin and need special treatment.)

Cassava can easily be recognised, being a regular cylindrical root, but much more slender than yam.

Cheese substitutes

Goat cheeses and sheep cheeses are available from good delicatessens and some health food shops. You can also buy them by post – see pp.432–3 for addresses. Not everyone who is sensitive to cow's milk can tolerate these. Note that goat's cheese is rather high in saturated fat.

Soya-based 'cheese' spreads are available in many health food shops. Tofu is another soya product that can also act as a substitute for soft cheese. Mashed or whipped tofu may be substituted for cottage and ricotta cheeses. Try livening it up with some fresh herbs or garlic. Be careful not to eat too much soya, as you can easily develop a sensitivity to it.

The following are useful substitutes for cheese in filling sandwiches or making quick snacks:

Peanut butter, other **nut butters** (p.218), sunflower seed spread.
Hummous (see p.212), if made to a thick consistency, is a very good sandwich-filling or spread.
Taramasalata (see p.223) makes a good sandwich filling, combined with tomatoes, cucumber or watercress.

Except for sheep and goat cheeses, most of these substitutes contain very little calcium. Tofu contains a little calcium, but far less than cheese: some types only contain 2% of the amount in Cheddar.

If you are avoiding milk as well, then you need to take a calcium supplement unless you can eat adequate amounts of other calcium-containing foods (see pp.196–7). Check that other nutrients found in milk (see p.197) are also being replaced by other foods.

Chestnuts

Dried chestnuts can be bought at some health food shops and large supermarkets, and from Chinese suppliers. They need to be soaked overnight and then washed. Boil them for an hour until they are quite tender, or cook them in a pressure cooker (for 15 minutes at about 15 lbs pressure). You can cook a large quantity and then freeze them in several meal-sized portions. Reheat them by frying slowly and serve with diced apple or other fresh fruit for an unusual breakfast.

In France, chestnuts are often eaten as a substitute for mashed potato. Mash the boiled chestnuts, dilute with a little warm water and add some milk (or a milk substitute) until you get a lighter consistency. Season to taste. This mash is rather sweet and is only eaten in small portions.

Chestnuts can also be made into soup, by cooking until soft then blending them with suitable flavourings, such as orange juice and a little fresh chilli pepper.

Chickpeas

Chickpeas are adaptable, filling and nutritious, with a far less 'beany' taste than other beans or lentils. They can be used in soups and casseroles, to make these dishes more filling, or mashed with a little butter and milk, as a substitute for mashed potato.

Pick out discoloured chickpeas, soak the rest overnight, then cook in twice their volume of water until soft (about 1–1 1/2 hours). Like other beans, chickpeas can cause flatulence: removing the skins after cooking can diminish this effect. To save on cooking, chickpeas can also be bought tinned from major supermarkets; these taste just as good, and are almost as rich in nutrients (see p.257).

Chickpeas can also be made into **hummous** by pulverising them (use a potato masher, or an electric blender) and adding plenty of olive oil, lemon juice and freshly crushed garlic – adjust the quantities to suit your taste.

Home-made hummous can be made stiffer and thicker than the dip commonly sold in restaurants and supermarkets, making it suitable as a sandwich-filling if you are unable to eat cheese. For a thick consistency, combine 280 gm (10 oz) cooked or canned chickpeas with 3 tablespoons of olive oil and 1 tablespoon of lemon juice, two pinches of salt and a small clove of garlic, crushed. Adjust the amount of lemon juice to suit your taste.

Because they are rich in protein, beans and chickpeas can be useful if you are avoiding meat. However, their protein is not as ideally suited to human needs as animal protein is, and does not contain sufficient amounts of certain amino acids. Fortunately these particular amino acids are found abundantly in grains, so combining chickpeas with wheat, rice or another grain creates a balanced meal that fulfils protein requirements (see p.349). If you are unable to eat grains, then nuts and seeds would help to compensate, or simply eat extra-generous helpings of beans and chickpeas which will supply adequate amounts of all the amino acids. Combining beans or chickpeas with a little animal protein (eg. cheese or yoghurt) will also overcome the problem.

Coco-yams – see *Dasheen*

Coffee substitutes

If you need to give up coffee, health food shops sell several coffee-substitutes such as dandelion coffee (from the roasted root) or Barleycup, Yarrow or Pioneer (made from roasted barley and chicory). Unfortunately these, too, may affect you if you drink them frequently.

Cornmeal or maize meal

Cornmeal can be prepared as polenta and served with fish, stews or casseroles. To make polenta:

1. Combine 115 gm (4 oz) maize meal with a level teaspoon each of salt and mild paprika, and a tiny pinch of cayenne.
2. Mix in 1/4 litre (1/2 pint) of water, adding the water slowly to prevent lumps forming.
3. Steam in a double-boiler, or put a small pan (containing the maize meal) inside a larger one containing an inch or two of water to get the same effect as a double boiler.
4. After 30 minutes, turn out into a greased baking dish and bake for 10 to 15 minutes at 170°C, (350°F, Gas Mark 4).
5. Pour a few spoons of juice from the casserole over the top, add a layer of grated cheese, then put under the grill to brown.

Dasheen

This root, and its close relatives, are variously known as dasheen, eddo, taro, cocoyam, tannia and yautia. There are actually two different species, but they are closely related. One has pink flesh, the other white, and they differ in size and shape, being either symmetrical and bulbous or rather knobbly and irregular. They make a very acceptable substitute for potato and other starchy foods. The texture is agreeable, and the flavour similar to potato but slightly nutty. The pink fleshed kind do turn a rather dismal blue-grey colour when cooked, but they taste just as good.

Peel and dice them, then boil in salted water for about 15 minutes. They can also be baked whole, at 180°C (375°F, Gas Mark 5) for about 1–1½ hours. The flavour is stronger when cooked in this way, rather like baked potato.

Dried fruit

Dried fruits are a good substitute for sweet snacks such as cakes and biscuits, if you need to avoid wheat, milk or eggs. Combine them with **nuts** (p.218) or **seeds** (p.221) for a tea-time treat, or to replace chocolate. If you have to avoid grapes, more exotic dried fruits are now available in some supermarkets, including mango, peaches, blueberries and pineapple. Figs and dates are also useful.

Unfortunately, drying fruit destroys almost all its Vitamin C, so you should also eat some fresh fruit as well.

Egg substitutes

If you react to hen's eggs, you may find you can tolerate those of other birds such as duck or quail. However proceed with caution and test them alone before putting them in recipes. If you have ever suffered symptoms suggestive of a true allergic reaction to hen's eggs (eg. tingling or swelling of the lips, nettle rash, difficulty in breathing) you should not try other types of egg.

There are various ways to substitute for eggs in baking. In biscuit recipes, try 2 tablespoons of water, 1 tablespoon of vegetable oil and ½ tablespoon of baking-powder to replace one egg. A little buckwheat flour mixed with water can replace the binding quality of eggs in some recipes. See also **cakes** (p.210).

In some puddings where eggs are used for setting the mixture, you can use gelatine instead. Dissolve one teaspoon in a little warm water to replace one egg.

You can also buy ready-made egg substitutes and egg-white replacers, by mail-order (see p.432 for addresses) or from good health food shops. These are intended for cake-making and do not reproduce the flavour of eggs.

Check that you are eating other foods capable of replacing the vitamins obtained from eggs (see p.195).

Flour

There are a number of flours now available to substitute for wheat flour, but these need to be used carefully as they do not have the same cooking properties as wheat flour. Basically, there are the white, starchy, low-protein flours and the darker high-protein flours. For breads and pastries you normally need a combination of the two, while each type is sometimes useful on its own. See also **thickeners** (p.224).

In the low-protein group are rice flour, potato flour, tapioca flour and sago flour. These can be used to thicken puddings, sauces, soups and stews. They are relatively tasteless, more or less interchangeable and uniformly low in protein. As protein is the element which causes doughs to bind and rise, all of these flours need help from one of the high-protein flours to make even the most rudimentary breads or biscuits.

The second group, the high-protein flours, are generally made from pulses (beans and lentils), with the exception of buckwheat flour. They include gram flour, chickpea flour, soya flour and lentil flour. Buckwheat flour has a dark greyish colour and a strong, smokey taste that needs to be well diluted with other flours. Soya and gram flour, though milder in taste, also benefit from mixing with the white flours. Finally, experiment with the sweeter flours like carob, chestnut and yam flours. Carob is very useful in desserts, biscuits and cakes where it gives a chocolatey flavour.

See also **biscuits** (p.206), **bread** (p.206), **cakes** (p.210), **pancakes** and **waffles** (p.219), **Pastry** (p.219).

Milk and cream substitutes

Some people who are sensitive to cow's milk find they are able to tolerate goat's milk or sheep's milk. Experiment cautiously with these, especially if you have not drunk milk for some time – you may well have stopped producing lactase, the enzyme that breaks down milk sugar (lactose). If you have, a sudden influx of milk will result in diarrhoea, because the lactose goes through to the intestine undigested and gives bacteria in the gut flora an unaccustomed feast. This bout of diarrhoea may give the impression of a true intolerance to the milk (that is, an intolerance to its proteins) rather than a temporary intolerance to lactose sugar. Your production of lactase enzyme can be built up again by drinking very small amounts of milk at first and gradually increasing the quantity consumed.

Goat's milk is sold in most health food shops and goat's milk powder is available by post. Unfortunately, suppliers are not covered by the same sort of health regulations that govern cow's-milk production, and it is a good idea to boil goat's milk before use, especially if giving it to children. There are some other drawbacks to this product. Firstly it has a very rank 'goaty' taste that takes quite a bit of getting used to. Secondly, it can easily provoke reactions in people who are already sensitive to cow's milk. Thirdly, it is rather high in saturated fat and, like goat's cheese, should only be used sparingly.

Sheep's milk may be found in health food shops in some areas. It has a much less pungent flavour than goat's milk and is pleasantly creamy. Unlike cow's milk, it freezes well, so you can buy it in frozen form. This milk can provoke cross-reactions in those sensitive to cow's milk, but it is less likely to do so than goat's milk.

Rice milk is a relatively new product that is now being sold in health food shops. It has a far more agreeable taste than soya milk (see below) although it is distinctively rice-flavoured. It is quite watery, and a dash of tinned coconut milk, or a little coconut powder (see below) will improve the consistency enormously. No calcium is added to rice milk, so it is a very poor source of this mineral: a calcium supplement may be advisable.

Soya milk is manufactured from finely ground soya beans, and its origin is evident in the strong, beany flavour. Most brands have some sugar added. It is obtainable from most health food shops and some supermarkets. To make your own, mix 165 gm (5 oz) of soya flour to a paste with a few spoonfuls of water. Gradually add 1 litre (1½ pints) of water, bring slowly to the boil, stirring continuously, then simmer for 20 minutes, stirring from time to time. Add a teaspoonful of honey, and vanilla essence if liked; store in the refrigerator.

Soya can readily provoke allergic/intolerant reactions, so it is not advisable to eat too much of any soya product.

Soya desserts and 'yoghurt' are also available. Sugar-free forms of soya milk, and concentrated soya milk, are both available by post. Ordinary soya milk is a poor source of calcium, but 'fortified' versions are now available (see p.317).

Creamed coconut is sold in supermarkets and Indian groceries, and in some health food shops. It can be used as a substitute for cream, if mixed with a small amount of warm water. Or you can just grate it directly onto fruit salad, chopped bananas etc. Unfortunately, it is loaded with saturated fat, but for an occasional treat it is quite acceptable. Delicatessens and some supermarkets now sell various Thai coconut products, including tinned 'coconut milk', and coconut powder which is made up with water to produce a milk-like drink. Again, these products are high in saturated fat.

Ground almonds can also be made into a cream substitute. Mix them to a paste with water and a little honey, then add more water until you get the right consistency.

Unroasted cashew nuts can be ground and mixed with water to form a cream substitute. Add honey and vanilla to taste. Dilute further to make cashew 'milk'.

'Milks' based on almonds and cashews contain a little calcium, but coconut cream does not. If using any of these substitutes, and eating no dairy products, you need to take a calcium supplement, or eat large helpings of other calcium-containing foods (see p.317). Check that other vitamins normally obtained from milk are not lacking in your diet (see p.197).

Millet

Millet is a tiny yellow grain. Although it can provoke cross-reactions with other grains, these are unusual, so it is a useful substitute if you are sensitive to wheat or rice.

Wash the grains well, soak overnight, wash again and cook in twice their volume of salted water. Bring to the boil and then simmer gently for about 20 minutes. Millet can be seasoned and served like rice as an accompaniment to various savoury dishes, or made into porridge for breakfast.

Cooked millet can be added to soups and casseroles to thicken them. Millet can also substitute for wheat flour in a cheese soufflé: make in the usual way, using 115 gm (4 oz) cooked millet, 3 eggs, 55 gm (2 oz) cheese, 140 ml (1/4 pint) milk, salt and pepper. Bake for 20 minutes with the soufflé dish in a tray of water.

If you are able to eat nuts, these 'millet burgers' are delicious. To make millet burgers:

1. Cook 225 gm (8 oz) of millet as above, but use a level teaspoon of salt.

2. While still hot, add half a jar (about 150 gm – 5$^{1}/_{4}$ oz) of sugar-free peanut butter (or another nut butter), and one level teaspoon of sesame seeds, already toasted (see p.221).
3. Mix the ingredients together well, using a potato masher to break up the millet.
4. Take a piece of the mixture – about the size of a small egg – roll it between your palms and then squash flat, pressing hard. It is vital to do this while the millet is still warm, as it becomes unworkable when cold. These quantities make about 30 burgers.
5. Fry the 'millet burgers' in oil over a low heat, turning them twice and allowing at least 20 minutes total frying time – this gives the outside a lovely crunchy texture. Use a non-stick pan or they may stick.

The burgers can be made in bulk and frozen unfried; they do not need to be defrosted before being fried. Although making a large batch is fairly time-consuming, it is well worth it as they are both delicious and filling. Four or five make the basis of a good breakfast or lunch.

Nuts and nut butters

If you have a true allergy to any kind of nut, including peanuts, you should not eat other nuts, because the chance of a cross-reaction is high, and nut allergy is potentially fatal. Those with *intolerance* to nuts, rather than allergy, may find that they can eat another type of nut, without ill-effects, but experiment cautiously, testing each kind of nut individually.

Unusual kinds of nuts may be worth testing, such as macadamia nuts, sold in many large supermarkets. Also look for pine nuts and unsalted pistachios, available in health food shops. Alternatively, try out some of the seeds, such as sunflower seeds. They are an excellent source of Vitamin E and some B vitamins.

Various novel kinds of nut butter are now on sale in health food shops, including almond butter, pecan butter, hazelnut butter and cashew butter. These are a good substitute for peanut butter, if you have peanut intolerance. Spreads made from seeds, such as tahini (sesame seeds) and sunflower seed spread, are also worth trying. See p.301 for information on their Vitamin E content which varies widely.

Nuts help to fill the gap left by biscuits and cakes if you find you must avoid wheat. They can be baked into flapjacks if you are able to eat oats (see **biscuits**, p.206.).

Do not eat too much of any one kind of nut: ring the changes.

If you are unable to eat *any* nuts or seeds, a Vitamin E supplement may be advisable. Check that other nutrients are not lacking (see p.198).

Pancakes and waffles

Pancakes and waffles can be made from rye flour if you are sensitive to wheat. Pass the flour through a fine sieve before making the batter, to remove some of the bran fragments and make the pancakes lighter.

Satisfactory pancakes can also be made with maize or barley flour, and taste good although they are slightly rubbery – beat plenty of air into the mixture just before frying to improve the texture. Buckwheat flour is fairly protein-rich and makes a good pancake batter, but should be mixed with other flours (see **flour**, p.215) to dilute the strong taste. Gluten-free mixes for pancakes can be bought by post (see p.432) and generally give excellent results.

Pasta

There are several sorts of non-wheat noodles that are not too difficult to come by. Chinese food-suppliers sell bean-thread or 'transparent' noodles which are made from mung beans. They also offer rice noodles but these may contain wheat starch so check the label carefully if you are sensitive to wheat. Neither of these products need cooking. Soak rice noodles in warm water for 15 minutes and bean-thread noodles for 5 minutes.

'Soba' noodles, made from buckwheat, may be bought from Japanese suppliers. Delicatessens or health food shops may also sell some of these products, and many stock buckwheat spaghetti. Some health food shops now sell rye pasta too.

Pasta made with gluten-free flour is obtainable by post – see p.432 for addresses.

Some health food shops now sell a new range of wheat-free pasta products, aimed specially at those with wheat sensitivity. Some varieties are based on maize or other cereals, others on bean flours making them suitable for anyone with a general sensitivity to grains.

Pastry

Pastry can be made with rye flour although it is heavier than pastry made with wheat, partly because rye flour is only available in wholemeal form. Putting the rye flour through a fine sieve first improves the quality by removing the larger pieces of bran from the flour. Adding some baking powder helps too. Alternatively, try the following recipe for pastry:

1. Mix together 113 gm (4 oz) rye flour, 57 gm (2 oz) ground almonds, 57gm (2 oz) cornflour, 85 gm (3 oz) hard margarine or butter, 1 beaten egg (use a duck egg, or an egg substitute if necessary), 1 teaspoon bicarbonate of soda and 1 teaspoon dried pectin powder (omit pectin if not available, but it makes the pastry lighter).
2. Mix all ingredients in a blender, adding as much cold water as needed to make a dough (about 1 or 2 tablespoons).
3. Roll out carefully between two sheets of greaseproof paper, as the dough is very fragile. Lift the pastry by draping it over a rolling pin.
4. Cheese can be added to make a topping for savoury pies.

Gluten-free mixes for pastry can be bought by post (see p.432 for addresses).

Plantains

Plantains look like large green bananas and may be bought from West Indian groceries. They are quite difficult to peel (use a knife) and need to be fried, boiled, or baked as for yams. They are savoury, not sweet, and can be used as a substitute for potatoes or rice.

Porridge

If you are unable to eat oats, a hot breakfast cereal based on maize meal can be bought in some health food shops. Alternatively, **millet** (see p.217) can be made into a porridge. Both these are grains, so watch for cross-reactions.

Pumpkin

Pumpkin is widely available from greengrocers in the autumn. It can be made into soups, or incorporated into pies and stews. Pumpkin can be used in place of potatoes, although it needs special handling to overcome its sweet, cloying quality: see the suggestions made for **sweet potatoes** (p.222). It can be baked whole, or chopped up and boiled in salted water.

Quorn

This is a new high-protein food, designed to act as a meat substitute for vegetarians. It is made from a specially cultivated type of fungus. Quorn is usually purchased in ready-made meals, with full cooking instructions on the package. If you are sensitive to yeast or mushrooms, you might experience a cross-reaction because these are also fungi.

Sago and tapioca

If you are sensitive to grains and miss rice or semolina puddings, these can be used instead.

Pearl sago and pearl tapioca are obtainable from many health food shops and from most large supermarkets. Both can be made into puddings with milk, or a milk substitute.

Seeds

These are a good source of many B vitamins, and sunflower seeds are especially rich in Vitamin E. **Sunflower seeds**, in particular, offer a simple and inexpensive way of boosting your nutrient and antioxidant intake. They are especially useful nutritionally in replacing nuts, for those who are allergic or intolerant of nuts.

If you have to avoid biscuits and crackers, seeds can help to replace such snacks. Wholefood shops generally sell sunflower and **pumpkin seeds**. Some sell sunflower seeds roasted in oil with soy sauce added: if you can eat soya, these are especially tasty.

Seeds can be added to muesli, or eaten with nuts and dried fruit for a tea-time snack.

Sesame seeds are rather small to eat as a snack but can be added to various baked items, both sweet and savoury. Toasting them under the grill before use gives them a strong and very special flavour that enhances most food: watch them carefully and remove from the grill as soon as they are golden brown. Unhulled sesame seeds are a very good source of calcium (see p.317). If you are of an allergic disposition do not eat sesame seeds too often, as they can provoke allergies. Note that they are *not* a good source of Vitamin E (see p.301).

Sorghum

This grain is not widely available, but can be bought by post (see p.432 for addresses). Cook it in the same way as millet.

Soya

Shops now offer soya-derived 'milk', margarine, 'yoghurt', dessert, meat substitute, flour, egg substitute and so on, but it is important not to eat too much soya. Unfortunately this bean can easily provoke intolerant or allergic reactions so it must not be seen as the ultimate solution to the problem of substituting for dairy products, wheat or meat. Watch out for the 'hidden' soya too (see p.201). Remember that tofu is made from it, as is textured vegetable protein (TVP). Check the ingredients of vegetarian burgers, risottos, sausage rolls and the pre-packed mixes for these – they are likely to contain soya.

Stock cubes

These usually contain yeast but some health food shops now sell a yeast-free vegetable 'bouillon' mix in the form of a powder or paste. This can also be obtained by post (see p.432). The paste can also replace spreads like Marmite.

You can, of course, make your own stock in the traditional way. Use the bones and other waste from meat or poultry. Boil them for about 1 hour with herbs and leave to cool, then skim off the fat, remove all the bones, strain, season and freeze.

Sweet potatoes

Sweet potatoes are available from West Indian and Chinese groceries, as well as from larger supermarkets. The skins range from white to yellow to red-purple, which is the most common variety sold in Britain. The flesh may be white or yellow: the yellow ones generally have a better flavour and are much richer in beta-carotene, an antioxidant (see p.339). Sweet potatoes are quite a good source of Vitamin E, useful for those who cannot eat nuts or seeds.

Peel them before cooking and keep them under water as they discolour instantly. They may be boiled, steamed, or deep-fried, and they cook surprisingly quickly. Alternatively, bake the roots whole in the oven at 190°C (375°F, Gas Mark 5), and peel when cooked. You can cook a large batch and then freeze portions to be reheated in different ways when desired. They have a sweet taste which is delicious when countered by a tart or acidic dressing. Try them with tomatoes, sharp fruit juices, a flavoured vinegar, mustard, sour cream or yoghurt.

Chinese cooks make a soup by boiling sweet potatoes in water or stock until they disintegrate and flavouring the liquid with root ginger.

The Chinese also make a delicious snack called deep-fried sweet potato balls. To make sweet potato balls:

1. Boil some sweet potatoes until soft.
2. Mash them and add rice flour (or wheat flour) to make a stiff dough.
3. Take a small piece of the dough, press it down flat, put a half-teaspoonful of peanut butter (or another nut butter) in the centre and seal the dough around it.
4. Roll in sesame seeds and deep fry in vegetable oil.

Tahini

This is a paste made from sesame seeds, sold in health food shops. It may be stiff or runny, light or dark. The darker tahini has a more pungent flavour, while the light, creamed tahini is quite mild-tasting and can substitute for butter. It is a very adaptable food but a poor source of Vitamin E given its content of polyunsaturated fat (see p.301) and needs to be combined with a good Vitamin E source, such as sunflower seeds or spread. Sesame can readily provoke allergy or intolerance, so it should not be eaten too often.

Taramasalata

This is a Greek dish, made with smoked fish roe, olive oil, lemon juice and garlic. It can be a useful sandwich filling in place of cheese. If you are wheat-sensitive, note that most taramasalata contains breadcrumbs. It also contains preservatives, and is often tinted a bright pink with artificial colourings. Some shops (eg. Sainsbury's) sell uncoloured taramasalata. To make wheat-free taramasalata:

1. Combine 125 gm (4 oz) smoked cod's roe with 120 ml (8 tablespoons) of olive oil and the juice of one lemon, adding a clove of crushed garlic for flavour.
2. Use a blender to turn the mixture into a creamy paste.

Tea substitutes

Try redbush or *rooibosch* tea, which contains little tannin and no caffeine. It tastes much like ordinary tea, with a good robust flavour and colour. 'Bancha' tea, sold as tea-bags, or as twigs which are boiled in water, is similar to ordinary black tea and contains very little caffeine. Any of these, however, may still affect those who are tea-sensitive. Explore the possibilities of herbal teas. Some are rich in vitamins (like rosehip tea), while others have sedative or digestive properties (like limeflower and peppermint respectively).

Thickeners

Sago flour can be useful as a thickener for soups, sauces and stews. If not on sale in your local health food shop, it is obtainable by post (see p.432 for addresses).

Arrowroot is increasingly difficult to find but it is sold in some delicatessens. This makes an excellent thickener.

Rice flour, potato flour, barley flour and rye flour are sold in some health food shops and can all be used as thickeners, although they need to be used with care as they tend to go lumpy more readily than cornflour. Gram flour, chestnut flour and yam flour can also be used.

Wild rice

This long dark grain is only distantly related to ordinary rice and should not cause cross-reactions, but be alert to possible adverse effects if you are depending on it a lot. It is rather strong and earthy in taste, which (along with the high price) tends to stop people eating too much of it. Wash the grains well and cook in salted water for 45 minutes. A small knob of butter and a little orange juice added to the cooked grain complement the strong flavour.

Yams

The yams sold in Britain are usually very large cylindrical vegetables (about the size of a vegetable marrow), although there are more bulbous or irregularly shaped varieties. All have white flesh and a thin dark brown skin. They can be diced and boiled in salted water for about 20 minutes, but are quite difficult to peel and chop even for those without arthritic fingers. One simple way around this problem is to bake the yam whole. Wash the root and cover the cut end, if there is one, with tinfoil. Bake at 190°C (375°F, Gas Mark 5) for 2–3 hours depending on the size of the root. Test the root with a blunt-ended knife to see if it is cooked right through. As soon as the yam is cool enough to handle, peel it and dice the flesh. If you have a freezer, the cooked yam can be frozen in small portions. For a quick meal, the pieces of yam can be fried slowly from frozen, or toasted under the grill. Try sautéed pieces dipped in a sauce.

For flavour and texture, yams are one of the best potato substitutes. They do have a slightly bitter aftertaste, but this is not unpleasant once you are used to it.

If buying from a small shop where the root vegetables are not labelled, make sure that you are buying yam rather than cassava. The latter is also cylindrical, but much more slender. Cassava (see p.211) must be boiled, not baked.

Yeast substitutes

See **bread** (p.206) for yeast-free alternatives. See also **stock cubes** (p.222).

Chapter 2.6

WEIGHT-REDUCING DIETS

It is a popular myth that you cannnot lose weight without vigorous exercise. This myth causes enormous suffering to many people with arthritis, especially osteoarthritis, because the degree of pain they experience is made much worse by being overweight, yet they feel they can do nothing to improve their situation.

Thousands of people with arthritis suffer unecessary levels of pain because the extra pounds they are carrying put extra pressure on their damaged joints. Even a few pounds of fat can make a big difference: when walking, as each foot hits the ground, the pressure felt by the knee and hip joint of that leg is equivalent to *four times* the body weight. So being ten pounds overweight puts forty pounds of extra pressure on each knee and hip joint. And it does so at every step. During certain actions, the load on one part of the knee is even higher: 7–8 times the weight of the body.

Being overweight seems also to have some other, more subtle effect on osteoarthritis, because it aggravates the disease in joints such as the fingertips, which are non-weight-bearing. So there is a second motivation for shedding weight and becoming slimmer. Less pain will mean more mobility, with general improvements in health and fitness – so it is well worth the effort. Apart from these benefits, the risks of heart disease, diabetes, and high blood pressure will all be reduced.

Gout sufferers are also well advised to lose weight, but it is important that they follow special guidelines, which are given on pp.244–5. Certain kinds of slimming diet can actually provoke gout attacks.

As for other forms of arthritis and arthralgia, anyone who is greatly overweight, and who has symptoms in the hips, knees or ankles, is likely to benefit from weight loss.

Anyone who is of normal weight, or underweight, should not embark on this diet. If you are not sure, consult Figure 1 which shows the range of weights that are considered 'normal and healthy' for someone of your height and build. Another rough-and-ready check is to see how much spare flesh you can grip on your midriff – just above the waist. Using your thumb and forefinger, take hold of this roll of flesh and see how thick the gripped layer is – it should be about 2.5 cm (1 inch) or less. If you can can 'pinch more than an inch' then you are probably overweight.

Should you be in any doubt about whether it is wise for you to undertake a weight-reducing diet, consult your doctor. (This is particularly important for anyone with rheumatoid arthritis or another form of inflammatory arthritis; see p.69)

Figure 1

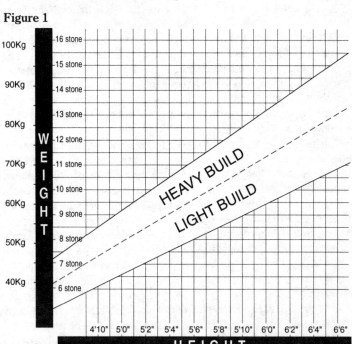

· *Slimming Without Exercise* ·

Women's magazines, exercise videos and popular diet books all advocate exercise as an important part of losing weight. In a sense they are right – vigorous exercise does burn off a lot of calories quickly, so it speeds up the slimming process. It also tones up muscles, and really strenuous exercise increases the metabolic rate even after the session is over, which means that more calories are burned just staying alive.

But the down side of all this publicity is that many people have become convinced that you can't lose weight without exercise. This is simply not true.

Everything we do uses up energy – walking around the house, turning over in bed – even the things we scarcely notice such as breathing, blinking and pumping blood round the body with the beats of the heart. Maintaining our bodies at a warm temperature day and night, which we all have to do even in the warmest house, uses up huge amounts of energy. Even thinking burns off the odd calorie or two!

All that is required to lose weight is that you reduce your calorie intake to slightly less than than your calorie requirement. The current recommendations are that you eat about 500–1,000 calories less per day than your energy requirements. This should produce a weight loss of 0.5–1 kg (1–2 lbs) per week. You may think it is nothing dramatic, but over a period of months it builds up to a substantial loss of weight.

There are two major advantages to losing weight in this gradual way rather than going on any sort of 'crash diet'. Firstly, after the initial shock of changing your eating habits has passed, you should find that you get used to the new regime and scarcely notice being hungry. Secondly, once you have reached your target weight, you wll find it easy to stay there because you have retrained your eating habits, over a long period of time, into healthier and slimmer habits which should be easy to maintain.

· *Losing Weight and Staying Thin* ·

The problem with losing weight is that, all too often, it goes straight back on once the 'diet' ends. This happens because a slimming diet is mistakenly seen as a short-term effort, a 'quick fix'. The truth is that excess weight is a long-term problem and it needs a long-term solution. After all, you probably put the weight on over a period of several years, perhaps even decades – it is unrealistic to expect to lose it all in a few weeks, then go back to your old eating habits (the habits that put the extra pounds there in the first place) without gaining weight once again.

Losing weight *for ever* should be the objective, and this requires a fundamental re-education of your appetite. This chapter explains how to achieve this, but it does not give you detailed menus and recipes, unlike the kinds of diets found in magazines. The reason is that strict menus can only ever be followed for a very short time. To stay thin you need a new set of instinctive eating habits that automatically keep you thin – not a fixed diet pinned to the kitchen cupboard that you follow religiously for a couple of weeks and then abandon.

· *Know Yourself and Know Your Food* ·

The two key steps to losing weight are knowing what you eat, and knowing how fattening different foods are. Before starting to diet, spend two or three days observing your normal eating patterns. Use a small notebook and make a note of everything you eat and drink – *absolutely everything*. For meals eaten at home, weigh your portions, or measure them out, so you have an exact quantity. Work out the calorie content of everything you eat and write this in the notebook. If you are unable to do it at the time, sit down each evening and fill in the calorie values. Then add up the total calories for the day.

Many packaged foods have the calorie content marked in a food information panel on the side. These can be very useful, but be careful to check whether the calories quoted are for the entire contents of the packet, or per 100 gm (3½ oz). Frequently, it is for 100 gm, and you can go badly wrong on calorie-counting if the packet contains 250 gm! For other foods, use Table 11, on pp.237–241, to obtain calorie values.

If the calorie values for the different days are not roughly the same, then continue with calorie counting for a few days more, to get a representative sample. Finally, calculate the average for the days recorded (by adding up the totals and then dividing by the number of days).

Magazines often give advice about the number of calories needed per day, but of course the actual value varies enormously, depending on how active you are, how well you absorb and process food, and whether you have a 'fast' or a 'slow' metabolism. Your best guide to how many calories you should eat is the average value you have calculated over the past few days: from now on you need to eat about *40% less* than this. Table 10 (p.230) can be used to work out your calorie target for the future. If, after a month of dieting, you have not lost any weight, then you should reduce your intake by a further 40%. Do not eat fewer than 800 calories per day.

Table 10: Calorie reduction levels

Present calorie intake	Reduction of 40%
4,000	2,400
3,900	2,340
3,800	2,280
3,700	2,220
3,600	2,160
3,500	2,100
3,400	2,040
3,300	1,980
3,200	1,920
3,100	1,860
3,000	1,800
2,900	1,740
2,800	1,680
2,700	1,620
2,600	1,560
2,500	1,500
2,400	1,440
2,300	1,380
2,200	1,320
2,100	1,260
2,000	1,200
1,900	1,140
1,800	1,080
1,700	1,020
1,600	960
1,500	900

· *Friendly Foods and Enemy Foods* ·

Keeping track of what you eat for a few days will give you some insight into the calorie content of different foods. When you begin to diet, you should continue the habit of checking calorie values for a while, until you get to the point where you know – without having to think too hard – which foods are the most fattening.

Try to think of these as 'enemy foods', and of the least fattening foods as 'friendly foods'. A piece of chocolate fudge cake or a bowl of ice cream is an enemy in disguise – like the Trojan horse, it looks very desirable, but hidden inside it is pain and increasing disablity. Long after the pleasant taste has faded from your memory, you will still feel the pain in your hips or knees, from carrying the extra pounds.

The principal enemies in food are fats and oils, which contain twice as many calories, weight for weight, as starch (the main constituent of potato, rice and pasta) or protein (the main constituent of lean meat, white fish and egg white). Many people avoid greasy chips and thick layers of butter on their bread, but fall victim to the 'hidden fats' in foods such as cake, cheesecake, mousses, other creamy desserts, biscuits, quiche and pies. Cheese, eggs, sausages, crisps, rich sauces or thick gravy, mayonnaise and salad cream are also full of hidden fat. Some types of yoghurt, such as Greek yoghurt, are extremely fatty. Again, looking at the labels on packaged food can be a real education. Note that most margarine contains just as much fat as butter: you need to buy a 'low fat spread' to get fewer calories.

The 'richer' something tastes, the more fat it contains. Beware of foods such as cookies, sold loose – they can contain much more fat than standard biscuits. Food sold loose may also come in larger portions than that in packets – if possible, weigh the item before estimating the calorie content. Cheating is all too easy – buying yourself a sumptuous giant double-chocolate cookie while out shopping, but reckoning the calories as if it was an ordinary biscuit for example. There is no point at all in cheating if the price you have to pay is pain.

When it comes to meat and fish, choose lean meat such as chicken or turkey breast, rather than fatty meat such as lamb. White fish is preferable to oily fish while you are slimming. When roasting meat or poultry, place it on a rack over a baking tray, so that the fat drains away. The toasting rack from a grill pan can be used for this purpose.

The other enemy, apart from fat, is sugar. Foods that contain a great deal of hidden fat, such as cakes and desserts, are often loaded with sugar as well, making them doubly fattening. Colas and other soft drinks are also full of sugar, and one or two cans a day will pile on a lot of extra calories. Sparkling water or 'diet' colas are a sensible alternative.

Quite apart from soft drinks, there may be a significant number of calories from drinks generally, especially if you take cream and sugar in coffee, for example. Be careful to note every cup and keep track of the calories they contain.

Friendly foods

Among the 'friendly foods' are fruits and vegetables, which, as well as being low in calories, are rich in vitamins, fibre and other nutrients. While cutting down on fattening foods, you can bulk up your main meals with extra servings of tasty vegetables – serve two or even three different kinds, rather than just one, to make meals more interesting and varied. The vegetables should not be cooked with oil, nor served with a knob of butter or margarine. If you boil them for a shorter time than usual, so that they are still quite crisp and crunchy, they will fill you up more (as well as being more nutritious).

Fruit makes an excellent alternative to calorie-rich snacks such as cakes and biscuits. If your teeth can cope with them, raw carrots or celery sticks are also extremely useful in warding off hunger pangs, by giving you something to chew on. Should you feel especially empty, a banana is very filling, but remember that it contains rather more calories than most fruit. Grapes, cherries and mangoes are rich in sugar, and should not be eaten in huge quantities, while avocado pears are almost entirely composed of oil, and therefore very fattening. Dried fruit such as raisins, and fruit tinned in syrup or cooked with sugar are also high-calorie foods. Other foods, often thought of as vegetables, which are actually high in calories, include baked beans, corn-on-the-cob, sweetcorn, parsnips and processed peas.

Surprisingly, perhaps, another type of 'friendly food' is anything that is rich in starch (also called 'complex carbohydrate'). Potatoes, rice, pasta and bread all fall into this category. Although they contain more calories than fruit or green vegetables, they are a useful part of any weight-reducing diet. The idea that such starch foods are 'fattening' is now considered mistaken and out-dated: as long as they are not smothered in butter, oil or rich sauce, they are relatively low in calories. One of their advantages is that they give a satisfactory 'full' feeling which ultimately helps with weight loss.

Choose your starchy foods carefully. Chips should be rejected in favour of boiled or baked potatoes (with a minimal scrape of butter). Plain rice is preferable to pilau rice, fried rice or egg fried rice. Fried bread is loaded with fat, whereas you can choose how much butter or margarine you spread onto toast. Slice your bread more thickly, and eat fewer slices: one thick slice spread with butter gives you less fat than two thin slices, both buttered.

· *Beginning the Diet* ·

Decide to start dieting on a particular day and stick to your decision as best you can. You should devise your own strategy for reducing your calorie intake by 40%, based on your present eating habits. This is far from being a 'crash diet' – it will give you slow, steady weight loss which is much the best kind.

For many people, cutting out sweet snacks is the answer – these supply a remarkable number of calories. Choosing low-fat foods whenever possible also works very well. Many supermarkets now sell low-fat alternatives to various foods although you should check how 'low' they really are by scrutinising the label. Diet drinks, artificial sweeteners and diabetic jams can be useful if you have a sweet tooth, but the type of jam sold in health food shops and labelled 'no added sugar' is actually sweetened with concentrated fruit juice and is just as sugary and fattening as ordinary jam. If you cannot live without chocolate, there are brands made for diabetics that are low in sugar, although they still contain plenty of fat, which is a major source of calories in chocolate. Just eat a small amount.

Continue recording everything you eat and counting the calories to check that you have achieved your 40% reduction. You can begin to phase this out when you find that estimating the calories in a portion of food has become second nature.

Make sure you eat enough protein while dieting (see pp.350–351). Most of us get more than enough, and this is only a cause for concern if you are eating very little meat, fish, milk products or eggs. If your protein intake is not adequate, the body will draw on protein in your muscles to compensate, and the muscles will become 'wasted'.

Weigh yourself about once a week to see how things are going. Bear in mind that your weight fluctuates from day to day owing to changes in the water content of the body. Daily weighing can therefore be alarming, and is not recommended.

· *Adjusting to Change* ·

If you have been used to eating hearty meals, you may have particular problems initially because your stomach does not experience its customary sensation of fullness. After a week or two, this passes, as your stomach and nervous system accept the change in the *status quo*, and no longer demand that the stomach be stretched to maximum capacity at each meal. It is certainly not 'natural' to fill the stomach in this way on a regular basis. Our hunter-gatherer ancestors needed to be able to gorge themselves when they found a particularly good crop of berries or nuts, or when they killed a large animal, and the maximal extension of the stomach allowed such golden opportunities to be exploited. But eating this well every day is inappropriate for the human body and inevitably leads to obesity.

Apart from the feelings of emptiness, you will also experience some genuine hunger – you cannot hope to lose weight without doing so. But the body has ways of mobilising its fat stores, and as it begins to do so, your hunger pangs should subside. The hunger is usually a temporary reaction to food deprivation, before the natural metabolic process starts up. When you feel hungry, try to focus on the positive aspect of the situation. Instead of thinking 'I'm so hungry' or 'I must have something to eat', think to yourself 'This feeling of hunger is a good sign – it means I'm going to lose weight and that will mean less pain'. Don't sit around focussing on your hunger. Go out if you can, or keep active, take up a hobby, watch something absorbing on television, or read a good book – whatever takes your mind off food.

Don't abandon your efforts to lose weight simply because you have lapsed briefly and given in to temptation. Many people give up altogether because this happens, instead of accepting it as a temporary setback and carrying on with their weight-reducing programme.

You may find that you lose quite a lot of weight initially, but then the rate of loss slows down. There are various reasons for this. Firstly, the liver has stores of a short-term energy reserve, known as glycogen. This is used up first, and its breakdown also releases water, which is expelled in the urine producing a sharp loss of weight. Once the glycogen has been used up, fat is broken down instead, and then weight loss is more gradual. Your overall metabolic rate may also decrease as a direct response to eating less, which will slow weight loss even further. Try not to be discouraged by this – you will still be shedding pounds, even if the pace is more gradual. If you can manage some exercise, such as swimming, this may help to increase your metabolic rate.

Once you have lost the pounds and are about the right weight for your height, you can increase your calorie intake a little. But be aware that you are now entering the most dangerous stage and if you go back to your old ways the fat will simply accumulate once more. Start strict calorie counting again for a while, to ensure that you avoid this pitfall.

Part of the secret of losing weight and staying thin is to change eating *habits*, and when one thinks how difficult it is to break *any* habit, however trivial, one realises why people so often fail to slim. But knowing that you are involved in breaking a habit is very helpful, because you then know that all this food which you crave is not actually necessary to your body – it's just a habit. If you can tell yourself this, you will find it easier to resist the temptation to keep on eating as before.

One habit that many older people need to change is the frugality that leads them to finish up leftovers rather than throw any food away. Such habits were essential in wartime and have persisted among the generations that remember rationing. In the modern era of plenty, this habit can lead to weight gain, because you tend to eat food that you neither want nor need. A useful maxim, if you have trouble throwing food away, is 'It has to be got rid of sooner or later, and sooner will be much easier'.

· *Reasons for Eating* ·

Human beings eat for many different reasons, not just out of hunger. Very often our cravings for food arise from boredom, loneliness, sadness or discontent with life. Tiredness or overwork may lead us to gulp down coffee and chocolate biscuits in the hope of keeping awake. Or we may eat to comfort ourselves, or to calm down – there are a thousand reasons.

Recognising that food is answering an emotional need, or filling a gap of some kind, is often essential before weight can be lost. Accepting this opens up other possibilities for dealing with the emotional problems in more direct and constructive ways. It may help to talk to a counsellor, to your GP, or to a close friend. Simply writing your feelings and thoughts down in a diary can be very therapeutic.

Getting out of the house and spending more time in company can also be beneficial in taking your mind off problems. But you must then resist the social pressures that lead to overeating – learn to be strong about turning down cakes and other treats if these are offered. Joining a 'slimming club' may help keep your morale up and provide at least one social outing each week where overeating will not be possible. Ask your GP, or the local hospital, if a slimming club is being run on the NHS. If not, there are private clubs, although these may cost a little more to join.

'Comfort eating' may be a difficult habit to break. One way to deal with it, if you need to lose weight, is to buy something small but especially nice as your 'treat', and to eat it very slowly savouring every mouthful. In this way, you get as much enjoyment but far fewer calories.

Table 11: Checklist for calorie-counting

FOOD	AMOUNT	CALORIES
Fruit		
Apple, one fruit	142 gm (5 oz)	49
Banana, medium size	100 gm (3¹/2 oz)	79
Orange, one fruit	198 gm (7 oz)	70
Tangerine, one fruit	100 gm (3¹/2 oz)	34
Grapefruit, one fruit	340 gm (12 oz)	143
Fresh strawberries, portion	100 gm (3¹/2 oz)	26
Grapes, portion	100 gm (3¹/2 oz)	57
Peach, one fruit	142 gm (5 oz)	50
Pear, one fruit	170 gm (6 oz)	78
tinned in juice, portion	100 gm (3¹/2 oz)	33
Plum, one fruit	70 gm (2¹/2 oz)	24
stewed with sugar, portion	100 gm (3¹/2 oz)	75
Raw cherries, 3–4 fruits	28 gm (1 oz)	11
Kiwi fruit, fruit	8 gm (3 oz)	35
Honeydew melon, one slice	227 gm (8 oz)	40
Prunes, tinned in juice	per prune	10
Dried Fruit		
Raisins, one handful	57 gm (2 oz)	140
Sultanas, one handful	57 gm (2 oz)	143
Dried dates	per dried date	15
Dried apricots	per dried fruit	10
Dried figs	per dried fig	30
Starters and Snacks		
Half an avocado	100 gm (3¹/2 oz)	202
Corn-on-the-cob (whole cob, without butter)	198 gm (7 oz)	117
Olives	per black olive	3
Crisps	28 gm (1 oz) bag	135
One medium sausage roll	57 gm (2 oz)	202
Nuts and Seeds		
Almonds	per whole nut	10
Brazil nuts	per whole nut	20
Cashew nuts	per whole nut	15
Hazelnuts	per whole nut	8
Peanuts, roasted	per whole nut	5

FOOD	AMOUNT	CALORIES
Pecan nuts	per half nut	15
Walnuts	per half nut	15
Sesame seeds	28 gm (1 oz)	170
Sunflower seeds	28 gm (1 oz)	163
Beans and Lentils		
Baked beans, tinned in tomato sauce	128 gm (4^1/2 oz)	118
Kidney beans, tinned	128 gm (4^1/2 oz)	154
Lentils, cooked	85 gm (3 oz)	84
Vegetables		
Broccoli, steamed or boiled	113 gm (4 oz)	27
Carrots	per carrot	15
Cauliflower, boiled	170 gm (6 oz)	19
Celery, raw or boiled	per stick	5
Lettuce	43 gm (1^1/2 oz)	5
Leeks, raw or boiled	100 gm (3^1/2 oz)	24
Mushrooms, raw or tinned	100 gm (3 ^{1}/2 oz)	13
fried in butter	100 gm (3 ^{1}/2 oz)	157
Onions, fried	57 gm (2 oz)	196
Tomatoes, fresh or tinned	100 gm (3^1/2 oz)	17
Spinach, steamed	100 gm (3^1/2 oz)	30
Sweetcorn, tinned	85 gm (3 oz)	66
Garden peas, tinned	85 gm (3 oz)	42
Potatoes, Pasta and Rice		
French fries	100 gm (3^1/2 oz)	280
thick cut chips	100 gm (3^1/2 oz)	189
Baked potato, small	198 gm (7 oz)	150
Pasta, cooked	100 gm (3 ^{1}/2 oz)	163
White rice, average portion	128 gm (4 ^{1}/2 oz)	157
Risotto, cooked with oil, butter and stock	57 gm (2 oz)	238
Breads and Flour		
Wholemeal/brown bread	28 gm (1 oz)	60
	100 gm (3^1/2 oz)	215
	1 thick slice	90
White bread	28 gm (1 oz)	66
	100 gm (3^1/2 oz)	235
	1 thick slice	100

FOOD	AMOUNT	CALORIES
Granary bread	100 gm (3$\frac{1}{2}$ oz)	235
	1 thick slice	100
French stick	100 gm (3$\frac{1}{2}$ oz)	270
	1 slice (57 gm/2 oz)	154
One croissant	57 gm (2 oz)	190
One pitta bread, white	70 gm (2$\frac{1}{2}$ oz)	185
Poppadums	per item	52
White flour	100 gm (3$\frac{1}{2}$ oz)	340
Wholemeal flour	100 gm (3$\frac{1}{2}$ oz)	310
Raw oats	57 gm (2 oz)	228
Milk and Cream		
Butter	100 gm (3$\frac{1}{2}$ oz)	737
	5 ml (1 tsp)	35
Whole milk	568 ml (1 pint)	375
Semi-skimmed milk	568 ml (1 pint)	261
Skimmed milk	568 ml (1 pint)	187
Single cream	15 ml (1 tbsp)	30
Double cream	15 ml (1 tbsp)	67
Cheese		
Cheddar cheese	57 gm (2 oz)	230
Edam or Gouda cheese	57 gm (2 oz)	186
Brie or Camembert	57 gm (2 oz)	172
Danish blue cheese	57 gm (2 oz)	200
Parmesan cheese	28 gm (1 oz)	109
Yoghurt		
Natural yoghurt, low-fat	85 gm (3 oz)	48
Fruit or nut yoghurt	85 gm (3 oz)	75
Greek yoghurt, with honey	85 gm (3 oz)	144
Eggs		
One egg, boiled or poached	size 3 (57 gm/2 oz)	80
One egg, fried		100
One Scotch egg	113 gm (4 oz)	340
Butter, Oil and Margarine		
Margarine – all types	28 gm (1 oz)	207
	5 ml (1 tsp)	35

FOOD	AMOUNT	CALORIES
Oil – all types	28 ml (1 fl oz)	252
French dressing (vinaigrette)	15 ml (1 tbsp)	84

Meat and Meat Products

Lean minced beef (cooked, drained of fat)	28 gm (1 oz)	65
Trimmed beef steak (lean only, grilled)	28gm (1 oz)	47
average steak, grilled	142 gm (5 oz)	238
Roast beef (topside, lean only)	85 gm (3 oz)	132
Roast shoulder of lamb, lean	85 gm (3 oz)	165
Roast leg of pork, lean	85 gm (3 oz)	156
Grilled bacon	one rasher	65
Chipolata pork sausage, grilled	one sausage	90
Lean ham	28 gm (1 oz)	42
Liver pâté	28 gm (1 oz)	88
One small pork pie	70 gm (2½ oz)	270

Poultry

Turkey breast, roast	85 gm (3 oz)	108
Roast chicken, without skin	85 gm (3 oz)	123
Roast duck, meat only	85 gm (3 oz)	159
Roast goose, meat only	85 gm (3 oz)	267

Fish

Cod fillet, crumbed, baked	142 gm (5 oz)	266
steamed or baked	142 gm (5 oz)	134
Smoked haddock, steamed	142 gm (5 oz)	141
Whole herring, grilled	142 gm (5 oz)	190
Kipper, grilled or baked	85 gm (3 oz)	180
Mackerel fillet, grilled	100 gm (3½ oz)	172
Plaice, steamed fillet	113 gm (4 oz)	105
crumbed, fried	113 gm (4 oz)	258
Whole sole, steamed	213 gm (7½ oz)	194
Trout, grilled or baked	284 gm (10 oz)	250
Tuna, in brine, drained	85 gm (3 oz)	105
in oil, drained	85 gm (3 oz)	246

Cakes and Biscuits

Digestive biscuit	each	70
Gingernut biscuit	each	50

FOOD	AMOUNT	CALORIES
Chocolate chip biscuit	each	55
Chocolate digestive	each	85
Chocolate brownie	each	300
Danish pastry	each	360
Mince pie	each	235
Scone, plain	each	183

Preserves and Condiments

Honey	5 ml (1 teaspoon)	40
Jam	5 ml (1 teaspoon)	35
Peanut butter	28 gm (1 oz)	175
Sugar	5 ml (1 teaspoon)	20
Mayonnaise, traditional	15 ml (1 tbsp)	150
reduced calorie	15 ml (1 tbsp)	44
Pickle	15 ml (1 tbsp)	40
Salad cream	15 ml (1 tbsp)	50
Soy sauce	15 ml (1 tbsp)	50
Tomato ketchup	15 ml (1 tbsp)	20
Tomato purée	15 ml (1 tbsp)	13
Yeast extract	5 ml (1 teaspoon)	26

Sweets and Chocolates

Butter toffee popcorn	28 gm (1 oz)	112
Butterscotch	each	25
Toffees	each	35
Chocolate, milk or plain	28 gm (1 oz)	150

Drinks

Orange juice, unsweetened	(1/4 pint)	55
Apple juice, unsweetened	(1/4 pint)	55
Tomato juice, unsweetened	(1/4 pint)	30
Cola and other soft drinks	(1/2 pint)	110
Mug of hot chocolate or malted drink made with whole milk	(1/2 pint)	200
Milk shake made with whole milk	284 ml (1/2 pint)	245

Single measures of:

Whisky, Scotch, Bourbon	25 ml	50
Liqueurs	25 ml	85

FOOD	AMOUNT	CALORIES
Standard measures of:		
Dry sherry	50 ml	58
Sweet sherry	50 ml	68
Martini Bianco/Rosso	50 ml	90
Gin and tonic	50 ml of spirit	145
Whisky and dry ginger	50 ml of spirit	180
An average glass of:		
Red wine	142 ml (5 fl oz)	95
Dry white wine	142 ml (5 fl oz)	94
Sweet white wine	142 ml (5 fl oz)	133
Beer, draught	284 ml (1/2 pint)	90
Cider, dry	284 ml (1/2 pint)	102
vintage	284 ml (1/2 pint)	285
Popular Meals		
Fish and chips, oven baked	340 gm (12 oz)	600
Macaroni cheese	284 gm (10 oz)	370
Quiche, cheese	85 gm (3 oz)	333
Onion bhaji (small)	each	85
Chicken tikka masala	one	400
Lasagne	one	525
Pizza – Margherita	227 gm (8 oz)	544
Yorkshire pudding	57 gm (2 oz)	122
Steak and kidney pie	170 gm (6 oz)	456
McDonalds:		
Hamburger	each	250
Cheeseburger	each	300
Big Mac	each	550
French fries	regular portion	290
Ice-cream, Cornish vanilla	57 gm (2 oz)	110
Lemon meringue pie	113 gm (4 oz)	216
Chocolate mousse	113 gm (4 oz)	192
Crème caramel	113 gm (4 oz)	148

DIETS FOR GOUT

The causes of gout are explained on pages 103–6. Briefly, most gout sufferers have too much uric acid in the blood, which leads to crystals of urate forming. These may form in the joint and then stimulate the immune system, which provokes a severe bout of inflammation, causing pain, redness and swelling.

The majority of gout patients (but by no means all) are overweight and drink a fairly large amount of alcohol. Both these factors contribute to the formation of crystals, as explained on pages 105. For such patients, the first form of treatment is to reduce alcohol consumption and lose some weight. Guidelines are given below.

There is also a tiny minority of patients for whom a low-purine diet may be worth trying. Instructions for this are given on page 245. However, modern drug treatments are so effective and so safe that they should make long-term low-purine diets unecessary for most people.

On the other hand, eating a large helping of purines all at once could trigger off an attack of gout, and should be avoided. Anyone who has suffered from gout, even if they have not had an attack for some time, should avoid meals that are unusually rich in purines. Fortunately the list of high-purine foods (see p.105–6) is not very long. Try to memorise it so that you can always be aware of the risks which certain meals might pose.

· *Reducing Alcohol* ·

Initially, all alcoholic drinks should be drastically reduced. (The idea that only port causes gout is a myth – see p.247.) The best plan is to stop drinking regularly, but to allow the occasional drink, up to about 3–4 units of alcohol a week. (A unit corresponds to one glass of wine, half a pint of beer, or a single measure of spirits.)

Why is alcohol so damaging? Firstly, it increases the rate of purine production by the body. Secondly, the processing of alcohol by the body also leads to some chemical changes in the blood. One effect is to release lactic acid, which makes the blood very slightly more acidic and can spark off the crystallisation process. This is why attacks of gout often follow heavy drinking sessions. Thirdly, the lactic acid also reduces the ability of the kidneys to extract uric acid from the blood.

If you are a heavy drinker it may be difficult to reduce or give up alcohol, especially at first. Sometimes there are withdrawal symptoms such as anxiety, shaking or insomnia. In general these clear up after a few days, so it is worth persisting. If you feel you need help with these symptoms talk to your doctor, who may be able to prescribe a sedative, on a temporary basis, to see you through the most difficult phase.

Taking a vitamin and mineral supplement may also be helpful at this stage. Alcohol has long-term effects on the body's supply of B vitamins in particular, and a yeast-free B-complex supplement, rich in thiamine, is worth trying. Eat regularly and aim for well-balanced meals. If you need to lose weight as well, advice is given on the next page.

Some studies have shown that evening primrose oil can reduce the symptoms of alcohol withdrawal. It appears that prolonged use of alcohol disturbs the way in which the body processes fatty acids. The special types of fatty acid found in evening primrose oil may be able to alleviate this problem.

Drinking is often an integral part of our way of life – particularly our social life. Simply absenting yourself from the situations where you usually drink – such as parties and bars – may be the key to success. This will be easier if you create some attractive alternative to such situations, so take up a hobby, develop an existing interest, or try a new sporting activity.

If you take no exercise at present, try a little swimming, bicycling or walking. Exercise can give a marvellous sense of physical well-being, a real 'high', especially if you are out in the fresh air as well. However, a body that has had no exercise for a long time will probably react with horror to the initial shock. You may well feel ghastly for the first fifteen minutes, but *keep going* – that feeling passes and is replaced by some very positive benefits, both mental and physical.

Whatever you do in the way of exercise, keep it *gentle* and build up *gradually*. A sudden burst of intense and unaccustomed physical activity can provoke a new attack of gout. An injury to a joint can also precipitate an attack.

Can you drink more alcohol once you have lost weight and have been free of gout attacks for some time? This is a difficult question to answer, and you should discuss the matter with your doctor. You may be able to drink in moderation, particularly if you avoid beer (which is rich in purines). However, if you suffered from any withdrawal symptoms on giving up alcohol, this indicates some degree of addiction, so there is an argument for staying entirely 'dry'.

· *Losing Weight* ·

Carrying too much weight around with you can cause all kinds of medical problems, not just gout. Losing weight will have multiple rewards, in terms of health, well-being and appearance.

The diet should begin when you are not actually suffering from an attack of gout.

Be warned that a starvation diet or 'crash diet' is not advisable for anyone with gout. Starvation forces the body to break down its fat reserves very quickly and this leads to a change in the body chemistry known as ketosis.

During ketosis the blood becomes slightly more acidic – the change is extremely small, but it can be sufficient to cause the uric acid to crystallise out more easily. There are several much-advertised commercial diets, which rely on a liquid food – these are very low in calories and not at all suitable.

To lose weight gradually, you need to reduce your total food intake, to cut out most sugary foods, and to reduce fats and oils. Weight-for-weight, fats and oils contain over twice as many calories as protein or starch. So a knob of butter is twice as fattening as the same weight of chicken (a high-protein, low-fat food) or the same weight of potato (a high-starch, low-fat food). Remember that there is a lot of 'hidden fat' in foods such as cheese, eggs, sausages, pastries, chips, potato crisps, gravy, sauces, mayonnaise, salad cream, biscuits and cakes.

Most prepared foods now carry a detailed chart of nutritional information on the label which shows calories and fat content. If you want to calculate the number of calories eaten each day you can refer to pages 236–241 for the calorific value of various fresh and prepared foods.

Vegetables and salads are useful when dieting because they provide bulk without contributing too many calories. Raw carrots or celery sticks can be chewed, instead of biscuits, chocolate or other fattening snacks. Fruit should be eaten too, but not to excess: the type of sugar found in fruit (fructose), may lead to an attack of gout if consumed in large amounts. For the same reason, do not drink too much fruit juice. Certain fruits and vegetables are higher in calories than you might expect, notably bananas, grapes and avocado pears.

In general you should try to fill yourself up with simple, starchy (complex-carbohydrate) foods such as bread, pasta, rice, potatoes and oatmeal. If you generally eat a lot of meat you should cut this down a little and choose less fatty types of meat, such as chicken, turkey, and lean cuts of pork. Always leave the fat and just eat the meat.

Non-oily fish such as cod and plaice can be eaten, but avoid any of the high-purine fish such as herrings. Indeed, it is wise to stear clear of all foods that are high in purines (see below for a full list) until you have lost weight and are free of gout attacks.

High-protein diets are not advisable, as they can provoke an attack of gout. Some of the weight-reducing diets recommended in books and magazines rely on cutting out most fats and carbohydrates, so that almost all of your energy comes from protein foods such as meat and fish. These 'steak-and-salad' type diets are not a good idea for someone prone to gout.

If you feel you need additional help with losing weight refer to Chapter 2.6 (p.226).

· Low-Purine Diet ·

Losing weight and strictly reducing alcohol will clear up gout in most sufferers. For the rest – or for those few who are thin and teetotal to begin with – modern drug treatments are generally effective and trouble-free.

A restrictive low-purine diet is, therefore, rather outdated. Because a lot of the uric acid in our blood comes from the breakdown of our own purines (p.105), reducing dietary purines only makes a small impact on the uric acid level. In those with a very high uric acid level, owing to an inborn error of metabolism (p.106), avoiding high-purine foods will make little or no difference. But for someone with gout whose uric acid level is only just above normal, a low-purine diet might well make a significant difference. If uricosuric drugs or allopurinol (see p.250) are out of the question, then this diet may prove useful.

The foods with the highest purine levels are:

Liver, kidney, sweetbreads, brain, heart and other offal
Meat extracts (Bovril, Oxo etc.)

Pâté
Sausages, if made with offal, as they often are.
Fish roe, herring, mackerel, shellfish, sardines, sprats, whitebait,
anchovies
Crab, shrimps
Alcoholic drinks, especially beer
Yeast extract and yeast tablets

Moderately high purine levels are also found in:
Pulses of any kind including split peas, lentils, haricot beans, baked
beans, chickpeas and soya beans
Soya flour, gram flour

As well as cutting out high-purine foods, do not eat excessive amounts
of any meat, fish or eggs, as these will boost your purine intake. You
should not take large doses of either Vitamin C or nicotinic acid (the
latter is also called niacin or Vitamin B3) although the amount of
nicotinic acid in a B-complex tablet would be safe. Do not have too
much fruit or fruit juice because of the fructose content (see pp.244–5).
If you need a painkiller, choose one that does not contain any aspirin
eg. paracetamol.

· *Low-protein Diets* ·

In Britain during World War II there was a marked reduction in the
cases of gout seen by doctors, due to the sharp reduction in the amount
of protein being eaten. No one would wish to return to the austere wartime diet, but there are a few gout sufferers who may find relief from
limiting not only their intake of high-purine foods but also the total
amount of protein eaten.

Such a diet is only needed by the very rare patient who cannot
tolerate the drugs prescribed for gout, and who continues to suffer
from gout attacks despite medical treatment, and despite losing
weight, cutting down alcohol and avoiding purines. It may be
particularly valuable for gout sufferers with these difficulties who also
have 'kidney stones' consisting of uric acid deposits. Needless to say,
your doctor should be consulted before beginning such a drastic diet.
And it must be carefully monitored to avoid the possibility of
malnutrition.

On this diet, the amount of protein eaten per day should be less
than 2 ounces (57 grams). A guide to the protein contents of food is
given on pp.350–351.

· Port, Plumbers and Old Lead Pipes ·

Gout has been linked with port drinking for over 200 years. Doctors in the 18th century noticed a connection, and this has passed into popular folklore to such an extent that 'gout' and 'port' are firmly linked in the minds of most people – most non-medical people, that is. Doctors now know that port is no more at fault in gout than any other strong alcoholic drink.

The observation probably *was* correct in the 18th century, however, when port contained a certain amount of lead, derived from the casks in which it was matured. Lead affects the kidneys, reducing their ability to get rid of waste products – including uric acid. So a mild form of lead poisoning can lead to gout, sometimes known as 'saturnine gout'. This type of lead poisoning may go undiagnosed because it does not produce symptoms like those of 'classic lead poisoning', which result from high levels of lead in the body.

Gout due to mild lead poisoning usually occurs in people whose work involves lead, mainly lead smelters, plumbers, people making or repairing stained glass, and those dealing in scrap metals. Soldering, battery manufacture and pottery glazing can also involve exposure to lead. Lead is absorbed through the skin and, because it can only be disposed of rather slowly, it tends to accumulate in the body. Oily substances encourage the absorption of lead by the skin, so handcream should *not* be applied before handling lead.

There has recently been a suggestion that it is not just those who work with lead that are at risk – mild lead poisoning might also occur in other people who have simply accumulated lead from the air, from food or from water. Again, gout may be the only notable symptom of this. Although this problem is thought to be very rare, there may be occasional cases.

Before considering the main sources of lead in the environment, bear in mind that it is only *very long-term* exposure which can result in a build-up of lead in the body. A brief exposure to these small amounts of lead will not cause any problems.

Exhaust fumes contain lead, unless a car is using unleaded petrol. Significant amounts of lead from this source only accumulate in people living near busy roads. White paint once contained lead compounds as pigments, so burning very old painted wood can release lead into the atmosphere. If battery casings are burned, this generates lead fumes, and there will also be some in the air near industrial lead smelters.

Lead in food is usually due to exhaust fumes: fresh fruit and vegetables sold from roadside stalls can be coated with a certain amount of lead, and should be avoided, or at least washed well. Picking blackberries or other fruit from roadside hedgerows is not advisable – find some at a good distance from the road. Vegetables grown in a garden by a busy road, or in a city centre, may also contain some lead. Lead-shot from rabbits, woodpigeons, pheasants or other game can also be a significant source, if some of the pellets are swallowed unnoticed.

Drinking water can contain moderate levels of lead but only if it is flowing through old lead pipes, and if the water is slightly acidic making the lead dissolve more readily. The main problem areas in the British Isles occur where drinking water flows from peaty land, as in the Highlands of Scotland and many parts of Ireland. In general, water authorities have replaced the old lead pipes in such areas. Lead pipes are safe in areas with 'hard' water because a protective layer of chalk will have built up inside the pipes over the years. Problems might occur if a centralised water softener is installed in an old house with its original lead pipes still in place, as the softened water would gradually remove the chalk layer. If you are concerned about your water you can ask the local water authority to test its lead content.

There are two other unusual sources of lead. One is the type of hair darkener much favoured by the former President Ronald Reagan. This contains a lead compound which can be absorbed and cause cumulative lead poisoning of a mild kind. The second source is in glazes used for pottery, which may contain lead-based pigments. In most western countries, any commercial pottery designed for food use will, by law, be coated with safe glazes. But pottery made at evening classes, or cheap pottery bought abroad where regulations are less stringent, might be a source of lead. Teachers of pottery-making should know which glazes are unsafe for use on tableware.

If mild lead poisoning is suspected, a simple test, analysing a sample of hair, can be ordered by a doctor. There are drug treatments available which speed up the clearance of lead from the body. It is important to also reduce current and future exposure to lead, having first identified the original cause of the problem. Anyone with a suspected problem with lead should not take supplements of Vitamin D unless absolutely essential, as this vitamin can enhance the toxic effects of lead.

· *Drugs used for Gout* ·

The drugs prescribed will depend on whether you are currently experiencing an attack of gout or not.

Short-term treatment during a gout attack

During a gout attack, all that can be done is to calm the inflammation and hasten the end of the attack. Non-steroidal anti-inflammatory drugs or NSAIDs (see p.418) may well be used for this purpose.

Alternatively, a drug prescribed solely for gout may be tried: colchicine. This drug first came into use in the late 18th century and has a prompt and dramatic action, relieving the pain and inflammation in just a few hours. It seems to work by blocking the signals that attract more of the immune cells called neutrophils (see p.104) into the joint. Because colchicine is so specific for gout, it is sometimes used to help with diagnosis: if the doctor suspects that a sudden attack of joint pain is caused by gout, colchicine will be prescribed to see if it works. The diagnosis is confirmed if colchicine proves effective.

Unfortunately, colchicine is rather toxic, and the doses that can be safely used are fairly small. Never take more than the dose prescribed and consult the doctor if side-effects such as abdominal pains, diarrhoea, nausea, vomiting, rashes, unusual bleeding or bruising, tingling or numbness occur. In the case of the first two symptoms, it is wise to stop taking the drug immediately. Severe vomiting and pain, or bloody diarrhoea should be regarded as an emergency and treated accordingly.

Once the diagnosis is certain, your doctor may prefer to prescribe an NSAID rather than using colchicine again. Few patients take colchicine on a long-term basis because of its toxicity. If you are given this drug as a preventive medicine, to be taken when a gout attack begins, take it as early as possible, because that is when it is most effective. Starting early keeps the required dose to a minimum. Avoid high-purine foods (see pp.245–6) so that you do not have to take the drug too often.

During an attack of gout, you should, preferably, rely on the drugs prescribed by the doctor and not take other painkillers as well. Aspirin can aggravate gout by blocking the clearance of uric acid from the blood, but the painkiller paracetamol (Panadol) is safe.

If both NSAIDs and colchicine fail to suppress the attack, corticosteroids (see p.414) such as prednisolone may be used. These are stronger anti-inflammatory drugs and must be used with caution. Occasionally, corticosteroids are injected straight into the gouty joint.

Long-term treatment to prevent gout attacks

If you suffer recurrent attacks of gout, and preventive measures such as losing weight and giving up alcohol have not helped, there are long-term drug treatments which can help. These aim to reduce the level of uric acid (see p.104) in the blood. Such treatments should only begin when you are *not* suffering from a gout attack.

The most popular drug is **allopurinol** (Aloral, Aluline, Caplenal, Cosuric, Hamarin, Zyloric) which blocks the production of uric acid entirely. It does so by interfering with an enzyme called xanthine oxidase, which converts xanthine (produced from purines) into uric acid. The chemical process then stops at xanthine instead of progressing to uric acid, and xanthine accumulates in the blood. Fortunately, xanthine is more soluble than uric acid (so less inclined to crystallise) and more easily disposed of by the kidneys. Allopurinol is technically known as a xanthine oxidase inhibitor. Most patients can take it for the rest of their lives with no ill-effects, although it is not suitable for everyone. There may occasionally be side-effects such as mild nausea or drowsiness which are nothing to worry about. Consult the doctor if these become severe, or if there are other effects such as headaches, a metallic taste in the mouth or tingling in the hands and feet. If you suffer a skin rash, stop taking the drug and see your doctor immediately.

Drink plenty of fluids when first taking allopurinol. As the level of uric acid in the blood falls, the urate crystals already formed around the body will begin to dissolve again. If there are tophi (large clumps of urate crystals – see p.104) these represent a substantial store of uric acid which is gradually dispersed into the blood as the drug takes effect. Consequently, the level of uric acid in the blood may actually *rise* in the first few weeks or months. Frequent glasses of water and other fluids are helpful in flushing the uric acid out of the body.

Because the uric acid level can rise at the outset, allopurinol may spark off a new attack of gout at this stage. Doctors are now aware of this problem, so they usually prescribe another drug as well during the first months. Either an NSAID or colchicine may be used, as for attacks of gout (see p.249). If you have tophi (on the rim of the ear, for example) these drugs should generally not be discontinued until the tophi have disappeared.

As an alternative to allopurinol, or in addition to it, there are drugs which encourage the kidney to dispose of uric acid more efficiently. These are called **uricosurics** and the three main ones are probenecid (Benemid), sulphinpyrazone (Anturan) and azapropazone (Rheumox). The last of these has a double action, being an NSAID as well.

Because they reduce the level of uric acid in the blood these drugs, like allopurinol, can cause existing crystals and tophi to dissolve, making the uric level rise once more (see above). Again, they can provoke a gout attack in the early stages, so other drugs must be given to avert this possibility.

There is an additional hazard with uricosurics, in that kidney stones may form, due to urate crystals depositing in the kidneys. Your doctor will probably prescribe other medicines to prevent this happening, and it is important to follow the instructions carefully. Should you experience pain when passing urine, or see blood in the urine, tell your doctor. Flushing of the face is also a side-effect that should be reported. If a rash or itchy skin develops, stop taking the drug and see the doctor as soon as possible.

. *Dietary Advice for Those Taking* . *Allopurinol*

The most important point is that you need to drink plenty of fluid, preferably water (see p.250). Try to drink at least 3.5 pints (2 litres) per day. If plain water gets too boring, try sparkling mineral water with a dash of some kind of cordial, or one of the ready-made flavoured waters now available. You could also use a little fruit juice to flavour the water, or drink it in the form of herb tea – peppermint tea is one that many people like.

It is not a good idea to boost your fluid intake with pints of tea or coffee – indeed, you may even need to cut down on these beverages. Caffeine and some of the other stimulants found in tea and cofffee, such as theophylline and theobromine, may cause problems for gout sufferers. They interact with the same metabolic pathway as allopurinol and can reduce its effectiveness. If allopurinol treatment does not seem to be working as well as it should for you, discuss with your doctor whether you should reduce your intake of tea and coffee. Note that chocolate also contains some substances of this kind.

Alcohol may increase the unpleasant side-effects of allopurinol, and you should limit how much you drink. Again this is something to discuss with your doctor. Finally, iron supplements should not be taken with allopurinol except for short periods, as this can lead to iron salts being deposited in the liver.

Chapter 2.8

HEALTHY EATING FOR EVERYONE WITH ARTHRITIS

Good food, with plenty of vitamins, minerals and other nutrients, is something that everyone needs to maintain their health. Such advice might seem obvious, but studies regularly show that some people with rheumatoid arthritis, osteoarthritis and other arthritic diseases are eating inadequate diets. So too are many people *without* arthritis – it is all too easy to slip into bad eating habits and miss out on certain crucial vitamins.

The fact that you have arthritis should not defeat your efforts to stay healthy in other ways, and a good balanced diet is essential for this. This chapter contains general guidelines on eating a healthy diet, plus special advice on the particular nutrients that may help with certain types of arthritis. If you are looking for more background information and detailed discussion of individual nutrients you will find it in Section 3 of the book – here we are simply concerned with straightforward advice.

If you have problems with chewing or swallowing, consult the section on page 266, as well as reading the general advice. Should you be about to undergo surgery – a hip replacement for example – look also at page 265.

The bulk of this chapter is intended for adults. A special section concerning children with arthritis can be found on page 263.

· *Overweight or Underweight?* ·

If you are either overweight or underweight, you should try to adjust your food intake so that you achieve a normal weight for your height. The diagram on page 227 will help you work out your ideal weight.

Arthritis of the knees, hips or ankles will be aggravated by carrying excess weight. Osteoarthritis in the finger joints also seems to be made worse by obesity, although the reason for this connection is not understood. Advice on losing weight is given in Chapter 2.6 (p.226). Gout sufferers will also benefit from losing weight but they need to be cautious about dieting (see p.244).

Being underweight is just as serious a matter. Some forms of arthritis increase the need for calories in general: the fever that often accompanies rheumatoid arthritis and systemic lupus erythematosus causes the body's metabolic rate to 'rev up', burning off extra calories. Unless you replace those calories you will eventually lose weight, and if your fat reserves become used up, the protein from your muscles will be utilised to make up the deficit. There is a danger of muscle wasting, and of going into a downward spiral of ill-health if you become this thin, so you need to make a real effort to eat more.

Make sure that the extra food you eat is good healthy food, because you may well be short of certain vitamins and minerals. Some high-calorie indulgences such as cake and ice-cream are useful in putting on weight, but do not eat too many of these 'empty calories' (see pp.259–260).

· *Who Needs Supplements?* ·

If we eat adequately, and choose our diet with care, we should not need vitamin or mineral supplements. This might seem self-evident, but the heavy advertising and promotion used for such supplements has created the widespread impression that human beings cannot survive without the help of tablets and capsules. The truth is that people are generally better off getting their vitamins and minerals from fresh foods, which also contain several minor nutrients *not* available in most supplements but now known to be useful (eg. fibre and carotenoids). It is conceivable that some foods contain other minor nutrients, so far unknown to science, which are valuable for health. In particular, taking Vitamin C tablets in place of fruit and vegetables leaves you short of several important nutrients (see p.295).

Nevertheless, vitamin and mineral supplements may have a useful role to play in certain situations. Firstly if someone has been eating an inadequate or unbalanced diet, and has developed deficiencies, their body's reserve store of a particular vitamin or mineral may be badly depleted. A supplement, providing a higher-than-normal dose of the nutrient concerned, will help to replenish the store.

Secondly, unusual demands on the body, such as the need to heal bed sores, or to recuperate after surgery, creates a need for certain extra vitamins and minerals. Again, a supplement may be the best solution: see p.265.

Thirdly, anyone who has a restricted diet that omits a major class of food (eg. dairy products) may run the risk of deficiency of certain nutrients. If other foods cannot fill the gap, supplements are required. Vegans and people following other restricted diets for personal reasons (eg. macrobiotic diets or strict Rastafarian diets) may need some supplements. For a summary of the nutrients that could be lacking in a vegan diet see p.392. Those with food sensitivities should consult the section on pp.194–204. For example, if you have to avoid dairy products, look up the 'Crucial nutrients' section for milk on pp.196–7, to find out what nutrients you are lacking by not eating this food group. If you dislike the alternative foods, or cannot eat enough of them to sustain the recommended intake of the missing nutrients, then you should take supplements.

Fourthly, some nutrients, when taken in doses above the normal intake, may have a beneficial effect on certain arthritic diseases. Whether they are acting as nutrients in this instance, or as drugs, is a debatable point (see p.277). In this chapter we will suggest ways in which levels of such nutrients can be boosted by means of dietary changes, rather than supplements: these suggestions are incorporated into the general recommendations for healthy eating given on pp.255–9. It is worth noting that, in almost every case, supplements were used in the experimental work which showed these nutrients could help with arthritic diseases. The doses in the supplements were generally higher than anything that could be achieved by food intake. So we cannot be certain that obtaining lesser quantities of the same nutrients by diet alone can benefit arthritic patients in the same way – but it is worth a try. If you are interested in going a step further and taking supplements of these beneficial vitamins and minerals (bearing in mind that the action may be that of a drug rather than a nutrient) turn to Table 15 on p.279 for a summary of the supplements that have proved beneficial. The experimental work involved, and the required dose of each nutrient, are described in the relevant chapter of Section 3.

Whatever your reasons for taking supplements, do not forget that they can have harmful effects if taken at the wrong dosage. Furthermore, even at the correct dose, some supplements are damaging to certain people with arthritic diseases. Before deciding to take any supplement, consult the 'Hazards' section for that nutrient in Chapter 3.2 (vitamins) or Chapter 3.3 (minerals).

Never take any supplement at a higher dose than that stated on the container or recommended by your doctor. Where higher doses have been tested experimentally, as described in this book, you can safely take that dose for the length of time it was taken in the experimental trial, but no longer. After that, you should continue at the recommended dosage. In particular, do not take an excess of Vitamins A and D, nor exceed the recommended dose for multivitamin tablets or cod-liver oil, both of which contain these vitamins. Do not combine cod-liver oil with vitamin tablets containing Vitamins A and D.

So far we have been talking only about supplements of vitamins and minerals. Go into any health food shop and you will also find other products described by the manufacturer as 'food supplements', usually based on a plant or animal extract, such as extracts of Devil's claw root, or extracts of green-lipped mussel. These products are actually unproven drug remedies, but they cannot be sold as drugs because they have not had the extensive testing required. *In particular, the manufacturers of these products do not need to have shown that they produce any benefit.* A loophole in the regulations allows them to be sold as a 'food supplement' with far less stringent testing. Such products rarely contain any significant amounts of nutrients that might actually be lacking in the diet, so they are not food supplements in any real sense. Chapter 4.8 (p.396) considers most of these products in detail. Some of the oils marketed in this way may be of benefit: these are described in Chapter 2.2 (p.143).

. *General Guidelines for Healthy* . *Eating*

Surveys of eating habits among those with rheumatoid arthritis or osteoarthritis have regularly found a poor intake of certain vitamins and minerals (as indeed have surveys of the population at large). The deficient nutrients are listed in Table 12, (p.256) along with the foods that are rich sources of each nutrient.

As a first step, look at each of these nutrients in turn, and think about how often you eat the foods listed. If the answer is 'infrequently' or 'never' to all the foods on a particular list, then you need to broaden your everyday diet to include one or more of these foods. You should pay special attention to Vitamin B5 or pantothenate, a vitamin that may be beneficial in rheumatoid arthritis (see p.29). Extra helpings of foods containing this vitamin may be worth trying.

Table 12: Nutrients often lacking in the diet of patients with rheumatoid arthritis or osteoarthritis

Nutrient	Foods that are rich sources
Zinc	Meat, especially lean red meat Shrimps, clams and oysters Eggs, cheese Nuts, seeds and wholemeal bread (see p.324 for exact amounts)
Magnesium	Shrimps Dark green leafy vegetables Peanuts and other nuts Lentils and peas Meat, fish and cheese provide lesser amounts (see p.328 for exact amounts)
Vitamin E or tocopherol	Sunflower seeds are the best source. Sunflower oil, safflower oil, almonds, hazelnuts and sunflower margarine are also very rich sources. Peanuts, avocados and sweet potatoes contain lesser amounts. Eggs and milk contain small amounts. Some foods 'use up' more Vitamin E than they supply (see p.301), including walnuts, pecans, pistachios, Brazil nuts, cashews and pine nuts, corn oil, soya oil, peanut butter and sesame seeds.
Folate or folic acid (a B vitamin)	Green vegetables, wholegrain cereals Nuts Yeast extract Eggs
Pyridoxine, (Vitamin B6)	Most meats, fish, egg yolk Wholegrain cereals, potatoes Bananas, red peppers, watercress, avocados Nuts and seeds Tempeh Most green vegetables are a moderately good source
Pantothenate (Vitamin B5)	Common in many foods. Meat, eggs, nuts and seeds are particularly good sources.

As will be clear from Table 12, nuts are a very good source of many of the vitamins and minerals most likely to be in short supply. Of the nutrients they contain, Vitamin E may be especially valuable to anyone with ankylosing spondylitis, rheumatoid arthritis, or another form of inflammatory arthritis because it acts as an antioxidant (see p.339). Osteoarthritis with an inflammatory component, (indicated by red, warm or swollen joints) may also be helped by Vitamin E. If you have any of these conditions, you should try to boost your intake of Vitamin E. For those who dislike nuts or have a sensitivity to them, seeds can be a useful replacement. Pumpkin seeds and sunflower seeds can both be bought in health food shops. Health food shops also sell nut butters made from a variety of nuts (almond butter and hazelnut butter for example) which are useful if you have difficulty in chewing nuts. Spreads made from sunflower seeds are also available. Some products may have Vitamin E added by the manufacturer as an antioxidant, and these are worth looking out for.

Next think about how often you eat fresh fruit and vegetables – and in what quantity. Most people in industrialised countries eat far too little vegetable matter, and what they do eat has often had its nutrient content reduced by overcooking, or by being cooked and then kept warm for long intervals, as often happens in cafeterias and canteens, or, sadly, in some hospitals and residential homes. Vitamin C, beta-carotene, Vitamin B6 and folic acid are the most badly affected by cooking and then being kept warm for long periods. Losses of these vitamins will also occur if cooked food is kept in a refrigerator for a day or more after cooking, so leftovers will be substantially less nutritious than fresh food.

At least some of your vegetables should be eaten raw in salads, or lightly cooked and served immediately for maximum nutritional value. Tinned and frozen vegetables are not ideal nutritionally and should not be your staple diet, but they are acceptable as an occasional fall-back when you cannot easily shop for fresh food. They are far better than no vegetables at all, and frozen green vegetables such as peas and green beans are generally better than green vegetables that have been bought fresh and then stored for several days at room temperature.

Dried vegetables, such as the carrots and peas found in packet soups, are very poor nutritionally. (Beans, chickpeas and lentils are always sold in dried form of course, but the important nutrients they supply, notably protein, are not affected by drying. Tinned beans and chickpeas are as rich in protein and almost as rich in vitamins as dried ones that have been soaked and boiled, and they save an enormous amount of time and effort in the kitchen.)

Remember to include some dark green leafy vegetables, such as broccoli or spring greens, for the magnesium, folic acid and Vitamin K they contain. If you have rheumatoid arthritis or another form of inflammatory arthritis, you should also include plenty of carrots, red peppers and other items, to benefit from the carotenoids which give them their colour. These pigments also act as antioxidants (see p.347). The best sources of carotenoids are listed in Table 13.

As far as possible, eat fresh raw fruits, rather than tinned or cooked fruits. They will be far richer in Vitamin C and carotenoids. Dried fruits, such as sultanas, raisins and dried apricots, lose almost all their Vitamin C, and more than half their carotenoids. Jams are generally low in Vitamin C, because of the prolonged boiling process required for jam making, but blackcurrant jam contains a little. Fruit juices sold in cartons or bottles are usually quite rich in Vitamin C.

Ideally you should consume fruit or vegetables with every meal, and eat some as snacks as well, to give a total of five helpings a day. Vitamin C tablets are *not* a good substitute (see p.295) although some extra Vitamin C in tablet form may be helpful if you have rheumatoid arthritis and bruise easily (see p.296) or if you are about to undergo surgery (see p.265).

Of course, painful hands and deformed finger joints can make it very difficult to eat fresh fruit and vegetables, because chopping and peeling are such daunting prospects. If this is a problem, refer to pp.269–271.

Anyone with rheumatoid arthritis accompanied by fever will have a high level of inflammation, and may benefit from making special

Table 13: Good sources of carotenoids

Carrots, eaten raw or freshly cooked, are by far the richest source.

Tinned carrots have about half the carotenoids of fresh ones, but are still an excellent source.

Swiss chard, kale and spring greens are very good sources, as are yellow-fleshed sweet potatoes and red sweet peppers.

Tomatoes, mangoes, canteloupe melons, passion fruit, guavas and papaya (pawpaw) are good sources.

Apricots, pumpkin, peas, green beans, courgettes, broccoli, okra and asparagus are all fairly good sources.

Note that oranges and tangerines are a not particularly good sources of carotenoids.

The carotenoid content of leafy vegetables is *substantially reduced* if stored at room temperature: storage in a refrigerator reduces losses.

Beta-carotene supplements are *not recommended* (see p.347).

---

efforts to eat plenty of antioxidants – this means lots of fruit and fresh vegetables, especially those rich in carotenoids, plus almonds, hazelnuts and sunflower seeds for their Vitamin E content. As well as helping with inflammation, antioxidants have many other benefits. They reduce the risk of heart disease and may protect against some forms of cancer.

A healthy diet should also include plenty of starchy (complex carbohydrate) foods, such as bread, pasta, rice and rolled oats. All these are made from cereal grains. Wholemeal bread is preferable to white bread, as it contains more B vitamins, but avoid unleavened bread, and products containing added wheat bran or oat bran which tend to block the absorption of minerals such as magnesium and zinc (see p.309). Starchy foods should comprise about a third of your food intake, according to current healthy-eating recommendations.

The diet described so far, with its combination of fruit and vegetables, some nuts or seeds, and starchy cereal foods, will also provide you with a good intake of dietary fibre. This is believed to be important in reducing the risk of heart disease and bowel cancer. As already noted above, it is inadvisable to eat bran as your daily fibre source because of its effects in blocking mineral absorption. The fibre found in fruit, vegetables, nuts, seeds and pulses (beans, peas and lentils) is now considered to be much healthier than either wheat bran or oat bran.

Few people in our society are lacking in protein, and most of us eat far more than we need. However, you should give some thought to the protein in your diet, especially if you are vegan or vegetarian. Consult the figures on page 350 if you are in any doubt about how much protein you need. Vegans should also check that the quality of the protein eaten is adequate (see p.349). Those with gout may need to avoid certain kinds of protein-rich food, which is also rich in purines (see p.245). Occasionally there are benefits in restricting total protein intake for gout sufferers (see p.246), or for patients with systemic lupus erythematosus whose kidneys are affected by the disease – your doctor's advice should be sought on this.

So much for the 'Dos' – now for the 'Don'ts'. *The main foods to be avoided are sugar and saturated fat.*

The main problem with sugar, apart from the damage done to our teeth, is that sugar represents 'empty calories': in other words, sugar provides plenty of calories with absolutely no vitamins, and no useful minerals (except in the case of brown sugar which contains some calcium, magnesium and iron). What is more, many sweet foods, such as cakes, biscuits and desserts, are also loaded with saturated fats.

This makes them doubly fattening. Even if you are not overweight, these foods may carry a nutritional risk, especially if your total food intake is low. Because they are 'empty calories', if you use these foods to satisfy your hunger, instead of nutritious foods such as fruit, vegetables, nuts and wholegrain cereals, then you run the risk of nutritional deficiencies.

Sugar is self-evident in food, thanks to our 'sweet tooth' or, more precisely, our sugar-seeking taste buds. Try to retrain your taste buds to prefer less sugary foods, and to demand them less often. It is an interesting experiment to eat no sugar-rich foods at all for a few weeks – just fresh fruit, but nothing with added sugar. As time passes, the fresh fruit begins to seem sweeter and sweeter, because it no longer has to compete with artificially sugary foods. On the other hand, when you next taste cakes, biscuits, and desserts again they will seem overpowering and unpleasant – far too syrupy and cloying. This shows that the taste buds *can* be re-educated.

Saturated fat is not as easily detected as sugar, and reducing your intake depends on knowing where such fat is found. Refer to Table 14 which shows the percentages of saturated fat in different foods. Try to minimise your consumption of foods near the top of the list, and be moderate about those in the middle.

Some of the dangers associated with saturated fat are now well known: most people are aware that eating a lot of saturated fat can increase the risk of heart disease. Less well known is the fact that saturated fat is far more important than the amount of cholesterol in the diet. The body manufactures its own cholesterol, and this is the source of most of the cholesterol in the blood. Provided you are not eating abnormally large amounts of cholesterol, the level in your bloodstream is independent of the amount eaten. But a high intake of

Table 14: Saturated fat in foods

Food	Saturated Fat
creamed coconut	87%
butter	55%
dripping	55%
lard or suet	41%
hard margarine	35%
double cream	31%
fresh coconut	31%
cream cheese	30%
whipping cream	25%

Food	Saturated Fat
Cheddar cheese	22%
peanut oil	19%
cheesecake	19%
chocolate	17–18%
Brazil nuts	17%
polyunsaturated margarine	16%
olive oil, soya oil	14%
most vegetable oils	10–12%
single cream, sour cream	12%
peanut butter	12%
grilled pork sausages	10%
pork pie	10%
cashew nuts	10%
Mars bar	10%
gateau	10%
roast lamb	9%
potato crisps	9%
digestive biscuits	9%
cream crackers	9%
Cornish pasty	9%
peanuts	8%
fatty roast pork	7%
grilled beef sausages	7%
hazelnuts, almonds, walnuts	5–6%
fruit cake	6%
ice cream	6%
Greek yoghurt	5%
roast chicken with skin	4%
lean roast lamb	4%
roast beef	4%
avocado pear	4%
egg	3%
Channel Island milk	3%
whole milk	2%
roast chicken without skin	2%
lean roast pork	2%
cottage cheese	2%
olives	2%
wholemilk yoghurt	2%
lean roast beef	1%
low fat yoghurt	0.5%
skimmed milk	0%
white fish (eg. cod)	0%

saturated fat causes the body to boost the level of cholesterol in the blood, and this increases the risk of a heart attack. Foods such as eggs, which are rich in cholesterol, are no longer considered to be quite as risky, whereas foods such as cream, which is loaded with saturated fat, are thought to be the major problem.

The role of saturated fat in some forms of cancer is also an incentive to reduce consumption. Cancer of the bowel (large intestine) is more likely among those who eat more saturated fat, particularly meat fat. There may also be a link between ovarian cancer and the milk fat found in dairy products. Diets rich in saturated fat and animal protein also increase the risk of kidney cancer.

Whether saturated fat intake has any effect on rheumatoid arthritis is a debatable question. At present there is too little evidence to decide, but it may play some small part. This topic is dealt with in detail on pp. 52–3.

All this advice about fat consumption should not be taken too seriously if you have a poor appetite. Not eating at all is the greatest risk for many with arthritis, especially the elderly. If you are underweight and eating little, then it is more important to keep your strength up than to worry excessively about the risks of heart disease. There is some truth in the saying 'a little of what you fancy does you good', and if you happen to fancy eggs and buttered toast, but have no appetite for cottage cheese or skimmed milk, you should follow your preferences rather than go without food. This is especially true of anyone over 75, where loss of interest in food and consequent malnutrition are major problems. Some fatty foods, such as eggs, cheese and meat, are an important source of nutrients, including those that older people frequently lack, such as Vitamin D and calcium. What is more, any damage to the arteries will already have been done by the age of 80 or so, and avoiding fats at this age is no longer a top priority.

Current opinion holds that, for the prevention of heart disease, it is better to replace saturated fats with mono-unsaturated fats, such as oleic acid, which is the principle constituent of olive oil, rather than with polyunsaturated fats, which are the main fats found in soft margarine and most vegetable oils. Along with this new advice goes a recommendation not to eat large amounts of trans fatty acids (see p.358).

To anyone with rheumatoid arthritis, the new recommendations on mono-unsaturates are especially good advice. There is a potential benefit from olive oil in relieving the symptoms of rheumatoid arthritis (see p.54) in addition to its value in preventing heart disease.

Another food recommended for the prevention of heart disease is likewise beneficial to people with rheumatoid arthritis. Oily fish, such as mackerel, sardines and herrings, reduce the risk of heart attacks when eaten regularly: current recommendations are to eat two or three helpings each week. The substances in the fish that are believed to reduce the risk of heart disease are called omega-3 fatty acids, the same substances that are thought produce benefits in rheumatoid arthritis, although the way they work is largely different in each case. A much higher dose of omega-3s is needed to have any effect on rheumatoid arthritis. It is possible to get the full dose for rheumatoid arthritis by eating fish, but you would need to eat oily fish every day, a diet which few people can sustain. If you are interested in trying fish oil for your joints, omega-3 fish oil supplements are probably the answer – or a combination of fish and supplements. Full details are given on pp.147–151.

· *Children with Arthritis* ·

Eating a healthy diet is particularly important for children with arthritis, because adequate supplies of energy, protein and nutrients are essential to sustain a child's growth. One survey of children with arthritis, carried out in Australia, found that they were not eating enough calories, and were short of calcium, zinc, and, in some cases, iron. Although some of the children were taking supplements, these tended to be Vitamin C, which they were all eating in abundance anyway, or other vitamins that were not deficient in the diet. None of the supplements contained calcium or zinc, the main missing nutrients. The researchers concluded that the children needed to eat more meat, fish, dairy products, nuts and pulses (beans and lentils).

Another survey, involving older children (12–14 years) in Norway, found low energy intake again, plus inadequate levels of calcium, zinc, iron and two of the B vitamins, thiamine and niacin. Vitamin C consumption was also below the recommended intake for these children. The same dietary recommendations made for the Australian children would correct these deficiencies, except for Vitamin C, which would require more fresh fruit and vegetables (see p.293 for the best sources). A study of American children with arthritis found deficient intakes of Vitamin E, zinc and iron. Those with systemic JRA (juvenile rheumatoid arthritis) were also eating too few calories. Of course, many children with arthritis have a poor appetite, and it is difficult to persuade them to eat, especially those with systemic JRA.

Nevertheless, it is important to try to coax them into eating as much food as possible, and to make sure that the food is highly nutritious.

The healthy eating guidelines for adults, given on pp.255–263 are largely applicable to children as well. It is even more important to ensure that calcium and Vitamin D intakes are adequate for children because deficiencies can lead to serious problems for growing bones (see p.298).

Surveys such as those described above regularly find some children who are not eating any dairy products, often on the advice of an alternative therapist, or a misleading self-help book. In most cases, no calcium supplement is given to these children, whose growth is put at risk by their calcium-deficient diet. Any child who is not eating dairy products should take a calcium supplement at the correct dosage for their age. Although it *is* possible to achieve an adequate calcium intake on non-dairy foods, it requires a knowledgeable and committed attitude to menu planning, and a cooperative and self-disciplined child who will eat plenty of lentils and broccoli and largely resist the temptations of crisps, sweets and soft drinks. Such children are rare. Even with a calcium supplement, the child who is avoiding dairy products may be at some risk of deficiencies in other vitamins (eg. some B vitamins), and needs to eat plenty of other good nutritious food.

This advice is intended for those who have a child *already on* a dairy-free diet for sound medical reasons. If you are thinking of taking your child off dairy products, we would advise you to consider this decision very carefully, in the light of the information on pp.191–2.

. *Why Some People Need More* . *Nutrients than Others*

Some medical conditions create an increased need for nutrients. If you have a serious problem such as fat malabsorption, you will undoubtedly be advised by your doctor, but the effects of more minor medical problems may be overlooked, so we will consider these here.

Anyone who has diarrhoea regularly, whatever the cause, may be short of some nutrients, and should eat a really good healthy diet to compensate – plenty of nutritious food and very few 'empty calories'. A multivitamin and mineral supplement may be advisable, but this is something to discuss with your doctor.

Those who are housebound, and rarely exposed to sunlight, need a regular supply of Vitamin D in their diet (see p.299), to replace that which is normally made by the skin. Inactivity can also lead to constipation, a particular problem for those who are bedridden. Eating more fibre can help to overcome this, but you should not resort to wheat bran or oat bran for your fibre (see p.259).

A more serious problem for those who are bedridden is pressure sores or 'bed sores'. Obviously, these have to be treated by relieving the pressure on the affected area, and this is the first priority, but improving nutritional status can help the sores to heal. Vitamin C intake should be at least 60 mg per day and supplements may be useful (but very large doses should not be taken). If there has been a shortage of zinc in the diet, this may have contributed to the development of pressure sores, and eating zinc-rich foods (see p.324) or taking a supplement may promote healing. An iron supplement may also be needed if there is anaemia – this can be diagnosed with a blood test. Sometimes deficiencies of A and B vitamins are also a factor, and a multivitamin and multimineral supplement may, therefore, be advisable. Protein requirements are high during wound healing, especially if there is a large, open sore, so extra helpings of protein-rich foods should be eaten. Calorie intake should be high in anyone who is underweight – one contributing factor in pressure sores is a lack of fat and muscle to provide an in-built 'cushion' between bones and mattress. Those who are confined to bed, but do not have bed sores as yet, should remember that maintaining a good diet can help to prevent this painful and unpleasant problem from developing.

If you are still in doubt about whether you are eating adequately, after reading this chapter, you can ask your doctor to make an appointment with a nutritionist or dietician. On the basis of your current diet, a nutritionist can assess your current intake of vitamins and minerals, and advise you on correcting any deficiencies.

Vitamins and surgery

Major surgery increases the body's requirements for many nutrients, and if you are about to undergo a hip replacement, or any other large operation, it would be advisable to take a multivitamin-and-mineral supplement. Begin this a week or two beforehand (or even earlier if you have been eating poorly) and continue for about two months after the operation. A supplement of Vitamin C is particularly useful in speeding up the healing process after surgery, and a little extra Vitamin C could be added to the multivitamin supplement but there is no value in taking more than 500 mg per day, and very high doses can be damaging (see p.295).

. *Overcoming Problems with Chewing* .
and Swallowing

Many patients with rheumatic diseases have difficulty eating a good diet precisely because of their disease. Chewing may be painful if the jaw joints are affected by arthritis. Those with Sjörgren's syndrome who have little saliva flow may find it hard to chew and swallow because their mouths are so dry. Swallowing is also problematic for some people with scleroderma.

Try to find ways around these problems rather than go without food. Saliva-substitute sprays can be prescribed for those with Sjörgren's syndrome and will make eating far easier and more pleasurable. If these have not already been prescribed for you, ask your doctor about them.

Using tasty herbs and spices in your cooking can also be a useful strategy, as this will stimulate the flow of saliva. Sauces and relishes, especially sharp fruity flavours, may also help. Choose the flavours you like best and try to make every meal a treat — you will probably still need help from a saliva spray or other artificial aids, but the added input from your own saliva will allow you to eat more and enjoy what you eat.

Another tactic is to use a food blender (liquidiser) to create soups and other easily swallowed foods. These can still be tasty and nutritious. If you do not have a blender, a potato masher can achieve similar results – apply it to solid foods such as cooked vegetables, then add water later. When you are too ill to cook, or too short of time, baby foods can be enormously useful: the range available is now very wide, and many suit adult palates, although you may need to experiment before finding the right ones for your taste.

Patients with problems in the jaw joints may be helped by some of the cutlery specially designed for arthritis sufferers, especially by spoons with a small shallow bowl. Suppliers of such cutlery, and other useful equipment, are listed on page 431.

Eating mostly liquidised food has a small disadvantage in that your teeth will be slightly more vulnerable to decay. This is because you produce less saliva if you do not chew, regardless of whether you have a normal or reduced saliva flow to begin with. Saliva contains protective elements that fight tooth decay, and with less saliva in the mouth, decay sets in more quickly. This disadvantage can easily be overcome by brushing the teeth more frequently.

· *No Appetite?* ·

People with arthritis often have a very poor appetite, which can cause nutritional deficiencies. Pain, drug side-effects, or depression are frequently at the root of the problem.

If pain is killing your appetite, tell your doctor this and ask if it is possible to prescribe more effective drugs. There may well be another drug that will suit you much better. Even if you have already tried several different kinds, it is worth trying again.

Drugs themselves can interfere with eating patterns, especially if they produce nausea among their side-effects. Some of the medications used for arthritic diseases have such effects, while others produce a general feeling of malaise which includes a loss of appetite. Should you suspect your drugs of causing such problems, ask your doctor about changing the prescription.

Depression is a natural reaction to the burden of an arthritic disease. Unfortunately, insomnia and lack of interest in food are common symptoms of depression, and can themselves lead to a further deterioration in health. If you are affected by depression, do not try to struggle with it alone, and resist the temptation to think that it is an inevitable state of mind for someone with arthritis. Seek help from your doctor. There are many new anti-depressant drugs which can have a very beneficial effect, and are not addictive. They may well be useful in lifting you out of your depression so that you can begin to rebuild your life. Counselling, and help with practical problems, may also be available.

· *Healthy Eating on a Low Budget* ·

Many of the foods recommended for a healthy diet are relatively expensive, and this can make it seem impossible to eat well on a low budget. But there are also some healthy foods that are very cheap, and by using these carefully you may be able to save money on other items, so that your overall food costs do not rise. For examples, pulses (i.e., lentils, dried peas, chickpeas and beans) are a cheap source of protein, which can replace meat to some extent. They are rich in many different vitamins and minerals, and will improve the overall quality of the diet. Some of the money saved by replacing meat with pulses could then be spent on items such as fresh fruit and vegetables. Some dried pulses are sold in supermarkets (although they may be hidden on a low shelf!) and a good selection can always be found in health food shops. They must be soaked thoroughly and cooked well. A pressure cooker is useful for cooking pulses with the minimum of gas or electricity. Canned pulses (such as baked beans) are also good value and nutritious. (If eating less meat, ensure your zinc intake is adequate; see p.324.)

Making your own muesli, using rolled oats, chopped nuts and dried fruit, will give you a cheaper and more filling breakfast than packeted breakfast cereals. It is also very rich in vitamins and minerals.

Foods such as peanut butter (preferably the sugarless kind), yeast extract (Marmite etc.) and wholemeal bread are all relatively inexpensive, filling and nutritious. If these are bought in preference to cakes, biscuits and desserts, they can bring the size of the weekly food bill down, while boosting the nutritional value of the diet enormously.

Jam, tinned vegetables and tinned fruit are items that can easily consume quite a high proportion of the food budget, and which are very poor value nutritionally. It is far better to spend money on fresh fruit and vegetables. An inexpensive and delicious jam with a higher nutrient content than normal jam can be easily made at home if you have a freezer. When strawberries are being sold cheaply in markets in the summer, buy a large quantity, wash and chop them, then mix with an equal weight of white sugar. Put into small plastic cartons or plastic bags in the freezer. The freezing process turns the mixture to jam. This jam only keeps for a week or so once defrosted, so make it in small portions and keep in the refrigerator when defrosted.

Some fish are very cheap and an excellent source of protein, as well as omega-3 fatty acids. Sardines, whether fresh or in tins, are a bargain, as are fresh sprats and pilchards. Herring and mackerel are also inexpensive. Fishmongers will often sell some items very cheaply or even give them away – salmon heads, for example, which have quite a bit of high quality salmon on them.

Some vegetables are far cheaper than others, such as spring greens, broccoli tops and carrots. All these are rich in minerals, vitamins and carotenoids (see p.347). Buying vegetables in a street market will reduce the cost substantially. Or do your supermarket shopping just before closing time on a Saturday and wait for the fresh produce to be marked down in price.

Check that you are getting all the Social Security benefits to which you are entitled. Every year, millions of pounds of benefit remain unclaimed, mainly because people do not know that they could receive them. Of particular interest to people with arthritis are certain benefits available to those with disabilities (see p.430).

· Problems with Preparing Food ·

Many people with arthritis in their fingers or wrists rely entirely on packeted food because it is too painful or difficult to prepare fresh food. This can be the beginning of a steady downward path into malnutrition and generalised ill health. Dried foods, in particular, are very low in many vitamins.

Fortunately there are many new gadgets and cleverly designed tools that can allow you to cook without so much pain, or which overcome the problems of deformed fingers. Some of the most useful are special cooking knives with a rocker action or saw-like action that have grip-handles and do not require you to press down on the blade with your forefinger. Other valuable items include ingeniously redesigned peelers and kitchen scissors that are far easier to use, chopping devices for vegetables, boards which hold bread while you butter it, tools for lifting saucepan lids, and devices that safely hold kettles or teapots and support them on a hinged platform while you pour. Addresses of suppliers can be found on p.431. It is also worth exploring your nearest department store for potentially useful aids: new gadgets come onto the market all the time. Social Services may be able to supply some useful items, such as spiked boards which hold food while you chop it up.

If your saucepans are of the heavy, solid-bottomed variety, it may be worth buying some lighter ones which will not strain your wrists so much. Alternatively, you can use a steaming basket, or a wire sieve that fits inside a saucepan, to cook vegetables, then lift them out when cooked, so that straining (of both the vegetables and your wrists!) is avoided. The wire baskets sold for blanching vegetables prior to freezing them are very useful for this purpose; department stores sell these. Smaller quantities of vegetables can simply be removed from the water with a perforated serving spoon.

Even lightweight pans are heavy when filled with water, and to avoid wrist strain (which can increase the risk of deformity) it is a good idea to use both hands when lifting pans. You can also slide pans along work surfaces to avoid lifting them. Use a plastic jug to fill electric kettles, as these are very heavy when full.

Existing tools such as cooking knives and peelers can be adapted to make them easier to grip by putting a piece of sponge rubber tubing over the handle to enlarge it. The tubing can be removed and washed when necessary. This is a cheap though temporary solution to food preparation problems, but in the long run you should aim to acquire some specially designed implements (see p.431).

If traditional style kitchen taps cause problems, consider having them replaced with lever-operated taps, which take the strain off your fingers completely. You can ask a plumber for an estimate of the cost without committing yourself. The reduction in pain will undoubtedly be worth the investment in the long run.

Electric tin-openers are remarkably inexpensive and well worth the money for anyone with painful arthritis in the hands. Devices for gripping the tops of bottles and jars are also invaluable: they are available in most hardware and department stores.

Another way to eat well despite painful hands is to buy vegetables that are peeled, washed, chopped and ready to cook. Most of the big supermarket chains now sell such products. Naturally they cost a little more, but if you can afford this extra expense, it is a good solution to cooking problems. Prepared and ready-washed salads are also available, as are fresh fruit salads and new potatoes, washed and ready to cook. If you cannot get to a supermarket because you do not drive, refer to p.271.

Although we have advised against convenience foods in parts of this chapter, there are a few modern convenience foods that are thoroughly worthwhile for those with arthritic fingers: ready-made pastry, often sold frozen, is one. It tastes as good as most home-made pastry and saves you enormous amounts of finger-work if you are a keen pie-maker. Fresh soups, sold in cartons or plastic containers, are also useful because they have not been 'cooked to death' like tinned or dried soups. (However you should add a handful of fresh parsley or chives to boost the nutrient content further.) Chopped nuts and toasted flaked almonds are available in large supermarkets, and will save you some effort. There may well be other such products, so look around.

Ready-made frozen meals are useful in providing tasty, easily prepared food. If they tempt your appetite when nothing else will, or allow you to eat a good hot meal when cooking is impossible, then they are obviously valuable. The unhealthiest thing you can do is to go without food altogether, or live on toast and biscuits.

Ring the changes with frozen meals rather than eating the same meal repeatedly. Try to combine each meal with a salad (it could be a ready-to-eat one – see above) or some freshly cooked vegetables to give a more balanced and nutritious meal. If you rely heavily on frozen meals, try to eat some seeds, nuts or nut butter (see p.218), some wholemeal bread, and some yeast extract, as well, to ensure that you get enough B vitamins and Vitamin E. Don't forget to have some leafy green vegetables regularly, and to eat plenty of fresh fruit.

The 'Meals-on-Wheels' service offers a daily hot meal which can be invaluable to elderly people. However, the food will be kept warm for some time after cooking, so, like canteen food, it may be deficient in some vitamins (see p.257). Some fresh fruits and salads should be eaten as well to make up for these deficiencies.

A commercial service offering frozen meals delivered directly to your door, is now available. The meals can be ordered by telephone from a printed menu, and include a main course and a dessert for about £2–3. They can be warmed up in an oven, a microwave or a special device supplied by the same company which is specially designed for use by the elderly. The company can also supply a small table-top freezer which will hold up to four weeks' meals. Vegetarian, diabetic, low salt, low fat and low calorie diets are all catered for. For the address and telephone number of this company, see p.432. As with Meals-on-Wheels, you should eat some fresh fruits and salads as well.

· *Problems with Cutlery and Crockery* ·

For those with severely deformed fingers and hands, even eating utensils may be problematic. There is now a wide range of specially designed cutlery and crockery which can help overcome such difficulties. Addresses of suppliers are given on p.431.

· *Difficulties with Shopping* ·

If you are eating less because shopping has become difficult, then it may be necessary to investigate other possibilities. Many local shops will deliver food to customers who have problems with walking, especially customers who have shopped there for some time: you should not feel afraid to ask. It may well be possible to telephone your order to the shop and pay on delivery.

Much as we may lament the decline of the corner shop, it must be admitted that large supermarkets offer many advantages to people with arthritis, including trolleys that save you from having to carry the goods around the shop, lower prices, a wider choice of fresh food, ready-peeled and chopped vegetables, and appetising frozen meals. Most now have wheelchair access as well.

If you do not drive and cannot get to a supermarket, consider whether there is anyone with a car who could take you there, or do your shopping for you. Ask Social Services if they can help, and enquire about local 'shopmobility schemes' (see below). If these options fail, see if a local taxi firm will offer you a concessionary rate for a regular weekly shopping trip.

'Shopmobility schemes' now operate in most large towns in the U.K. where there are modern shopping centres. The scheme provides an electrically powered scooter or wheelchair, or a manual wheelchair, free of charge to anyone who needs it, for use within the shopping centre. You do not need to be an orange-badge holder, or to be permanently disabled, so if you have 'bad times' and 'good times' you are quite entitled to use the scheme during your bad periods. The scheme is available to anyone who wishes to use it, and all you need to do is telephone the shopmobility office and book a vehicle. In most towns, there are arrangements for people arriving by bus or car, and everything is made as easy as possible as regards getting from the bus stop or car park to the shopmobility office where you pick up the vehicle. Trained staff will show you how to use the electric vehicles, and in some towns an escort can be provided during your shopping trip, if you need extra assistance. To find out if there is a shopmobility scheme in operation locally, telephone the city council. Not all shopping centres have food supermarkets, so check before you set off.

NUTRIENTS AND ARTHRITIS

Chapter 3.1

HOW NUTRITION AFFECTS ARTHRITIS – AND VICE VERSA

Four quite separate issues are discussed in this section of the book pp.275–346, and it is important not to confuse them.

The *first issue* is whether vitamin or mineral supplements can either cure or alleviate arthritis. The answer to this is: 'On the whole, no'. However, there are instances where a particular vitamin or a mineral has been shown to help in some small way, for certain forms of arthritis. These are summarised in Table 15 (see p.279).

Because there are so many extravagant claims for vitamins and minerals made in the popular press, this section deals individually with each vitamin and mineral that is (or has been) the subject of such claims in relation to arthritis. The primary aim of this section is to supply the background information which will allow a rational assessment of such claims.

When vitamins, minerals and other nutrients are recommended in magazine articles, leaflets or popular books, one or two scientific trials are often quoted, supposedly showing that the nutrient works. Very often there is careful selection of evidence involved – only those scientific studies that gave positive results are quoted, while studies that showed no benefit are not mentioned. This is misleading. Sometimes the studies that gave positive results were only pilot studies, where patients were not treated 'double-blind' (see p.27). It is well known that such studies often get positive results, thanks to the enthusiasm of both the researcher and the patients, whereas follow-up trials, that are conducted in a double-blind way, show no benefit from the treatment. In the chapters that follow, we quote all the scientific studies available to us at the time of writing, and give an assessment of how good they were.

A special note is required here on our decision to include

osteoporosis in this book. Osteoporosis is not a form of arthritis, it is a disease of the bones. However, people with rheumatoid arthritis are more susceptible to osteoporosis, and the same is true for some other arthritic disorders, such as ankylosing spondylitis. Vitamin and mineral supplements, or an improved diet, can be very helpful indeed in preventing osteoporosis, or in arresting its progress once it has begun, which is why we have included it in the chapters that follow. Much more is involved than simply taking a calcium supplement or drinking milk, and Chapters 3.2 and 3.3 give background information on all the individual vitamins and minerals involved. A checklist of the nutrients concerned is given in Table 16 (see p.279). If you are just looking for straightforward advice on dietary measures to prevent or treat osteoporosis, turn to Chapter 2.3 (p.161), which summarises the recommendations given here.

The *second issue* is whether people with arthritis might be lacking in vitamins or minerals as a direct or indirect *result* of their disease. The evidence available does suggest that patients with arthritis are slightly more vulnerable than others to nutritional deficiencies, but on the whole these tend to be mild deficiencies.

Loss of mobility, or stiffness and pain in the hands, can make shopping and cooking difficult, and some arthritics eat less as a result, or rely on convenience foods which may lack certain nutrients, notably Vitamin C, folic acid (a B vitamin), Vitamin K, boron and carotenoids (see p.347). This problem can affect patients with osteoarthritis and any other disabling arthritis, as well as those with rheumatoid arthritis who often have little appetite to begin with. It is particularly common in elderly people living alone.

With rheumatoid arthritis there are also two special factors that can actually increase the need for vitamins and other nutrients. Firstly, during periods of active joint inflammation and fever, the body's metabolic rate is higher and this can create an increased need for some nutrients. Secondly, the effects of drugs may be to reduce the absorption of some nutrients, or to increase the body's requirement for particular items. (A list of drugs that may affect nutrient requirements is given in Table 17 – see p.280).

Nutritional deficiencies that are a result of arthritis do not, in general, make the arthritis worse, but they could produce other symptoms. These are sometimes rather vague symptoms, such as tiredness or depression, bad skin, a sore tongue or cracked lips, irritability or mental confusion. Such symptoms might not be recognised as a real illness, or they might just seem to be part of the arthritis itself. Arthritis sufferers at risk of nutritional deficiencies need to improve their diet or take a supplement.

Anyone who is concerned about this and simply wants some straightforward practical advice on healthy eating should turn to Chapter 2.8 (p.252) where all the general recommendations made in this chapter are summarised.

The *third issue* concerns anyone who has successfully completed an elimination diet and is now following a restricted dietary regime. If you are avoiding certain key foods there may be some risk of vitamin or mineral deficiencies. This topic is considered on a food-by-food basis in Chapter 2.5. Consult the section on pp.194–204, looking up any food or group of foods you are avoiding to see what vitamins or minerals may be lacking in your diet as a result. There is also advice on how to obtain these nutrients from other foods.

Vegetarians, and more especially vegans, are often at risk of nutritional deficiencies, and they will find a summary of the potential deficiencies on p.392, with more details in the relevant sections of Chapters 3.2 and 3.3.

The *fourth issue* is related to the first. It is the assertion that nutritional deprivation results from some aspect of the modern Western diet, and that this is the actual *cause* of arthritis. This assertion is made by many proponents of popular dietary treatment, notably Dr Dong (see p.365) and Dr Campbell (see p.384). Refined flour and other processed foods are often singled out for blame, although the theory varies from one author to another. The subject is considered in full on pp.408–410.

. *Vitamin or Drug? 'Megavitamin'* . *Therapy*

A vitamin is, by definition, a substance required in very small quantities which, when lacking, causes a distinctive and recognisable set of symptoms – the **deficiency state** characteristically associated with that vitamin. The aim of researchers and nutritionists is to establish exactly how much of a vitamin is needed, per day, to prevent this deficiency state from developing.

With several vitamins there is still controversy about the recommended dose, and about identifying the deficiency state. Sometimes, with closer observation of patients, or more precise methods of measuring vitamin levels in the blood, it becomes clear that there are also *marginal* deficiency states for a vitamin which often have more subtle and elusive symptoms than the *major* deficiency state first identified. Vitamin K (see p.306) provides a good example of this, and Vitamin E may also come into this category (see p.302).

If a patient is clearly in a deficiency state, then the vitamin is usually given in high doses for a while, often at several times the recommended daily allowance. The objective is to overcome any absorption problems that may have led to the deficiency state in the first place, and to replenish the body's stores of the vitamin. After a few weeks or months, the dose is reduced to more normal levels, as long as the deficiency symptoms have been cured.

Using vitamins as drugs is a different matter entirely. This involves giving high doses, many times the recommended daily allowance, to people with no sign whatever of a deficiency of the vitamin concerned. The vitamin is not correcting a deficiency under such circumstances; it is acting (if it has any effect at all) as a drug. When Vitamin C is taken by ordinary healthy people at doses above 500 mg per day, it is being used as a drug (although a largely ineffective one – see p.295).

Drugs can have side-effects, and so do vitamins at high doses. The fat-soluble vitamins (A, D and E) are particularly toxic, but the prolonged use of any vitamin at high doses could be risky. The general 'megavitamin' treatments sold in some health food shops are most unlikely to help anyone with arthritis, and they could produce ill-effects for some people. Before deciding to take any vitamin supplement you should read the 'Hazards' section concerning that vitamin in Chapter 3.2 (p.282). The same also goes for mineral supplements, which are covered in Chapter 3.3 (p.309). The hazards of certain supplements are summarised in Table 18 (see p.281).

Some of the studies reported here, which produced benefits for patients with certain forms of arthritis, did use vitamins or minerals at levels above the daily recommended allowance. They may have been acting as drugs in some of these trials, but since the trial will also have looked for side-effects in a thorough and systematic manner, we can be reasonably sure that taking a supplement at the same dose *for the same length of time* is unlikely to produce any ill-effects.

Table 15: Nutrients that affect arthritis

Vitamin B$_5$ (pantothenic acid) may be helpful in rheumatoid arthritis (see p.291).

Vitamin B$_6$ (pyridoxine) may help some people with carpal tunnel syndrome (see p.98).

A special form of **Vitamin B$_{12}$**, called methylcobalamin, may help with rheumatoid arthritis (see p.291), but this is not available commercially.

Vitamin E may help with rheumatoid arthritis (see p.304), and could also be valuable for other forms of inflammatory arthritis. The same is true of carotenoids (see p.345). Combining **Vitamin E** with a good intake of carotenoids and selenium may be especially valuable (see pp.345–6).

Vitamin E may be of help in ankylosing spondylitis (see p.305). (**Vitamin K** may also be advisable for patients with this disease – see p.307).

Those who have an inflammatory component in their osteoarthritis, could possibly benefit from **Vitamin E** supplements (see p.305).

Vitamin C may help with the 'easy bruising' that sometimes accompanies rheumatoid arthritis (see p.296) but see Table 18 (p.281) for potential hazards.

Vitamin D supplements are essential in osteomalacia and rickets (p.288–9). **Calcium** may also be needed. Cases of 'refractory rickets' require **magnesium** as well (see p.326).

Those on a **low-calcium** diet may develop secondary hyperparathyroidism, which resembles rheumatoid arthritis (see p.313).

Gout can be affected by intake of **purines** (see p.245) and by **total protein** in the diet (see p.246)

Some fatty acids may improve the symptoms of rheumatoid arthritis (see Chapter 2.2 pp.143–160)

Table 16: Foods and nutrients that may be relevant to osteoporosis

Calcium	(see p.314)
Vitamin D	(see p.301)
Vitamin K	(see p.307)
Folic acid	(see p.292)
Vitamin B6 (pyridoxine)	(see p.292)
Magnesium	(see pp.326–7)
Manganese	(see p.332)
Phosphorous	(see p.319)
Potassium	(see p.330)
Boron	(see p.333)
Zinc	(see p.325)
Copper	(see p.338)
Protein, particularly its sulphur content	(see pp.406–7)
Fibre	(see p.353)

For dietary advice on reducing the risk of osteoporosis, see Chapter 2.3 pp.161–169.

Table 17: Drugs and nutrients

Note that the drug names given here are the official names, or general drug categories, not the brand names by which you probably know your drugs. To check whether you are taking any of these drugs, look at the leaflet inside your drugs pack, which may say what type of drug it is; if not, ask your pharmacist or doctor.

Penicillamine can sometimes produce copper deficiency which in turn leads to a type of anaemia called hypochromic anaemia.

Penicillamine also acts against Vitamin B_6, pyridoxine (see pp.292–293).

Aspirin and other **salicylate drugs** can induce a deficiency of potassium (see p.329–330)

Aspirin and other **salicylate drugs** can create a deficiency of folic acid, a B vitamin (see pp.292–293)

Prolonged use of **aspirin** can lead to a depletion of Vitamin C in the body.

Those who have suffered bleeding from the stomach, due to taking **NSAIDs** (non-steroidal anti-inflammatory drugs), may be anaemic and require an iron supplement (see p.320).

Corticosteroids can induce a deficiency of potassium.

Corticosteroids increase the losses of both calcium and zinc in the urine.

Cyclosporin A can induce a low level of magnesium in the blood (see p.326).

Methotrexate affects the metabolism of the B vitamin folic acid, and a folic acid supplement should be taken, but only under close medical supervision (see p.293).

Those taking **Methotrexate** should not drink alcohol, as this substantially increases the risk of liver damage.

Table 18: Potential hazards of supplements for those with arthritis

Sarcoidosis patients should never take **Vitamin D** supplements except under close medical supervision (see pp.300–301).

Very occasionally, **iron supplements** make rheumatoid arthritis worse (see p.321).

High doses of **Vitamin C** can sometimes make both gout and rheumatoid arthritis worse (see p.246 and p.295).

Stopping high-dose **Vitamin C** suddenly can cause 'rebound scurvy' (see p.295).

Patients with Sjögren's syndrome may react badly to **niacin** or **Vitamin B$_3$** (see p.291).

Long-term supplements of **Vitamin D**, at high doses, can lead to calcification of the kidneys and other soft tissues (see p.411).

All the **fat-soluble vitamins (A, D, E** and **K)** tend to accumulate in the body and are potentially toxic if taken in amounts greater than the recommended intake.

Most **vitamins** are harmful if taken in excessive doses.

Some **amino acid** supplements, such as **tyrosine,** may make rheumatoid arthritis worse (see pp.351–2). Others (eg. **tryptophan**) are dangerous for anyone, and have caused some deaths (see p.352).

Alfalfa tablets, sold in some shops as a 'food supplement' may be very damaging to those with systemic lupus erythematosus (see pp.138–9).

Those taking **fish oil** supplements might need to take additional Vitamin E (see p.151). (Anyone eating oily fish or taking cod-liver oil must also have a high intake of Vitamin E – see p.150.)

Omega-3 fish oils are not recommended for those with certain medical conditions, or taking certain drugs – (see p.152).

Chapter 3.2

VITAMINS

Vitamins were big news in the 1930s. Their importance in human nutrition had just been realised, and doctors were itching to try them out on every puzzling and frustrating disease they could think of. Naturally, the various forms of arthritis were prime candidates.

Patients with rheumatoid arthritis were given blood tests and urine tests for vitamin levels and many seemed to be short of a particular vitamin. But further investigation showed that this was often illusory – the patients were not actually deficient in the vitamin, they just lacked any substantial reserves of the vitamin stored in the body. Some of the tests used then could not distinguish between these two states. Only a few patients had genuine deficiencies.

Vitamin supplements were given to all these patients – whether they had a genuine deficiency or just a lack of stored vitamin – to see if there was any improvement in the arthritis. There was none, although other symptoms did clear up in those patients with a genuine deficiency. The vitamins studied included Vitamin A, the Vitamin B-complex and Vitamin C.

Vitamin D, which has a role in the healthy development of bones (see pp.296–7), was also studied extensively in the 1930s. There was great enthusiasm, among some doctors, for giving very large doses to treat several different forms of arthritis. The amounts used were much higher than the daily requirement for this vitamin, so it was really being used as a drug rather than a vitamin. Unpleasant side-effects were common (Vitamin D is toxic in large amounts) and there seemed to be no sustained benefit as far as the arthritis was concerned. For some people the arthritis did seem to improve, but the effects ceased soon after the treatment was stopped – and it had to be stopped because of the side-effects.

Despite these early disappointments, interest in vitamins as a possible treatment for arthritic diseases (and many other ills) has remained strong. Vitamins seem to have an irresistible lure: they are 'natural', they are cheap to buy, and they are full of a magical promise of glowing health. This, of course, is exactly the image promoted in advertisements for vitamins, and clearly they are good business for the people making and selling them. Yet most of the supplementary vitamins taken in developed countries are totally unecessary, because the people taking them are already eating a more-than-adequate diet. These extra vitamins are literally 'going down the drain', excreted from the body because they are unecessary.

Having said that, there may sometimes be a case for using vitamin supplements in particular patients with arthritis. The disease process itself can lead to an inadequate diet, or increase the need for nutrients, as described on pages 276–7. In such cases, the object of taking a supplement is not to alleviate the arthritis itself, but to avoid symptoms of vitamin deficiency.

Furthermore, there are a few deficiencies that probably begin as a result of the arthritic disease, but then actually contribute to the complications of the disease. One of these 'vicious circles' has been observed in rheumatoid arthritis, and tends to involve elderly patients eating a very poor diet: if there is a deficiency of Vitamin C this can add to the 'easy bruising' that sometimes occurs in rheumatoid arthritis (see p.296). Similarly, if a patient is not eating milk, butter, eggs or margarine, and is housebound, Vitamin D deficiency could develop and contribute to the loss of bone density (osteoporosis) that is associated with the disease (see p.298).

Recent research has also revealed a few other roles for vitamin supplements in the direct treatment of arthritis or related conditions. One study showed a benefit from Vitamin E supplements to patients with rheumatoid arthritis (see p.304). Another appeared to confirm reports that Vitamin B_6 can help some people with carpal tunnel syndrome (see p.98).

In general, however, vitamin supplements are not a miracle cure for arthritis. 'Megavitamin' tablets, giving high doses of all vitamins, have been suggested for arthritis, and frequently tried by patients, but there is little justification for taking these, and a real risk of toxicity from too much Vitamin A or Vitamin D.

The individual vitamins, and their relevance to arthritis (if any), are considered below.

Weights and Measures

When looking at the recommended doses of vitamins it is important to note that some are given in milligrams, which is written as 'mg', while other doses are given in micrograms, which may be written as 'mcg' or 'µg'. (The 'µ' is a Greek letter 'mu', pronounced mew.) Confusing milligrams with micrograms could be dangerous as a microgram is very much smaller: there are a thousand micrograms in a milligram.

Some vitamins are measured in IU or international units, a completely different system of measurement that cannot easily be translated into milligrams. It is used to allow direct comparison between different forms of the same vitamin, where the different forms have different strengths. In general, IU are a more useful and reliable measurement than mg or µg.

· *Vitamin A* ·

This vitamin, also known as retinol, is of primary importance for vision. It is sometimes claimed to have antioxidant (see p.339) properties as well, but in fact it is only a very weak antioxidant.

Natural sources of Vitamin A

These include milk, butter, eggs, kidney and liver. In the U.K., margarine has Vitamin A added to it by law. Vitamin A can also be manufactured, in the body, from a substance called beta-carotene (see p.347) which occurs abundantly in carrots, red peppers, mangoes, and dark green leafy vegetables. Beta-carotene acts as an antioxidant, unlike Vitamin A itself.

Deficiencies of Vitamin A

Vitamin A can be stored in the body for many months ahead, so that a temporary lack of the vitamin in the diet is no cause for concern. It is present in a very wide range of foods, and as a result Vitamin A deficiency is extremely rare in developed countries, except in people with diseases that cause malabsorption of food eg. pancreatic disease or small-bowel disease. In such cases, a doctor should be involved in prescribing a supplement and supervising the effects.

The main symptoms of marginal Vitamin A deficiency are poor vision in dim light and dryness of the eyes (although this last symptom can also be due to various other causes – consult your doctor if this is a problem.). A low level of Vitamin A in the blood may be a consequence of mild zinc deficiency (see p.325).

How much Vitamin A is needed?

Recommendations in different countries range from 500–1000 μg (micrograms, see p.284) of Vitamin A (retinol) per day for adults, with 700 μg as a generally acceptable figure.

Since 6 μg of beta-carotene can substitute for 1 μg of retinol, the daily dose of beta-carotene is 4,200 μg (4.2 mg). This could be obtained from 70 gm (2½ oz) of cooked carrots, 142 gm (5 oz) of cooked red peppers, 198 gm (7 oz) of cooked spring greens, or 284 gm (10 oz) of cantaloupe melon. The daily dose when expressed in IU (International Units) is 2,300 IU of retinol. Avoid taking supplements of beta-carotene – see p.347.

Hazards of Vitamin A

Toxicity generally occurs when doses exceed 7.5-10 mg (7,500–10,000 μg) per day of retinol, but it is wise not even to approach this level: Vitamin A is very toxic, and the risk is cummulative because this is a fat-soluble vitamin which is retained by the body (unlike Vitamin C for example, where an excess is excreted in the urine). An overdose is most unlikely to occur on a normal diet, but could happen with supplements. This sometimes results from too much cod-liver oil or other fish-liver oils being taken (there is the additional hazard, with these oils, of too much Vitamin D). The problem does not affect omega-3 fish oils (see pp.50–51), which are made from the flesh of the fish rather than the liver.

If newly pregnant women take high doses of Vitamin A (7.5 mg per day or more) this can cause deformities in the child. The first three months of pregnancy are the high-risk period. Beta-carotene is safer than Vitamin A in this and other situations where a supplement is required, because it is only converted to Vitamin A in response to the body's needs. However, you must not take high doses of beta-carotene supplements as this has other serious risks attached (see p.347) and it is much better to derive it from natural food rather than supplements.

Vitamin A and rheumatoid arthritis

Vitamin A supplements have been tried for rheumatoid arthritis without effect, as described on p.282.

· *Vitamin B-Complex* ·

There are eight vitamins included in this 'family' (listed in Table 19) and they serve a variety of functions in the body, many to do with the health of the nervous system or the blood. Some of the B family interact with each other, one B vitamin modifying the absorption or action of another B vitamin. Because of this, supplementing one B vitamin and not another can sometimes cause problems. This is why the B vitamins are generally supplemented as a whole, in a 'Vitamin B-complex' tablet.

Table 19: The B vitamins

Vitamin	Daily requirement (for adults)	Food sources
Vitamin B_1 (Thiamin)	0.8–1.2 mg	Found in many foods. Pork and beef are good sources. So are wholegrain cereals, beans, peas and lentils. Levels can be reduced by prolonged cooking.
Vitamin B_2 (Riboflavin)	1.2–1.8 mg	Milk and milk products, meat, cereal grains, yeast extract and some green leafy vegetables. Levels can be reduced by prolonged cooking.
Vitamin B_3 (Also called Vitamin B_7, Nicotinic acid, niacin, niacinamide or nicotinamide)	12 – 20 mg	Meat, especially beef, fish and milk are good sources. Yeast extract and wholegrain cereals, other than maize, are also valuable. This vitamin can also be made from tryptophan, an amino acid found widely in protein-rich foods, so deficiency is unlikely on most diets.

Vitamin	Daily requirement (for adults)	Food sources
Vitamin B$_5$ (Pantothenic acid or pantothenate)	3–7 mg	Common in many foods. Meat, eggs, nuts and seeds are particularly rich sources.
Vitamin B$_6$ (Pyridoxine)	1.2–2 mg	Most types of meat and fish are good sources. So are egg yolks, wholegrain cereals, potatoes, bananas, red peppers, watercress, avocados, nuts, seeds, and tempeh (a soya product). Most green vegetables are a moderately good source. Levels are somewhat reduced by cooking and steadily decline in food kept hot after cooking.

Vitamin B$_7$ – see Vitamin B$_3$

Vitamin	Daily requirement	Food sources
Vitamin B$_{12}$ (Cobalamin or cyanocobalamin)	1.5–2 µg	Meat is the best source. Fish, eggs and milk supply smaller amounts. No useful amounts in vegetable foods (see p.288). Readily destroyed by cooking.
Folic acid, folate or folacin (*No number*)	180–200 µg	Eggs, nuts, yeast extract, wholegrain cereals and green vegetables, especially leafy vegetables. Levels are greatly reduced by cooking and continue to fall if food is kept hot. Tinned vegetables lose much of this vitamin.
Biotin (*No number*)	15–70 µg	Widely found in meats, milk products and wholegrain cereals.

Natural sources of B vitamins

These are different for each member of the complex, but generally speaking a diet that includes whole grains, green leafy vegetables (raw or lightly cooked) and eggs will provide adequate amounts of all the B vitamins. Meat will boost the supply, as will yeast extract or brewer's yeast tablets. Other foods, such as milk, beans, nuts and fish, also contain certain B vitamins. Highly refined foods such as white flour and white rice are deficient in many B vitamins so it is important not to rely too heavily on these foods.

Vitamin B_{12} is the one that causes most concern among doctors today, because it can be in short supply for vegetarians, and a deficiency may cause irreversible damage to the nervous system. The deficiency can go unnoticed until it is too late, for reasons that are explained below.

Vegans (strict vegetarians who do not eat eggs or milk products) are at particular risk of developing a Vitamin B_{12} deficiency because this vitamin is mainly found in meat, with lesser amounts in fish, milk, and eggs. There are no sources other than animal products – unlike many other B vitamins, B_{12} is not found in yeast (although a synthetic form of the vitamin is added to some brands of yeast extract – see p.289). Claims to the contrary are frequently made by proponents of vegan diets, so it is worth going into this subject in more detail. Vitamin B_{12} can be made by certain bacteria, certain fungi and certain algae (microscopic plant-like cells), but it is definitely not made by yeasts, crop plants or animals. The bacteria living in our digestive systems (the 'the gut flora') do make this vitamin, but because we cannot absorb it through the wall of the large intestine (the final part of the digestive system, where the vitamin is made) this source is of no benefit to us. Animal foods are rich in Vitamin B_{12} only because animals have absorbed and accumulated the vitamin from bacteria in their own digestive systems (which are organised differently from ours), or from soil bacteria.

The belief that Vitamin B_{12} can be found in other foods (such as yeast, tempeh and other fermented soya products, spirulina and seaweeds), arose because the test for B_{12} used until recently was inaccurate. It did measure B_{12} but it also measured some related substances called 'noncobalamin corrinoids', which are of no value to humans as vitamins. A more accurate test has now been developed, which only measures Vitamin B_{12}. This test shows that yeast, tempeh, spirulina and seaweed only contain very small and variable amounts of Vitamin B_{12}, which are probably due to bacterial contamination. They do contain plenty of noncobalamin corrinoids, which accounts for their good showing in the earlier, less discriminating, test.

If vegans are not eating foods that have been 'fortified' with Vitamin B_{12}, then supplements will be necessary. For vegans who are yeast-sensitive, there are yeast-free B-complex supplements.

Fortified foods include some brands of soya milk (currently, Plamil and Unisoy Gold, in the U.K., but others may become available in future, so check labels), soya cheese, several brands of yeast extract (Tastex, Barmene, Natex), some brands of textured soya protein (Protoveg) and one breakfast cereal (Grape-nuts). (Another B vitamin that may be lacking in vegan diets, riboflavin, is also found in most of these products.) If you are relying on fortified foodstuffs, you should check that you are getting enough B_{12}. Initially, check the quantity of Vitamin B_{12} in the product and divide by the daily requirement (1.5–2.0 µg) to work out how many days' worth it represents. If you are not eating the product within that time span you are obviously not going to meet your daily requirement, and should consider adding another fortified foodstuff to your diet, or taking a supplement in tablet form. Note that the amount of Vitamin B_{12} needed rises to 2.5 µg per day for breastfeeding mothers.

Eggs and milk both contain Vitamin B_{12}, and the daily requirement can be obtained from three cooked eggs, 426 ml ($^3/_4$ pt) of milk, 156 gm ($5^1/_2$ oz) of most hard cheeses, or 85 gm (3 oz) of Edam or Emmenthal cheese. Yoghurt and cottage cheese are not very good sources.

Boiling milk destroys most of its Vitamin B_{12}.

Deficiencies of B vitamins

There may sometimes be a need for Vitamin B supplementation in arthritis, not to treat the joints themselves but to promote more general health. Anyone suffering from arthritis may be at risk of marginal nutritional deficiencies – these tend to occur quite often as a result of the disease process itself. Furthermore, studies of people with rheumatoid arthritis or osteoarthritis have shown that their diets are often lacking in one or more B vitamins because their disabilities prevent them from eating enough good food.

The signs and symptoms of a Vitamin B deficiency may include cracking of the skin at the corners of the mouth, greasy or reddened skin on the face generally, and a sore red tongue. However, there may be a deficiency without any of these obvious signs – and there can be other causes for signs and symptoms such as these so do not jump to hasty conclusions. Some types of Vitamin B deficiency affect the nerves and brain, producing irritability, memory loss, emotional instability, and other symptoms.

A special word is needed about Vitamin B_{12} and vegetarian diets. In general, vegetarians who eat milk and/or eggs are not likely to be short of Vitamin B_{12}. However, problems can arise if there is a medical condition that affects the stomach or other parts of the digestive system (eg. Crohn's disease) and so reduces the ability to absorb the vitamin. If intake is low, as it often is in vegetarians not taking supplements, poor absorption can lead to deficiency. Unfortunately, with advancing age the stomach and intestines may become less efficient, so older vegetarians are at risk unless taking a supplement. Anyone who has had part of the stomach removed – to treat an ulcer for example – would be at particular risk. Vegans, of course, are at a much higher risk. There is good reason for vegetarians and vegans to take special care over this vitamin. If their diet includes a lot of green leafy vegetables, then the characteristic initial symptoms of B_{12} deficiency – a type of anaemia called megaloblastic anaemia – will not appear immediately. This is because green leaves are especially rich in folic acid, another B vitamin, which 'covers' for Vitamin B_{12} temporarily, and prevents the anaemia from showing up. However, folic acid cannot replace Vitamin B_{12} in another of its roles – one which concerns the nervous system: as a result the B_{12} deficiency can cause lasting damage to the nerves before it is noticed and treated.

The early signs of nerve damage include loss of sensation in the feet and legs (with consequent unsteadiness when walking, especially in the dark), confusion, depression, and numbness or tingling in the hands and feet. Unfortunately, such symptoms are often disregarded in elderly people, who are at particular risk of B_{12} deficiency because they do not absorb nutrients from their food as efficiently as younger people. The body is very efficient at conserving its stores of vitamins when one is in short supply in the diet, so a Vitamin B_{12} deficiency may take a long time to develop. People who have been apparently healthy on a vegan diet for 20 years may then begin to show signs of Vitamin B_{12} deficiency as their stores of the vitamin are finally depleted. Those on macrobiotic or strict Rastafarian diets are also at risk. Breastfed babies of vegan mothers have sometimes suffered deficiencies, with damage to the nervous system as a result.

How much is needed?

See Table 19 (p.286). In general, if supplements are needed, a B-complex tablet should be taken (see p.286), and the recommended dose on the package should be followed. With certain rare exceptions (see p.291) B vitamins are not toxic, because they are water-soluble and any surplus is easily washed out of the body in the urine.

Hazards of B vitamins

If you suffer from Sjörgren's syndrome, you should be aware that you may react in an unusual way to Vitamin B supplements. Niacin or Vitamin B_3, when given at a dose of 75 mg per day (1000 times the daily requirement) has caused side-effects of hot flushes and racing heartbeat, in half those with Sjörgren's syndrome. Such side-effects would only be seen at a much higher dose among healthy people.

Vitamin B_6 should not be taken in high doses – more than 100 mg – for prolonged periods. One study found that people taking 200 mg per day (100,000 times the daily requirement) for a month became dependent on ('addicted to') this vitamin.

B vitamins and arthritis

In the 1930s, supplements of the Vitamin B-complex were tried out as a cure for arthritis, but with little success, as described on p.282. More recently some of the individual B vitamins, such as pyridoxine, have again been tested by medical researchers to see if they were of use in rheumatoid arthritis: again the results were negative.

A few of the B vitamins do have a little evidence in their favour. One of these is pantothenic acid or pantothenate, also called Vitamin B_5. Levels of this vitamin are reported as being low in the bloodstream of people with rheumatoid arthritis, although this is true of many nutrients and does not necessarily mean that a supplement can help. In the case of Vitamin B_5, there is a single scientific trial, carried out by general practitioners from different parts of the U.K. , which suggested that a supplement of 2 gm (2,000 mg) of calcium pantothenate per day, taken for eight weeks, might alleviate some symptoms of rheumatoid arthritis including pain and morning stiffness. The same trial showed definitively that the supplement was of no value to those with osteoarthritis.

Because only one good trial has been carried out with this vitamin, we cannot firmly recommend its use. However, it is relatively non-toxic and even at this high dose (about 500 times the recommended daily allowance) is unlikely to do any harm. There are no reports of it interfering with the absorption or action of other B vitamins. If you are keen to try this vitamin, there is probably no harm in doing so provided your doctor agrees.

Researchers in Japan have recently investigated a particular form of Vitamin B_{12}, known as methylcobalamin or methyl B_{12}, which is alleged to help people with rheumatoid arthritis. There seems to be some limited evidence in favour of methyl B_{12}, but it is far too soon to say. The substance is probably not acting as a vitamin in this instance, but as a drug.

It is rare for a vitamin to actually alleviate any form of arthritis, or any related disorder. However, one of the exceptions to the rule occurs with Vitamin B_6. This vitamin, also called pyridoxine, has proved helpful in some cases – but not all – of carpal tunnel syndrome (see p.98). If you want to try this supplement you should talk to your doctor first. This vitamin should generally be taken as part of a B-complex supplement, for the reasons given above (see p.286). It should not be taken at high dose for more than 2–3 weeks (see 291).

B vitamins and osteoporosis

There are good reasons for thinking that a deficiency of folic acid might contribute to the development of osteoporosis, and that rather more folic acid is needed by women after the menopause. Folic acid is important in the breakdown of a toxic substance called homocysteine, derived from food. The levels of this substance increase after the menopause, and can be lowered by giving a folic acid supplement. The evidence linking homocysteine with osteoporosis comes from another source: medical studies of people with an inherited disorder that leads to large amounts of homocysteine accumulating in their bodies. Such individuals develop severe osteoporosis while still quite young. This is tenuous evidence, and the theory that homocysteine might play a part in osteoporosis among older women has not yet been tested, but it seems that increasing intakes of folic acid might be a sensible strategy. Folic acid deficiency occurs in almost a quarter of 65-year-olds.

A different line of evidence suggests that Vitamin B_6 (pyridoxine) could also be relevant to osteoporosis. When rats are fed diets lacking in B6 they develop osteoporosis. This again is rather weak evidence, but since blood tests show that about half of the (apparently healthy) population has a deficiency of this vitamin, increasing the amount eaten would seem to be warranted.

Advice on boosting the intake of both these vitamins is given in Chapter 2.8 (p.252).

Drugs and B vitamins

Several B vitamins are opposed in their action by drugs that may be used for arthritis treatment. In most cases, this calls for B-complex supplements.

Penicillamine, which is often used for rheumatoid arthritis, acts against Vitamin B_6. Anyone on long-term therapy with this drug should take a B-complex supplement. You will probably have been advised to do this by your doctor. If you have not received such advice, talk to your doctor before starting the supplement.

Aspirin and related drugs in the salicylate group can create a deficiency in folic acid, one of the B vitamins. Some doctors believe that anyone on long-term therapy with such drugs should take a B-complex supplement.

In the case of one drug, methotrexate, it is now considered particularly important to replace the vitamin concerned (folic acid), as this will reduce the toxicity of the drug, but the dosage of the vitamin and the time when taken, in relation to the methotrexate, must be *exactly right*, or the vitamin could prevent the drug from working. Methotrexate is used as a second-line drug against rheumatoid arthritis, and is believed to work by blocking the rapid growth and multiplication of cells in the synovium (see p.421). It probably achieves this by interfering wtih the cells' ability to use folic acid. Your doctor should prescribe a folic acid supplement for you and tell you exactly when to take it. Do not take any other Vitamin B complex or multivitamin supplements that contain folic acid or folate. The dose of folic acid in foodstuffs will not interfere with the action of methotrexate.

· *Vitamin C* ·

Vitamin C is involved in the repair and maintenance of healthy connective tissue, among other functions. It is essential for the production of collagen, the vital ingredient in articular cartilage (see p.413) which lines the joints. Early researchers believed that this made Vitamin C deficiency a strong candidate for the underlying cause of arthritis, and in the 1930s Vitamin C supplements were enthusiastically tried out, but the results were disappointing.

It seems that, once the articular cartilage is in place, Vitamin C plays no further part in its health, so a lack of Vitamin C does not lead to either osteoarthritis or rheumatoid arthritis.

Natural sources of Vitamin C

Most fruits are a good source of Vitamin C, particularly oranges, grapefruit, blackcurrant, strawberries and kiwi fruit. Avocado pears and fresh parsley are also rich sources of Vitamin C. Certain salad vegetables are rich in Vitamin C, notably watercress, cress or rape seedlings, green or red sweet peppers and raw cabbage.

The vitamin is destroyed by heat, so cooked fruits are less useful than fresh fruits. Jam is usually very low in Vitamin C because it is boiled for so long.

Vitamin C is soluble in water, so it leaches out of vegetables if they are left to soak before cooking. Cooked cabbage and other 'greens' do have a certain amount of Vitamin C, provided they are cooked lightly and served promptly once ready, but if they are overcooked the Vitamin C is all destroyed.

Potatoes are also a good source of Vitamin C, as long as they are not soaked before boiling, not boiled for any longer than is necessary, and eaten as soon as they are cooked, rather than being kept warm. New potatoes cooked in their skins are the best source.

Since canteen food is often over-cooked and kept warm for long periods of time, the Vitamin C content of the vegetables is likely to be very low. Vitamin C deficiency occurs most often in elderly people eating a diet of 'convenience foods'. It can also occur in institutions unless there is careful supervision of meals – not just what is served up, but what is actually eaten.

Deficiencies of Vitamin C

Scurvy, the deficiency disease caused by very low Vitamin C intake, can include joint pain among its symptoms – but this is not arthritis. Blood vessels throughout the body are weakened in scurvy, and the joint pains come about because tiny blood vessels around the joint rupture – blood then seeps into the joint space causing increased pressure and ultimately pain.

Scurvy is only likely to occur in someone living almost entirely on tinned and packeted food with no fresh fruit or vegetables in their diet. The characteristic symptoms of scurvy are swollen, bleeding gums, a dry scaly skin and unusual susceptibility to bruising (a bruise is due to tiny blood vessels breaking, causing leakage of blood into the surrounding tissue). Severe scurvy needs to be treated promptly as the loss of blood can prove fatal.

A *marginal* Vitamin C deficiency produces a rather different picture from scurvy. There may be mental symptoms such as depression and hypochondria, and an accumulation of skin scales around the roots of hairs on the arms and legs. The hairs themselves may be wavy or coiled. In addition, cuts may take a long time to heal, bruising may occur more readily, and there is less resistance to infections.

Long-term use of aspirin at high doses can deplete the levels of Vitamin C in the body.

Hazards of Vitamin C supplements

Vitamins such as folic acid and Vitamin K, minerals such as boron and potassium, flavonoids, antioxidants such as carotenoids, and other valuable ingredients such as fibre – all these are found in fruits and vegetables, and make a Vitamin C tablet seem like a very poor substitute. It is a serious mistake to think that you can neglect fruit and salads because you are taking Vitamin C.

If you do decide to take Vitamin C, avoid the chewable tablets which can be devastating to tooth enamel. No more than 500 mg per day of Vitamin C is necessary.

The idea that Vitamin C is an utterly harmless health-giving substance that everyone should swallow in huge quantities is a rather strange myth, and one that can cause problems. Sometimes the very high doses of Vitamin C obtained from supplements seem to make rheumatoid arthritis worse, for reasons that are not understood. They can also cause problems for people with a tendency to gout.

The very high doses of Vitamin C that some people take to prevent colds are generally disposed of in the urine and do not cause any further problems, but some people suffer disturbed sleep on these high doses, and there is a risk of oxalate-type kidney stones developing. Sadly, there is also little evidence that they actually prevent colds or flu. However, some evidence suggests that colds may be less severe and not last as long if Vitamin C supplements are taken.

Cases of 'rebound scurvy' have been reported when people who were taking high doses of Vitamin C suddenly stopped taking the supplement completely – clearly their bodies had become used to the high intake and they continued to excrete Vitamin C in large amounts even when the supplement was discontinued. To avoid such problems, anyone who has been taking high-dose Vitamin C supplements for some time should reduce the dose gradually over a period of weeks before stopping the supplement altogether.

Vitamin C and inflammation

Many popular books on diet and arthritis point out that Vitamin C levels in the blood are often low in patients with rheumatoid arthritis, and recommend a Vitamin C supplement on the strength of this observation. It is indeed correct that levels fall, probably as a result of inflammation processes which use up Vitamin C and other antioxidants (see p.339) whose role is to protect tissues from the damaging products of inflammation. Some studies have found that the higher the concentration in the blood of the chemicals which accompany inflammation, the lower the levels of Vitamin C. Unfortunately adding more Vitamin C to the diet does not help to quell the inflammation or fever of rheumatoid arthritis as researchers initially hoped. Even injecting Vitamin C into the joint space does nothing to combat the inflammation there.

Nevertheless the fact that Vitamin C is needed for other purposes in the body is a good reason to try to compensate for the deficit that inflammation creates. The best plan is to eat plenty of fruit, salads and fresh lightly-cooked vegetables. If this is difficult, a supplement of Vitamin C can be taken, but this is not a real substitute for fruit and vegetables, which contain so many other nutrients besides Vitamin C.

Vitamin C and spontaneous bruising

So far we have only been talking about Vitamin C in relation to general health maintenance, not as a potential treatment for arthritis. However, there is just one symptom of rheumatoid arthritis itself which might improve in response to a Vitamin C supplement. Patients with rheumatoid arthritis sometimes have a tendency to bruise at the slightest knock, or even to suffer spontaneous skin bruising, when no obvious injury has occurred. This happens because the walls of tiny blood vessels (called capillaries) are weak and rupture easily. For anyone on an inadequate diet, Vitamin C deficiency could be contributing to the problem. Researchers have shown that giving a supplement of 500 mg of Vitamin C per day may reduce or eliminate the bruising.

· Vitamin D ·

Bones have two vital ingredients: firstly, a complex network of microscopic collagen fibres and other proteins which form a strong, rubbery framework, and secondly, crystals of calcium phosphate salts, laid down on this framework, which add hardness to the collagen. The collagen is always laid down first, and the addition of calcium salts is known as calcification. The main salt involved is tricalcium phosphate or hydroxyapatite.

Calcium and phosphorous are needed to make this salt, and Vitamin D is responsible for controlling the absorption of these two elements from foods. It also prevents them from being lost in the urine. As well as ensuring the supply of calcium and phosphorous, Vitamin D helps with the actual process of calcification.

Natural sources of Vitamin D

Vitamin D is found in fatty fish, egg yolks, milk (in small amounts), butter, cheese and margarine. (This refers to the U.K., where both Vitamins A and D are added to margarine by law. The situation is different in some other countries, and you should check the package for details of added vitamins.) Although fatty fish can be a very rich source, the amounts present vary greatly from one catch to another, making it a somewhat unreliable source. Cod-liver oil is particularly rich in Vitamins A and D and has traditionally been used as a supplement; the content of both vitamins is standardised. Vegans are often very short of Vitamin D in the diet and may need a supplement, or a fortified food, eg. margarine or one of the brands of fortified soya milk that contain Vitamin D (check labels).

No supplement of Vitamin D – nor any dietary intake – is needed if you spend time out of doors in the sunlight, because the action of sun on the skin enables the body to make this vitamin for itself. About 20 minutes of sunlight per day is needed to make all that the adult body requires, although children may need more, especially those with dark skins whose skin pigments absorb some of the sunlight. Elderly people do not make Vitamin D as efficiently and they are advised to spend 1–2 hours outdoors daily. In the U.K., and other regions at the same latitude, no ultraviolet light reaches ground level between October and March, and since it is the ultraviolet that creates Vitamin D, none is formed during the winter. However, Vitamin D can be stored for up to six months so any surplus made in the summer will sustain you through the cloudy winter months. Research shows that, even in an overcast country such as the U.K., 70% of Vitamin D in the blood comes from sunlight exposure.

If you are in the habit of using sunblock creams, you should regularly allow about 20 minutes in the sun without cream, so that your body can stock up on Vitamin D. Only some areas of skin need to be exposed, so you can still apply sunblock to the places where you burn most easily. Glass blocks ultraviolet light, so sitting in a sunny window or conservatory will not allow Vitamin D to be produced.

Of course, you should be sensible about exposure to sunlight, especially if you are in the tropics, or in areas where the ozone layer is thin, because of the risks of melanoma (one type of skin cancer). However regular and moderate exposure to the sun is probably beneficial on balance as long as there is a good intake of antioxidants such as Vitamins C and E, carotenoids and selenium in the diet. These antioxidants protect against the free radicals that are generated by sunlight (see p.342); it is free radicals that are largely responsible for the carcinogenic effects.

Unfortunately arthritis often keeps people indoors. Researchers in Denmark who studied more than 100 patients with rheumatoid arthritis found that many of the more severely disabled were lacking in Vitamin D, probably because they did not get out into the sunshine often. If you are housebound, a Vitamin D supplement may be advisable, but discuss this with your doctor first. You could also enquire from Social Services about the possibility of voluntary help to get you out more – to a nearby park where you could sit in the sun, for example.

Vitamin D deficiency in children

Children are far more susceptible to Vitamin D deficiency than adults, because they are growing and laying down new bone rapidly. An ordinary diet may not give them enough of the vitamin unless they also get plenty of exposure to sunlight. There is insufficient Vitamin D in breast milk for a baby, so it must have some sunshine to augment this, or take a Vitamin D supplement. Because Vitamin D is toxic if taken in excess, it is vital that the dose given is approved by a doctor or midwife. Premature babies are particularly vulnerable to Vitamin D deficiency.

A shortage of Vitamin D in children results in rickets, a disease that is relatively rare today but can still occur. The symptoms of rickets include aching of the legs, knees and sometimes other joints. There may also be poor growth and development, tender swelling of ankle and wrist joints, swelling at the ends of long bones and vulnerability to infections.

Those most often affected are children of Asian parentage living in northern climates. It is possible that darker skin makes less Vitamin D than light skin when exposed to the same amount of sunlight. (It seems plausible that lighter skin evolved in European populations as a result of the need, in pre-agricultural times, for Vitamin D formation in winter.) Anyone of Caribbean origin following a strict form of Rastafarian diet could also be at risk.

The traditional Asian diet is often a factor in rickets, because it may not include items such as fish, eggs, milk or butter which supply Vitamin D. The flour used to make chapattis adds to the problem. It contains substances known as phytates (see pp.309–310) which bind calcium and make it less easily absorbed; the lack of calcium, in addition to the lack of Vitamin D, makes the children more vulnerable to rickets.

Other groups of children at risk of rickets are those fed on a vegan diet or a strict macrobiotic diet. Such children often need a Vitamin D supplement: there is a synthetic form that is not derived from animals (see p.300).

Breast milk from vegan mothers may have so little Vitamin D that rickets develops unless the baby is given another source of Vitamin D; however, regular exposure to sunlight will reduce the need for Vitamin D in the milk.

Rickets can be readily treated with supplements of Vitamin D, plus calcium where needed. It is important that treatment begins as early as possible, to avoid deformities such as the characteristic bowing of the legs. Some cases of rickets require magnesium as well as Vitamin D and calcium (see p.326).

Vitamin D deficiency in adults

In adults, lack of Vitamin D results in a condition known as osteomalacia. The bones are already formed in an adult, of course, but they still have to be repaired and maintained: small areas of bone are broken down and remade all the time. When this happens in someone with insufficient Vitamin D, the bone is remade without adequate calcium salts. Bones become weakened as a result, and the earliest symptoms are vague aches and pains in the bones which may well be dismissed as 'psychosomatic' or 'just a bit of rheumatism'. If the condition goes untreated the bones may become so weak that they can break easily. There may also be partial breaks which are then repaired, and these show up on X-rays as faint lines across the bones.

The muscles are also weakened in osteomalacia, particularly the muscles around the hips which may make it difficult to get up out of an armchair or climb stairs. Deafness can be another of the symptoms.

Cases of osteomalacia have occurred among elderly women on vegan diets or very low-fat diets. It can also develop in women of Asian origin living in countries such as the U.K., and in those who are housebound and get little sunlight. One study in the U.S.A. concluded that even healthy older women living at northerly latitudes and eating a normal diet, might come close to Vitamin D deficiency in the winter.

Various conditions interfere with the absorption or metabolism of Vitamin D, making osteomalacia more likely. These include coeliac disease, surgery of the stomach or bowel, liver or kidney disease, alcoholism, prolonged use of drugs for epilepsy and a high intake of aluminium (eg. in some antacid medicines used for indigestion).

Osteomalacia is distinct from osteoporosis. In osteomalacia, calcium salts are lost from bone without any loss of cartilage, whereas in osteoporosis there is a general loss of bone mass ie. a loss of both cartilage and calcium salts. However, someone with advanced osteomalacia may develop osteoporosis as well.

How much Vitamin D is needed?

If a Vitamin D supplement is needed, for example in a housebound person who is getting little sunlight, and whose appetite is poor, then a dose of 100 IU (international units) per day is enough. This is equivalent to 2.5 µg. To obtain this from food, you would need to eat two eggs and 57 gm (2 oz) of butter or 14gm (1/2 oz) of fortified (U.K.) margarine per day. Alternatively, 42 gm (11/2 oz) of margarine would suffice. For someone who has been on a poor diet for some time, and is just starting a supplement, then 400 IU or 10 µg per day should be taken for a while. Your doctor can advise you on when to reduce the dose to 100 IU per day. A teaspoonful of cod-liver oil provides 8.4 µg of Vitamin D.

One form of Vitamin D, known as ergocalciferol or Vitamin D_2, is not derived from animals, and can therefore be taken by vegans.

Hazards of Vitamin D

Do *not* take excessive amounts of Vitamin D as these can be toxic. This is a fat-soluble vitamin and it therefore accumulates in the body with time. The symptoms of overdose include malaise and drowsiness, nausea, pains in the abdomen, constipation and excessive thirst. There is no risk of overdose of Vitamin D from long exposure to sunlight, as the body regulates the amount produced.

Over a prolonged period, even a non-toxic dose of Vitamin D can cause problems because it encourages the absorption of calcium from food, and calcification of soft tissue can occur (see p.318). Regular monitoring is essential.

A Vitamin D supplement should never be taken by those suffering from sarcoidosis, as they convert the vitamin to its active form at too high a rate and are therefore particularly vulnerable to absorbing too much calcium. It may be necessary to restrict the intake of Vitamin D from foods.

Vitamin D and arthritis

Because of the involvement of Vitamin D in bone formation it was an obvious candidate for early experiments (mostly carried out in the 1930s) using vitamin therapy for arthritis. These trials, some of which involved very high, toxic doses of Vitamin D, were largely unsuccessful, as described on p.282.

Vitamin D and osteoporosis

If there is a deficiency of Vitamin D in the diet, and little exposure to sunshine, this may contribute to osteoporosis.

· Vitamin E ·

This is actually a group of different several substances, called tocopherols. They are antioxidants which are believed to protect the body from the damaging effects of substances known as free radicals (see p.340).

Natural sources of vitamin E

The best sources of Vitamin E are sunflower seeds and sunflower oil, safflower oil, polyunsaturated margarine (if made from sunflower oil), hazelnuts, almonds, wheatgerm and sweet potatoes, with lesser amounts of useful Vitamin E in peanuts, avocados, eggs and milk products. The amount required varies depending on how much polyunsaturated fat (see p.357) is eaten and on several other factors such as smoking, drinking alcohol, exposure to air pollution and time spent in the sun (see p.342). Foods high in polyunsaturated fatty acids and low in Vitamin E, such as oily fish, create an increased demand for Vitamin E which must be met in some way (see p.150). Some nuts and cooking oils, although rich in Vitamin E, do not contain enough to match the amount of polyunsaturated fatty acid they contain. The worst foods in this respect are walnuts, sesame seeds and sesame spread (tahini), corn oil and soya oil. Pine nuts, Brazil nuts, cashews, pistachios, pecans and peanut butter are also inadequately supplied with Vitamin E, but to a lesser degree.

Deficiencies of Vitamin E

Vitamin E deficiency produces no unique set of signs and symptoms so it is difficult to diagnose. There is sometimes damage to the nervous system in the arms and legs, with a resultant loss of coordination and sensation, particularly the ability to detect vibrations. Most doctors believe that deficiency of this vitamin is rare, except among people with diseases such as cystic fibrosis which prevent the absorption of oils and fats from food – Vitamin E is a fat-soluble vitamin.

While true deficiency may be rare, there is evidence that people with higher intakes of Vitamin E and other antioxidants (see p.339) are less susceptible to several types of cancer. Furthermore, recent research has shown that Vitamin E supplements may be useful in preventing heart attacks.

Levels of Vitamin E in the blood are sometimes below normal among people suffering from rheumatoid arthritis, and levels within the affected joints may also be reduced. This is thought to be a result of ongoing inflammation, which depletes the body's supply of antioxidants (see p.339).

Whether this low level of Vitamin E actually constitutes a deficiency state is debatable. Nor is it known if Vitamin E supplements will reduce the symptoms of inflammation in rheumatoid arthritis. Remarkably little research has been done on this important topic, and no large-scale controlled trials have been carried out.

How much Vitamin E is needed?

The amount of Vitamin E required depends on the quantity of polyunsaturated fatty acids (PUFAs) eaten, because Vitamin E is needed as an antioxidant for these fats (see p.342). Current recommendations are 0.4 mg of Vitamin E per gram of PUFA. The average intake of PUFAs in western diets is about 18 gm per day, although individuals vary tremendously depending on their eating habits. If 18 gm of PUFA is consumed, then about 7 mg per day of natural **alpha-tocopherol** (the most potent form of Vitamin E) are needed, as a minimum intake. This is equivalent to 10 mg of synthetic alpha-tocopherol, or 10 IU (International Units).

International Units (IU) are useful in assessing Vitamin E because the different forms of the vitamin vary so much. Compared to natural alpha-tocopherol, beta-tocopherol is 50% as effective, and gamma-tocopherol only 10% as effective. Synthetic alpha-tocopherol is 67% as effective, but less readily absorbed.

If you eat more than 18 gm of PUFAs per day then you should ensure that your Vitamin E intake is increased to match. This is particularly important if you are eating a diet rich in oily fish (see p.150). When capsules of fish oil or evening primrose oil are taken, there is less need to worry about Vitamin E because it has already been added. For example, a supplement of 10 gm of omega-3 fish oil (see pp.50–51) would generally contain about 22 mg of alpha-tocopherol. However, in a study which compared patients taking fish oil and Vitamin E with those taking coconut oil and Vitamin E, the levels of Vitamin E in the blood did not rise among patients taking fish oil, whereas they did among those taking coconut oil. This suggests that the fish oil 'used up' absolutely all of the Vitamin E added to it, in which case a little more Vitamin E might be beneficial.

Many people who are trying to eat a healthy diet have very high intakes of PUFAs, notably linoleic acid. Some may eat as much as 40 gm of PUFAs per day, which would necessitate a Vitamin E intake of 16 mg per day.

As long as sunflower oil or safflower oil are used for cooking, the Vitamin E requirement will be easily met, with some to spare for other foods that are low in Vitamin E but high in polyunsaturates. Corn oil and soya oil should not be used. Walnuts should balanced by equal quantities of almonds or hazelnuts, or by some sunflower seeds or sunflower oil. Other nuts, such as Brazils, cashews, pecans and pistachios, can be mixed with lesser amounts of almonds or hazelnuts: a ratio of 6:1 is about right. If peanut butter is part of your diet, the deficit should be easily offset by the surplus Vitamin E in sunflower or safflower oil: the deficit in 57 gm (2 oz) of peanut butter is matched by the surplus in 7.5 ml (1 1/2 teaspoonfuls) of sunflower oil or 15 ml (1 tablespoonful) of safflower oil. If you are not using cooking oil, then 7 gm (1/4 oz) of sunflower seeds, or 9 gm (1/3 oz) of sunflower margarine will match 57 gm (2 oz) of peanut butter. Tahini should be used sparingly, or alternated with sunflower spread.

Hazards of Vitamin E

Vitamin E is toxic if taken in excess and as it is a fat-soluble vitamin, like Vitamins A and D, it is not easily excreted and tends to accumulate in the body over long time periods. No one should consume more than 400 IU – that is 400 mg of synthetic dl-alpha-tocopherol or 270 mg of natural d-alpha-tocopherol, as there have been occasional reports of toxicity at higher doses. Some authorities do suggest that higher doses can be taken – up to 3,000 IU per day – but we believe that such high doses are unnecessary, and that caution should be the rule with all fat-soluble vitamins.

Anyone taking anti-coagulant drugs (eg. for pulmonary embolism or for thrombosis) should not take Vitamin E supplements without the agreement of their doctor. This includes the Vitamin E used as a preservative in fish oil capsules or in any other preparation: always read the labels on any 'alternative remedy' before you take it. Because it is naturally occuring, Vitamin E is favoured as a preservative in wholefood products with a high oil content (where it acts as an antioxidant) – again, check the label.

High intakes of Vitamin E can make the effects of a deficiency of Vitamin K (due to poor diet, reduced fat absorption, or anticoagulant drugs) much worse.

Vitamin E and rheumatoid arthritis

There are only a few trials involving Vitamin E supplements. One was designed to investigate the possibility that Vitamin E was responsible for the improvement seen in rheumatoid arthritis sufferers taking fish oil – the Vitamin E is added to preserve the fish oil, and there had been suspicions that it was the Vitamin E producing the improvements rather than the oil itself. The trial therefore compared patients taking fish oil with others taking coconut oil as an inactive placebo; both oils had the same amount of Vitamin E added.

All the patients improved, but those taking fish oil did better. This trial gave a useful answer as regards fish oil, clearly indicating that it had some real benefits, separate from both placebo effects and Vitamin E. Unfortunately the question of whether Vitamin E itself was useful remains unanswered, because the improvement in the group taking coconut oil could have been either placebo effect or a benefit from Vitamin E. The researchers should have included a third group taking coconut oil only (without Vitamin E) as they themselves regretfully pointed out in their report on the trial.

One small-scale trial of Vitamin E used supplements of 400 IU per day (270 mg of alpha-tocopherol) for 6 weeks. The researchers asked patients to try to reduce their dosages of non-steroidal anti-inflammatory drugs (NSAIDs; see p.418), and found that the patients taking Vitamin E were able to achieve much greater reductions than those given a placebo tablet.

Another small trial, carried out at a hospital in Austria, used a much larger dose of Vitamin E and found that patients with rheumatoid arthritis suffered less pain after three weeks of supplements. Those showing the greatest rise in blood levels of Vitamin E were those whose pain decreased the most. A similar improvement was seen in morning stiffness.

Our provisional advice, based on these fragments of evidence, would be that a supplement of Vitamin E is probably worth trying for rheumatoid arthritis, especially if you have prominent signs of inflammation, such as fever and malaise, or warm red swelling around the joints. Combining Vitamin E with carotenoids and selenium may be worthwhile (see p.345–6).

Vitamin E and osteoarthritis

The same Austrian research team, whose work is described above, later studied people with osteoarthritis, and found that a high dose (400 mg of natural alpha-tocopherol, equivalent to 600 IU) was as effective as a standard NSAID drug in controlling the pain. There seems to have been some degree of inflammation in the joints of these patients, which may account for the benefits of Vitamin E. The trial was only continued for three weeks, and it is inadvisable to take such a high dose of Vitamin E for a prolonged period (see p.303 for maximum doses).

Further evidence comes from a study at an Israeli hospital where a high-dose supplement of Vitamin E was tested for osteoarthritis and turned out to be somewhat better than placebo. Unfortunately, this trial had some flaws and cannot be taken as firm scientific evidence. Another trial in which a combination of Vitamin E, Vitamin A, Vitamin C and selenium was given to people with osteoarthritis showed no benefits (see p.335); in this case the dose of Vitamin E was not reported.

Doctors in Germany have conducted two double-blind trials of Vitamin E, at a dose of 400 IU for six weeks, among patients with osteoarthritis. In both instances, pain was said to be reduced but neither trial has been fully described in scientific journals, so it is difficult to assess these claims. Overall, we would provisionally conclude that there is probably little to be gained from taking Vitamin E, unless there are clear signs of inflammation occuring as a result of the osteoarthritis – signs such as redness, tenderness or warmth around the joint.

Vitamin E and ankylosing spondylitis

Only one trial using Vitamin E has been carried out in this disease. The vitamin was compared with a standard drug treatment (an NSAID) and apparently found to be just as good. The results of this trial have not been published in full, so it is difficult to assess its value. There is probably no harm in trying Vitamin E if you have ankylosing spondylitis, but keep to the recommended dose (see p.302) and do not discontinue prescribed drugs without your doctor's agreement.

· *Vitamin K* ·

Until quite recently, this vitamin was only thought to be important for blood clotting. Deficiencies were considered to be very rare except in newborn babies.

Recent research has shown that Vitamin K is needed to make osteocalcin, one of the proteins which form the rubbery framework of the bones – the framework around which calcium phosphate crystallises. Osteocalcin is thought to be important in bone repair. In women with osteoporosis, the osteocalcin found in the blood is only half as efficient as normal osteocalcin at binding calcium phosphate, and this is probably due to mild Vitamin K deficiency.

Natural sources of Vitamin K

The foods that are rich in this vitamin include parsley, cabbage, broccoli and other 'greens'. The greener the leaves, the more Vitamin K they contain. Liver, margarine and vegetable oils (especially soya oil) are also quite good sources, and milk supplies small amounts of Vitamin K. Some is also produced by the bacteria that normally live in the intestine (the 'gut flora') and this boosts the supply.

Deficiencies of Vitamin K

More sensitive tests for Vitamin K have recently been developed and these have shown that a mild deficiency is probably quite common. This is not sufficient to have any bad effects on blood clotting, but may be a contributing factor in osteoporosis (see p.307).

Anyone who does not eat green vegetables regularly is at risk of Vitamin K deficiency.

Repeated courses of antibiotics increase the risk because they may kill off the bacteria in the intestine which manufacture Vitamin K.

Poor absorption of fat from the diet, or the use of anticoagulant drugs, can also lead to Vitamin K deficiency; note that high doses of Vitamin E will make matters worse.

How much Vitamin K is needed?

This depends on body weight. The amount recommended at present is 1 µg per kg (2.2 lb) so someone weighing 63 kg (10 stone; or 140 lb) would need 63 µg. With increasing knowledge about Vitamin K (see p.306) it is possible that the recommended intake will be increased. The *average* daily intake in the U.K. is only 50–100 µg, so some people are clearly at risk of deficiency.

A serving of broccoli weighing 56 gm (2 oz) would supply 75–100 µg of Vitamin K, thus meeting the daily requirement for most people. A generous garnish of chopped parsley, weighing 14 gm (1/2 oz) would supply 70–85 µg of Vitamin K.

Supplements of Vitamin K are now made by at least one company, although not many shops stock them. As with all vitamins, it would be much better to get your requirement from foods rather than supplements, if you can.

Hazards of Vitamin K

This is a fat soluble vitamin, so, in theory, it could be toxic, but because it has not been widely available as a supplement, and because it would be difficult to get high intakes from food, there are no data at present on toxicity. If supplements are taken they should be treated with caution, and the dosage on the package should not be exceeded.

Vitamin K and osteoporosis

When patients with osteoporosis were assessed for Vitamin K, the levels in the blood were about one third of those in people of the same age who did not have osteoporosis. After Vitamin K supplements were prescribed for women past the menopause, losses of calcium in the urine — which are associated with osteoporosis – declined sharply. Osteocalcin levels rose and the osteocalcin also became more efficient at binding calcium phosphate. Other experiments have shown that broken bones heal more rapidly when Vitamin K intake is boosted, even though the intake had apparently been adequate.

Vitamin K and ankylosing spondylitis

A study of osteocalcin levels in patients with ankylosing spondylitis showed that levels were substantially reduced. Men with ankylosing spondylitis had about 50% of normal levels of osteocalcin, while women with ankylosing spondylitis only had about 25% of normal levels. This finding may explain why people with ankylosing spondylitis are particularly vulnerable to osteoporosis. The researchers showed that levels of Vitamin D products and parathyroid hormone (both of which can affect osteocalcin) were normal. Unfortunately, they did not check Vitamin K levels.

More research is urgently needed in this area, but in the meantime it might be advisable for those with ankylosing spondylitis to improve their intake of Vitamin K-containing foods in the interests of preventing the development of osteoporosis.

Chapter 3.3

MINERALS

The term 'minerals', in nutrition, refers to substances such as iron, calcium and zinc. These are simple elements that the body needs in order to make larger and more complex substances. For example, iron is needed to make haemoglobin, a large protein molecule that incorporates iron. Haemoglobin can bind oxygen and carry it around the body in the bloodstream. Without iron, haemoglobin cannot be made in sufficient quantities, and this leads to one form of anaemia.

Some minerals are needed in substantial amounts, others in very small amounts – the latter are known as 'trace elements'. Many minerals are important because they form part of an enzyme or coenzyme – a molecule that makes particular chemical reactions happen within the body.

Deficiencies of certain minerals can play a part in some forms of arthritis. However, the extravagant claims made for minerals such as selenium in the treatment of arthritis are misleading.

Mineral Blockers

Plant foods contain certain substances that bind to some minerals and prevent those minerals being absorbed by the body. The main offenders are known as phytates, oxalates and tannin. The minerals affected include calcium, magnesium and manganese, which all play a part in the repair and maintenance of bones, and are therefore important in the prevention of osteoporosis. Absorption of iron, zinc and copper also suffers. Some research has found a link between shortages of these minerals and susceptibility to osteoporosis. Hence the special importance of this topic to those arthritis sufferers at special risk of osteoporosis (see pp.120–121) – although it is of general relevance as well, because many people are lacking minerals such as iron, zinc and magnesium with adverse effects on their health.

Phytates (also referred to as phytic acid) are found in the most fibrous outer layers of cereal grains, particularly wheat and oats. Unleavened bread (bread made without yeast), such as soda bread and pitta bread, chapatis, phulkas, parathas and nan bread, contain the most phytates, especially if the bread is made with wholemeal flour. Phytates are also abundant in wheat bran, oat bran, wheat-based and oat-based breakfast cereals, muesli containing wheat or oat flakes, and in anything made from wholewheat flour without the use of yeast: wholemeal pasta, wholemeal cakes, pastry, biscuits, cookies, crackers, crispbread etc. Some wholemeal crackers and crispbreads have extra bran added which boosts their phytate content. Phytates are largely broken down by yeasts when leavened bread — the ordinary Western loaf – is made, and do not usually cause problems.

If there is plenty of calcium in the diet, consuming a certain amount of phytate is not harmful, but in the diet of Asian communities living in cloudy northern climates, the phytates in chapatis, combined with a low level of calcium and Vitamin D in the diet, and the lack of sunshine, can lead to rickets in children or osteomalacia in adults (see pp.298–9). Vegans eating a lot of unleavened wholemeal food items could also be at risk of calcium deficiency.

Although a high-fibre diet is desirable, the widespread use of wheat bran to add fibre to the Western diet is also a cause for concern. This can greatly reduce the absorption of minerals. For example, if milk is consumed alone, 38% of the calcium is absorbed, but when added to a high-bran breakfast cereal, only 26% of the calcium is absorbed. The same sort of reduction occurs for magnesium, a mineral that is far more likely to be lacking than calcium in the average diet.

Evidence for the health-giving effects of wheat bran is far less convincing than most people imagine, and fibre is best obtained from fruit and vegetable sources (see p.353). Other whole grains, such as brown rice, sweetcorn (maize), rolled oats, oat bran and rye also bind minerals and reduce their absorption. Oat bran, now widely promoted as part of a healthy diet, binds minerals even more fiercely than wheat bran. Corn bran is three times as effective as wheat bran in binding the calcium from other foods, and so making it unavailable to the body.

Soyabeans, soya flour, soya milk and soy protein (often used as a meat substitute) also bind some minerals. However, these dietary items are not generally thought to cause any mineral deficiencies, except for soya protein which may produce problems for vegetarians if their mineral consumption is already low.

Oxalates are similar to phytates, and they too reduce calcium absorption. Rhubarb, beetroot and sweet potatoes all contain large amounts of oxalate but the richest source is spinach, which is as effective as wheat-bran cereal in reducing the uptake of calcium from milk. The calcium in spinach itself is so strongly bound by oxalates that only 3–5% is absorbed.

(Spinach's reputation as a healthy vegetable is thoroughly undeserved. As well as blocking the absorption of calcium and magnesium, it also binds manganese, which, like the other two minerals, is important in the maintenance of strong bones. In the interests of avoiding osteoporosis in later life, spinach and related vegetables (swiss chard, chard, spinach beet) should not be eaten often, particularly by vegans. Nor is spinach a rich source of iron — Popeye was wrong! This popular myth originated as a typing error: in a table showing iron content of vegetables, the decimal point was typed in the wrong place for the figure relating to spinach, which made it seem ten times richer in iron than it actually is.)

Other foods rich in phytates and/or oxalates include almonds, cashews, sesame seeds and dried fruits.

Tannin is found mainly in tea – it is the stuff that makes the inside of the teapot brown. Drinking tea with meals is inadvisable for vegans or anyone on a dairy-free diet, since the tannin will greatly reduce the amount of calcium obtained from other foods and could easily create a calcium deficiency. Manganese, magnesium and iron absorption will also be adversely affected.

Certain foods block the mineral blockers and counteract their effects. These include Vitamin C, citric acid (found in oranges, lemons and other citrus fruits) and protein, especially animal protein. If any of these are eaten at the same time as a mineral blocker, such as bran, it will result in far better mineral absorption for iron, although there is less beneficial effect on calcium absorption.

Most people eating a healthy mixed diet with plenty of fruit and green leafy vegetables, some meat and milk products, and other foods such as cereals and nuts, need not worry about mineral blockers. Those who should be careful are people with little appetite who are not eating well, the elderly (who absorb nutrients less efficiently), vegetarians (who might be short of iron and/or zinc), anyone avoiding milk products (who might well be short of calcium) and anyone eating few green vegetables (who might be short of magnesium). Vegans or those on macrobiotic diets might be lacking manganese, in addition to iron, zinc and calcium. If you fall into one of these groups, you need to avoid eating large quantities of wheat bran, unleavened bread and other unyeasted wholemeal products. Do not drink tea with meals or directly afterwards – orange juice would be a good substitute as the Vitamin C and citric acid will improve mineral absorption, particularly that of iron. It may also be wise not to habitually drink red wine or coffee with (or immediately after) meals: these contain polyphenols, another group of substances that block the absorption of non-heme iron (the kind of iron found in vegetarian foods).

· *Calcium* ·

This mineral is involved in the calcification or hardening of bone.

Calcium nutrition is affected by the diet as a whole. On the one hand, some foods contain substances that block the absorption of calcium. Known as phytates, oxalates and tannins, they occur in foods such as unleavened bread, wheat-bran cereals and crackers, wholemeal pastry and cakes, spinach and tea (see pp.309–311).

On the other hand, high-protein foods increase losses of calcium from the body (see pp.405–7). Those most at risk in this respect are people eating a diet containing plenty of cheese, eggs, meat or fish, but not many fruits and vegetables. This is the typical Western diet, and its effects, in terms of losses of calcium, cannot be remedied by taking in more calcium. These topics are dealt with in more detail on pages 164–5.

Natural sources of calcium

Dairy products such as milk, yoghurt and cheese are the main source of calcium in the Western diet. (Because of the acidifying effect on the urine – see above – and consequent calcium loss from the body, cheese is not a particularly good source unless combined with a large portion of salad or fruit.)

Some nutritionists are concerned about the emphasis on dairy products as a calcium source because they are low in magnesium, and the ratio of the two is important. They believe that plant sources should provide more of our calcium, since they also contain a good supply of magnesium.

The main plant sources are broccoli, nuts (especially hazelnuts), seeds, oats, lentils and beans. Certain fruits will supplement the calcium supply, notably figs, blackcurrants, oranges and raisins. However, fairly large amounts of these vegetables and fruits (see p.317) are needed to supply the daily requirement (see p.314).

Bread contains some natural calcium, plus a certain amount added by law (in the U.K.) to all except wholemeal loaves. Soya milk and tofu may also be fortified with calcium, but check the packet to be sure.

Fish with small soft edible bones, such as sardines, are an excellent source of calcium if eaten whole, but a poor source of magnesium.

In hard-water areas, some calcium is obtained from tap water. In the U.K., the contribution from tap water is about 15% of the daily requirement on average, but much lower percentages will be achieved where there is soft water. If you currently have hard water, using water filters or installing a water softener will obviously reduce this source.

The quantities of available calcium in different foods are given on p.317.

Deficiencies of calcium

Insufficient calcium absorbed from the diet can contribute to rickets in children (see p.134) and osteomalacia in adults (see p.119), conditions whose fundamental cause is a lack of Vitamin D.

A severe shortage of calcium and/or Vitamin D in the diet, if allowed to continue for several years, can lead to a condition known as secondary hyperparathyroidism. For some with this condition, the early symptoms look remarkably like rheumatoid arthritis, and are easily misdiagnosed. If you have been eating a dairy-free diet for some time, and have recently developed what appears to be rheumatoid arthritis, it would be wise to tell your doctor about your eating habits, so that the possibility of secondary hyperparathyroidism can be considered. The disorder is easily treated, so this could lead to a prompt recovery.

For people on restricted diets owing to food allergy or intolerance, calcium deficiency is the most common nutritional problem, because milk and milk products are often excluded entirely, and these are important sources of calcium. Alternative calcium-containing foods are listed on page 317.

The most worrying situation is when children are on a diet that lacks sufficient calcium. Such a deficiency can seriously affect their growth and development. It is most important that children either eat dairy products, or take a suitable calcium supplement (see pp. 314 and 318). Women who are breastfeeding also need to ensure that their calcium intake is adequate (see p.314).

A shortage of calcium in the diet is also thought, by many medical authorities, to be one risk factor for osteoporosis, the thinning of the bones which occurs mainly in older people, especially women who have gone through the menopause or 'change of life'. However the exact role of calcium is still unclear, and the dose needed per day is hotly debated. Many medical researchers believe there is far more to osteoporosis, in nutritional terms, than simply a lack of calcium. For more on this, see below, and for practical advice about avoiding osteoporosis, turn to Chapter 2.3 (p.161).

How much calcium is needed?

This is an extremely tough question to answer, as regards the group most at risk of osteoporosis: women who have gone through the menopause ('post-menopausal' in medical terms), as well as those who are currently going through the menopause or are coming up to the age when it can be expected (45–55 years). It is dealt with fully in the next section.

Calcium requirements for children are set at 400–800 mg per day by the WHO (World Health Organization) and most countries, rising to 600–1200 mg per day for teenagers and young adults (11–24 year olds). Breastfeeding mothers need 1000–1200 mg per day. Adult men and premenopausal women are advised to take 400–500 mg per day by WHO, but 700–800 mg per day by the U.S. government and most European countries.

Corticosteroids increase the losses of calcium in the urine, and anyone taking such drugs should keep their calcium intake high. The overall composition of the diet also has a profound effect on calcium losses in the urine, as described below.

Calcium and osteoporosis

High-calcium diets, or calcium supplements, are commonly regarded as the standard preventive measure against osteoporosis or 'thinning of the bones'. The most generous estimates put the amount of calcium required by menopausal and post-menopausal women at 1,500 mg per day (roughly equivalent to drinking 1.2 litres or 2 pints of milk). Other estimates of requirements for this age group range from 525 mg per day upwards.

There may be a case for not supplementing calcium at very high levels such as 1,500 mg/day. When on a diet with a *lower* calcium content than this, the body adjusts itself accordingly and is more efficient in absorbing and utilising the calcium that *is* available. What is more, on a lower calcium intake, the absorption of other minerals such as magnesium is greatly improved. There is concern in some quarters that magnesium may be lacking in the Western diet.

Other aspects of the modern Western lifestyle are probably contributing to our epidemic of osteoporosis. Important factors so far identified include lack of regular, strenuous physical activity (which stimulates bone growth and repair), and various dietary habits which encourage calcium loss from the bones, such as eating large amounts of salt, and drinking alcohol and caffeine. Cigarette smoking is also believed to increase calcium loss.

Well known among medical researchers, but less well publicised, is the fact that eating a high-protein diet, especially when combined with high intake of cereal grains and few vegetables or fruits, causes a substantial increase in the amount of calcium lost from the body in the urine. The reasons for this are explained on pp.405-7.

Laboratory studies in which people are fed varying amounts of protein and calcium show that, as protein consumption increases, more calcium is needed to outweigh the losses in urine. But at a certain level of protein consumption, the extra calcium simply cannot compensate for what is being lost. The body goes into 'negative calcium balance': more calcium is going out than is coming in, which means that the bones are being depleted.

These laboratory findings may explain why other studies – ones that look at the effect of calcium intake on osteoporosis in Western women eating their habitual diet – give such varying and contradictory results. Some of these studies seem to show that higher calcium intakes reduce the risk of osteoporosis, while others find no benefit from extra calcium. This can be explained if we think of the high protein diet (plus lack of physical activity and other lifestyle factors) causing steady losses of bone mineral: extra calcium may be able to compensate, or it may not, depending on how great the protein-induced losses are for the particular group of women being studied. So some trials find that calcium helps – others do not.

In addition to a high protein intake, other factors of the modern Western diet may also be contributing to the problem of osteoporosis. These include low levels of Vitamin K, folic acid and magnesium in the diet – all nutrients that are found in green leafy vegetables. Other vitamins and minerals may also be lacking and may encourage the development of osteoporosis.

A great deal more research needs to be done to confirm these findings and to establish exactly how much calcium is required, but it seems certain that, to reverse the present trend towards ever-increasing rates of osteoporosis, we must do far more than just take calcium supplements. Recommendations for a comprehensive dietary approach to preventing osteoporosis are given in Chapter 2.3 (p.161).

Assessing calcium intake

Calcium is one of the minerals where intake may well be deficient for many people, and it is therefore useful to calculate the amounts in the foods you eat. Vegans, and those avoiding dairy products, are particularly at risk of not getting enough calcium. The question of how much calcium is actually absorbed from the food is relevant, and care should be taken to avoid phytates and other mineral blockers (see pp.309–311) if your diet is low in calcium.

Even foods that are rich in calcium may contain other substances that block absorption, a fact that is often ignored in popular books on nutrition. For example, spinach is frequently listed as a good source of calcium for vegans. In fact it is so loaded with oxalates that only 3–5% of its calcium is absorbed, making it virtually worthless as a calcium source.

Other foods differ considerably in the percentage of their calcium that can actually be absorbed. Only about 37% of the calcium in milk is absorbed, while the figure for soya products is lower still, at 31%. Green vegetables of the cabbage family, such as broccoli and spring greens have better absorption, 50–68%.

The official recommended intakes for calcium refer to the total amount eaten, not the amount absorbed. It is assumed that people are eating a mixed diet, with three-quarters of their calcium derived from dairy products, and that the overall absorption will probably average out at 30–40%. If this is the case, the different absorption rates of non-dairy foods do not matter too much when calculating the total amount of calcium available from the diet. However, the differences may be very important to vegans and anyone else avoiding dairy products: the calcium in cauliflower, for example, is four times as useful as that in haricot beans ('baked beans'): absorption rates are 68% and 17% respectively.

In the tables below, we have adjusted the figures for total calcium content to take account of absorption rates, using milk (37%) as the standard. You can add up the totals and compare them directly to the recommended daily allowance. For example, if you were to eat 200 gm (7 oz) of Chinese cabbage a day this would supply 300 mg of calcium or 25–50% of the daily requirement for a young adult.

Unfortunately, figures are not yet available for the absorption rates from bread or cheese, so we have used estimates of 50% and 37% respectively. Note that this refers to leavened bread (made with yeast) and figures will be much lower for unleavened bread (see p.309–310).

As these figures clearly show, dairy products can be very useful in supplying a large part of the calcium requirement, but bear in mind that they are extremely poor sources of magnesium which must therefore come from other foods (see p.328). Vegetable foods that are rich in calcium, such as broccoli, have the advantage of providing magnesium as well, and providing them in the correct ratio – two parts calcium to one part magnesium. Where calcium is obtained from dairy products, a magnesium-rich food such as hazelnuts, peanuts, walnuts or oat flakes should be consumed regularly as well.

Table 20: Amount required to supply 300 mg total calcium: (adjusted to allow for different absorption rates)

Whole or skimmed milk	250 ml (just under $^1/_2$ pint)
Cheddar-type cheese	43 gm ($1^1/_2$ oz)
Reduced fat cheese	36 gm ($1^1/_4$ oz)
Yoghurt (whole milk)	150 gm ($5^1/_4$ oz)
Cottage cheese	410 gm (15 oz)
Cream cheese	330 gm (12 oz)
Camembert-type cheese	85 gm (3 oz)
Ice-cream	230 gm (8 oz)
Evaporated milk	100 ml (7 tablespoonfuls)
Milk chocolate	150 gm ($5^1/_4$ oz)
Sardines, tinned, including the bones	57 gm (2 oz)
Wholemeal bread	400 gm (14 oz)
Brown or white bread (if fortified with calcium)	200gm (7 oz)
Fortified soya milk (*Unisoy Gold*, *Plamil*)	*378ml ($^2/_3$ pint)
Unfortified soya milk	7 litres ($12^1/_2$ pints)
Soya beans, white haricot beans, and 'baked beans'	550 gm (19 oz)
Red-skinned beans	2400 gm (5 lb $4^1/_2$ oz)
Pinto beans	1079 gm (2 lb 6 oz)
Tempeh, tofu made with nigari	*255 gm (9 oz)
Soya cheese, tofu made with calcium chloride or calcium sulphate	*75–150 gm ($2^3/_4$– $5^1/_4$ oz)
Almonds	156 gm ($5^1/_2$ oz)
Unhulled sesame seeds	50 gm ($1^3/_4$ oz)
Hulled sesame seeds	340 gm (12 oz)
Radishes	460 gm (1 lb)
Watercress	125 gm ($4^1/_2$ oz)
Parsley	100 gm ($3^1/_2$ oz)
Chinese cabbage	200 gm (7 oz)
Cauliflower	510 gm (1 lb 2 oz)
Spring greens	255 gm (9 oz)
Turnip greens	137 gm ($4^3/_4$ oz)
Purple broccoli	170 gm (6 oz)
Green broccoli, cabbage	460 gm (1 lb)
Brussel sprouts	630 gm (1 lb 6 oz)
Dried figs	120 gm ($4^1/_4$ oz)
Black treacle	57 gm (2 oz)

* may depend on brand purchased: look for the calcium content on the package.

Hazards of calcium supplements

Too much calcium could be damaging, and calcium supplements should not be over-used, especially the kind which also contain Vitamin D. If there is excessive calcium in the blood (usually a result of too much Vitamin D) it is likely to become deposited in soft tissues where it does not belong. The main site of this damaging calcification is usually the kidney. However calcification can also occur in other soft tissues. Anyone taking a high-dose supplement of Vitamin D should be tested regularly for the level of calcium in their blood, to ensure that it has not risen too high: if you have been prescribed Vitamin D, ask your doctor to confirm that your calcium levels are being monitored. Do not take non-prescribed Vitamin D supplements unless you are sure you need them, and keep well within the recommended dose; if in any doubt consult your doctor.

Calcium supplements need to be selected carefully. Calcium citrate is one of the best, although not the cheapest. Calcium carbonate is inexpensive and is absorbed well as long as it is taken at mealtimes, when the stomach acid can act on it. People who produce too little stomach acid (a common problem with advancing age) would be better off taking calcium citrate. Bonemeal and dolomite are sometimes sold as calcium supplements. However they are not recommended, as they may be contaminated with toxic metals.

Taking high-dose calcium supplements while also taking non-steroidal anti-inflammatory drugs (NSAIDs – see p.418) might lead to an increase in blood pressure, because the drugs suppress the regulatory mechanism in the kidney which usually comes into play to deal with large calcium loads. If you are concerned about this, ask your doctor to check your blood pressure.

· *Phosphorous* ·

This mineral is a crucial ingredient in calcium phosphate, the crystalline substance that makes bones hard. All the phosphorous consumed in our food is in the form of phosphate (which consists of phosphorous and oxygen). Once absorbed by the body it is combined with calcium to make calcium phosphate crystals.

As well as its hardening role in the bones, phosphate is important in various chemical reactions in the body. It is also used in the chemical 'buffers' which control the acidity of the blood (see p.405).

Sources of phosphorous and phosphate additives

Phosphorous is found in many foods, but is particularly plentiful in hard cheeses, sardines, egg yolks and wheat bran. Nuts, beans and lentils, wholemeal bread and pasta, rye crispbread, wholewheat cereals and rolled oats are also rich sources, while levels are fairly high in meat and most fish.

Various phosphates are used as food additives, denoted by the following E numbers: E338–341, E450–452 and E1410–E1414. They are used in colas and other soft drinks, for example, and in frozen chickens to bulk out the meat.

Baking powder is made with phosphate, which makes self-raising flour a rich source. This type of flour is used mainly for cakes and sponge puddings.

Deficiencies of phosphorous

Deficiencies of this mineral are extremely rare – the average Westerner far exceeds the daily requirement for phosphorous. Very occasionally phosphorous deficiency occurs in elderly people taking diuretics (drugs that increase water loss from the body), in people taking a lot of indigestion remedies, or in alcoholics. The symptoms include muscle weakness and increased susceptibility to infections.

How much phosphorous is needed?

Calcium and phosphorous are needed in roughly equal amounts. Current U.K. recommendations are to eat about 540 mg per day.

In fact, the average daily intake in the West is between 1,200 mg and 2,000 mg – far in excess of the amounts recommended. It is unlikely that this excess causes any problems, but a few doctors are concerned about the impact on osteoporosis (see below).

Phosphorous and osteoporosis

Some doctors have suggested that the high intake of phosphate in the Western diet might interfere with the uptake and utilisation of calcium. However, a scientific trial comparing low intakes of phosphate with high intakes of phosphate (up to 2,000 mg per day) showed that there was no adverse effect on uptake of calcium, and in fact the phosphate seemed beneficial because less calcium was lost in the urine. Although calcium absorption is apparently unaffected, high phosphate intake could still affect bone density in some other way. An American study of osteoporosis which looked at bone density in elderly women, showed that those with the highest intakes of phosphorous in their diet had a somewhat lower bone density. This has not yet been confirmed by other studies, and it is unclear how phosphate intake might have this effect, but it would seem sensible to avoid eating large amounts of phosphate.

· *Iron* ·

Iron is an essential part of the red substance, haemoglobin, which carries oxygen in the blood.

Natural sources of iron

All red meat is a good source of iron, but liver, kidney and heart are especially valuable (and inexpensive). Poultry and fish supply some iron, while shellfish and egg yolks are particularly good sources. In the U.K., most bread other than wholemeal bread must be fortified with iron by law, but wholemeal bread is still a richer source. Oats and millet are good sources, as are beans and lentils, molasses and parsley. Spinach, despite its reputation, is not rich in iron and may block its absorption (see p.111).

The iron in meat is known as **heme iron**, while that in eggs, milk and plant foods is **non-heme iron**. Heme iron is much better absorbed by the human body than non-heme iron, putting vegetarians at some risk of iron deficiency.

Mineral blockers such as phytates, oxalates and tannin (see pp.309–311) interfere with iron absorption, especially non-heme iron. Drinking tea with meals is therefore inadvisable for vegetarians. Orange juice and other sources of Vitamin C, greatly improve the absorption of non-heme iron by opposing mineral blockers.

Deficiencies of iron

A lack of haemoglobin, known as anaemia, can be due to deficiency of iron although there are other causes as well. Tiredness is one of the major symptoms.

Anaemia and rheumatoid arthritis

Patients with rheumatoid arthritis quite often suffer from anaemia even though their diet contains adequate amounts of iron.

Occasionally this is due to taking NSAIDs (non-steroidal anti-inflammatory drugs, see p.418) which can cause damage to the lining of the digestive tract. If this damage is severe there may be loss of blood in the faeces, sufficient to lead to anaemia. Any sign of blood in the stools should be reported to your doctor. Generally the bleeding occurs in the stomach or the part of the intestine just beyond the stomach, and by the time the blood is passed in the stools it is black in colour, rather than red. If your stools look black or 'tarry', let the doctor know as soon as possible. It is important to emphasise that any serious degree of bleeding is fairly unusual even among those who have been taking NSAIDs for a long time.

Far more common is an anaemia that results directly from the disease process of rheumatoid arthritis. Exactly how this occurs is not clear. It seems that the reticuloenothelial system may be at fault – the part of the immune system which is responsible for mopping up debris and dead cells, (including red blood cells) and breaking them down. Instead of releasing the iron from dead red cells, as it should do, the reticuloendothelial system of patients with rheumatoid arthritis apparently retains the iron, causing a shortage in the blood. Iron may also be taken up and retained by the joint synovium, which is greatly enlarged in rheumatoid arthritis.

Another possibility is that the diet is lacking in folic acid (see p.187), a B vitamin that is needed for the efficient utilisation of iron.

If you are lacking in iron, your doctor may suggest a supplement, although taking extra iron does not always correct the deficiency since there are often reduced levels of iron-transporting proteins in the blood of those with rheumatoid arthritis, as well as a reduced iron supply. The insufficient quantities of transporting proteins cannot be remedied except by drugs such as corticosteroids which treat the underlying disease. Nevertheless you should take whatever iron supplements are prescribed (unless you have a serious adverse reaction to them – see below).

Hazards of iron supplements

Occasionally patients with rheumatoid arthritis find that iron supplements make their symptoms worse. This is rare but when it does happen it can produce quite a sharp deterioration. If you began to get worse about the time you started taking iron tablets, and think the two might be connected, stop taking the supplement for now and discuss the matter with your doctor or rheumatologist.

Patients with gout who are taking the drug allopurinol should avoid taking iron supplements at the same time, except for short periods (see p.251).

Iron supplements can lead to zinc deficiency if the intake of zinc is already low.

How much iron is needed?

The amounts recommended for adult males and post-menopausal women range from 6 mg to 10 mg per day, with more needed by teenagers.

Until the menopause, women need more iron per day than men because they lose blood every month during menstruation. Recommended amounts range from 11.5 mg to 22 mg per day, but women with especially heavy periods may require even more. Pregnancy may further increase the requirement, but opinion is divided on this point; in the U.S.A. the authorities set the requirement at 30 mg per day during pregnancy.

Since vegetarians and vegans are most at risk of iron deficiency, they should calculate whether their diet is providing enough. The following vegetarian foods are valuable sources:

To obtain 1 mg of iron you would need to eat:

Wheatgerm	14 gm ($1/2$ oz)
Wholemeal bread	43 gm ($1\,1/2$ oz)
Fortified breakfast cereals	14–28 gm ($1/2$–1oz)
Eggs	50 gm ($1\,3/4$ oz)
Sunflower seeds, pine kernels, cashew nuts	18 gm ($2/3$ oz)
Pumpkin seeds	10 gm ($1/3$ oz)
Unhulled sesame seeds	7 gm ($1/4$ oz)
Parsley	14 gm (1 oz)
Watercress	50 gm ($1\,3/4$ oz)
Seaweeds	7 gm ($1/4$ oz)
Haricot beans, 'baked beans', chickpeas, peanuts, peanut butter	43 gm ($1\,1/2$ oz)
Soya beans, tempeh, lentils	35 gm ($1\,1/4$ oz)
Soya flour	14 gm ($1/2$ oz)
Peas, split peas	57 gm (2 oz)
Prunes	35 gm ($1\,1/4$ oz)
Raisins, dried figs, dried apricots	28 gm (1 oz)
Black treacle	10 gm ($1/3$ oz)

· *Zinc* ·

Zinc is one of the most controversial topics in nutrition, with some people maintaining that deficiency is very common, while others disagree. This controversy cannot easily be resolved because it is very difficult to measure the levels of zinc in the body accurately.

Natural sources of zinc

Muscle meats such as beef, lamb and pork are a good source, with lean meat containing the most zinc, and red meat (eg. beef) being superior to white meat (eg. pork or chicken). Fish is not a particularly good source, although shrimps and clams are, and oysters (if you can afford them!) are one of the richest sources available. Cheese and egg yolks supply some zinc.

Wholegrains (wholewheat, rye, oats, maize and brown rice) are also quite rich in zinc, whereas refined foods such as white flour are not. However, the phytate found in un-yeasted wholewheat products (see pp.309–310) blocks zinc absorption, so that only 10–15% of the zinc eaten is absorbed from a diet based on unleavened bread, bran, and other wholewheat foods, compared to 20–40% absorption on a highly refined diet. Eating animal protein, especially meat, partially counteracts the effect of phytate and thus improves zinc absorption. Soya protein tends to block absorption. Nuts, parsley, carrots, lentils and beans, buckwheat, and potatoes are fairly good sources of zinc, although the amounts vary tremendously in all vegetable foods depending on the soil and the crop variety grown. In view of the difficulties in ensuring an adequate zinc intake from vegetable food, vegetarians and vegans should consider taking a small zinc supplement.

Deficiencies of zinc

There are no unmistakable signs of zinc deficiency. The signs and symptoms claimed range from diarrhoea, skin conditions, poor taste and smell, sleep disturbances and hair loss, through to impaired growth, slow healing of wounds, impotence, low sperm count and infertility. Of course, all these can be due to other causes. The usual approach in diagnosing zinc deficiency is to give a zinc supplement and see if the symptoms clear up – something that falls far short of sound scientific medicine! The only reliable indicator of zinc deficiency – and even this is debatable – is the appearance of white flecks or spots on the fingernails.

How much zinc is needed?

An intake of 15 mg per day for men and 12 mg a day for women is generally recommended. An extra 1 mg a day during pregnancy and 2 mg a day when breastfeeding is suggested. Men lose 1 mg of zinc in semen with each ejaculation.

Taking an iron supplement increases the need for zinc by reducing zinc absorption. Corticosteroid drugs increase the losses of zinc in the urine, and a high zinc intake is advisable to compensate for this.

Since vegetarians and vegans are most at risk of zinc deficiency they should attempt to calculate how much zinc their diet provides.

To get 1 mg of zinc without eating meat you would need to consume:

Wholemeal bread	57 gm (2 oz)
Fortified breakfast cereals	50 gm (1³/₄ oz)
Wheatgerm	7 gm (¹/₄ oz)
Brown rice	142 gm (5 oz)
Eggs	77 gm (2³/₄ oz)
Cheddar cheese	28–50 gm (1–1³/₄ oz)
Soya cheese, tempeh	57 gm (2 oz)
Almonds, peanuts	28 gm (1 oz)
Walnuts	43 gm (1¹/₂ oz)
Sesame seeds, pumpkin seeds, sunflower seeds, cashew nuts	21 gm (³/₄ oz)
Watercress	142 gm (5 oz)
Baked beans, haricot beans, soya beans	100 gm (3¹/₂ oz)
Lentils, chickpeas, split peas	70–85 gm (2¹/₂–3 oz)

Bear in mind that all values for zinc are highly variable, and these figures are only a general quide. Err on the generous side with zinc-rich vegetable foods to ensure you get enough, or take a supplement.

Hazards of zinc supplements

To correct a deficiency, no more than 20 mg a day is needed. Doses of 50 mg a day affect iron and copper levels adversely. Even at lower doses, if taking zinc for longer than six months, blood tests for iron, copper and histidine should be carried out from time to time, since depleted levels have been reported in response to zinc.

Zinc and inflammatory arthritis

The levels of zinc in the blood of people with rheumatoid arthritis may be slightly below normal. This in turn reduces the level of a substance called retinol binding protein (RBP) whose job it is to transport Vitamin A from the liver to the bloodstream. Since Vitamin A levels are reduced in rheumatoid arthritis owing to a reduction in RBP, researchers have speculated about the possibility of giving zinc supplements to improve Vitamin A status and perhaps relieve some of the symptoms of rheumatoid arthritis. However, the results have been disappointing.

Several studies have looked at the effects of high-dose zinc supplements on rheumatoid arthritis. The results seem rather contradictory, but overall the weight of evidence is against zinc. It looks as if this mineral supplement may produce some short-term benefit but that this disappears after about six months, and patients may then begin to deteriorate, *sometimes ending up with more severe symptoms than at the outset*. The side-effects of zinc at the very high doses used in these trials (135 mg per day) were also unpleasant, especially the lingering and obtrusive taste of the zinc.

A study of zinc in patients with psoriatic arthritis produced far more encouraging results. The same dose was used, and apparently reduced joint pain, morning stiffness and joint swelling. Despite the improvement in their arthritis, the patients saw no benefit to the psoriasis itself. It should be noted that these patients showed no apparent deficiency in zinc before the trial began, so the supplement was not correcting a deficiency: zinc sulphate seemed to be acting as a drug in this instance. For this reason you should not try out a course of zinc without the full agreement of your doctor.

Zinc and osteoporosis

Some studies have found that zinc levels are unusually low in the blood and bone of elderly people with osteoporosis. Zinc is thought to be important in the formation of healthy bone. Consuming a little more zinc, as well as other vitamins and minerals, may be beneficial in warding off osteoporosis – see Chapter 2.3 (p.161).

· *Magnesium* ·

This mineral plays various important roles in the body, including several that relate to bone maintenance.

Natural sources of magnesium

Magnesium is often in short supply when people eat a diet of highly refined foods, since the important sources are dark green leafy vegetables (but not spinach or chard where absorption is blocked by oxalates – see p.310), peanuts and other nuts. Shrimps are also a good source. Drinking water is an important source of magnesium in hard-water districts, and by installing a water-softener, using water filters or drinking bottled water, you may reduce your intake. People living in softwater districts need to eat more magnesium-rich foods.

Phytates and tannin (see pp.309–311) block the absorption of magnesium.

High or even moderate alcohol consumption increases the loss of magnesium in the urine, and can lead to magnesium deficiency. This may contribute to the development of osteoporosis in alcoholics. The regular use of diuretics can deplete magnesium levels in the body.

A high consumption of sugar, fat, calcium and/ or Vitamin D all increase the need for magnesium.

Magnesium and rickets

Magnesium is vital for the action of Vitamin D, so a severe deficiency can result in disorders such as rickets not responding to Vitamin D supplements. This problem, known as 'refractory rickets', only clears up when a magnesium supplement is given in addition to Vitamin D.

Magnesium and inflammatory arthritis

Some research suggests that magnesium deficiency leads to increased levels of pro-inflammatory messenger molecules, or cytokines (see p.415) which could contribute to the inflammation of rheumatoid arthritis and other inflammatory forms of arthritis.

Patients with rheumatoid arthritis taking the drug cyclosporin A tend to show depleted magnesium levels in their blood.

Magnesium and osteoporosis

Magnesium is involved in the proper absorption of calcium from food, and it is also found in small amounts in the calcium phosphate crystals of the bones: if there is too little magnesium, the crystals form in a different way and the bone is more brittle as a result. Various studies have shown a link between mild magnesium deficiency and osteoporosis.

One scientific trial of magnesium supplements has been carried out in Israel. Thirty women with symptoms of osteoporosis and low levels of magnesium in their blood were given 250–750 mg of magnesium per day for six months, followed by 250 mg per day for another 18 months. In 71% there was an increase in bone density – a reversal of the osteoporosis. Another 16% suffered no further loss of bone density, whereas women with osteoporosis who had not been treated (the control group) continued to lose bone mass at a steady rate. The women who did not respond to the magnesium supplement all had a disorder of the thyroid or parathyroid gland which was responsible for their osteoporosis. Although this trial has been criticised because the control group was not exactly comparable with the treatment group, the finding of an increase in bone density is so impressive that it outweighs the criticism.

Another trial of magnesium gave 600 mg per day, combined with 500 mg calcium and a wide range of other nutrients: most of the vitamins and eight other minerals. There was an improvement in bone density among those taking the supplement, who were all women past the menopause with some early signs of osteoporosis. Because there were so many different ingredients in the supplement, this trial does not provide any conclusive evidence about magnesium.

How much magnesium is needed?

The current recommendations for magnesium intake in the U.S.A. and northern Europe (about 270–350 mg per day) are much too low, according to some researchers, who think that we should be consuming over 500 mg per day. Actual intakes fall far short of this – about 70–160 mg per day on average. One study in the U.S.A. showed that 85% of women were getting less than 300 mg per day.

Pregnancy increases the need for magnesium and calcium. Women who have had a large number of children may have developed a long-standing deficiency of both magnesium and calcium. Diabetics are also vulnerable to magnesium deficiency.

After the menopause, women lose more magnesium in their urine, but this can be corrected by Hormone Replacement Therapy (HRT). Elderly people often have poor absorption of magnesium combined with increased losses in the urine, so they need a higher intake.

High calcium intake can block the absorption of magnesium, a fact that worries many doctors given the meagre supplies of magnesium in Western diets and the large intake of calcium, whether from dairy products or calcium supplements. The ideal ratio of calcium to magnesium is 2:1, whereas average Western diets provide ratios as high as 4:1, even without calcium supplements.

To obtain 100 mg of magnesium, you would need to eat:

Sardines	200 gm (7 oz)
Peanuts	57 gm (2 oz)
Hazelnuts, walnuts	70 gm (2¹/2 oz)
Lentils	100 gm (3¹/2 oz) (dry weight)

These are foods with the highest content of absorbable magnesium. Other foods will provide much lesser amounts.

You would obtain 25 mg of magnesium from the following:

Lean meat	100 gm (3¹/2 oz)
Most fish	100 gm (3¹/2 oz)
Cheese	100 gm (3¹/2 oz)
Milk	250 ml (¹/2 pint)
Peas	70 gm (2¹/2 oz)
Broccoli, courgettes, spring greens, dark green cabbage	114 gm (4 oz)
Potatoes	150 gm (5 oz)
Cauliflower, sweet peppers, aubergine, carrots, mushrooms	250 gm (9 oz)
Most other vegetables	500 gm (1 lb 2 oz)
One small banana	70 gm (2¹/2 oz)
Blackcurrants, kiwi fruit, pineapple	150 gm (5¹/4 oz)
Most other fruits	300 gm (10¹/2 oz)
Chocolate	43 gm (1¹/2 oz)
White rice	70 gm (2¹/2 oz)
White bread	100 gm (3¹/2 oz)
Pasta	43 gm (1¹/2 oz)

Popular books on nutrition frequently recommend wholegrains and bran as good sources of magnesium. It is true that the outer layers of cereal grains, the bran, are rich in magnesium, but they are also rich in phytates (see p.309) which bind the magnesium and make it unavailable. Research has shown that wheat bran and oat bran both retain their own magnesium, and remove magnesium from other foods eaten at the same time. Exposure to yeast does not cancel out this effect, so wholemeal bread will not contribute any absorbable magnesium to the diet, even though its magnesium content is quite high. No research has yet been carried out on brown rice, as far as we know, nor on rye and barley, but it seems likely that their bran layers will have the same properties.

In view of the uncertainties currently surrounding magnesium absorption from cereal grains, and the low levels in most foods, it may be advisable to rely on a supplement if you are concerned about your intake of this mineral.

Hazards of magnesium supplements

Some laxatives contain magnesium, as do some indigestion remedies. If you regularly take medicines of this kind, check their constituents for magnesium before taking a magnesium supplement – as with any mineral, it is possible to take too much. Excessive magnesium produces a loss of calcium phosphate from the bone similar to that seen in osteomalacia (see p.119).

· *Potassium* ·

Potassium, in conjunction with sodium and chloride (the last two are both found in table salt), plays a vital role in maintaining the body fluids, such as the blood, in a stable state, so that the body functions efficiently. Potassium tends to make the blood slightly more alkaline, ie. able to neutralise acids (see p.404).

Natural sources of potassium

Many foods contain potassium, but if they also contain substances such as sulphur that produce acid when the food is broken down by the body, the benefits of the potassium are cancelled out. Fruits and vegetables are rich in potassium, but low in acid-forming minerals, and their overall effect on body fluids is to make them more alkaline, which reduces calcium loss from the bones (see pp.403–7).

Deficiencies of potassium

Serious potassium deficiency is very unusual, except among the elderly (see below), but most people in industrialised societies should probably eat more more potassium, which is found abundantly in fruits and vegetables. Increasing the intake of these foods leads to a more alkaline blood and urine, as explained on p.406, offsetting the effects of our high-protein diets. This reduces the loss of calcium from the body and may therefore help in the prevention of osteoporosis.

Taking aspirin or corticosteroids increases the need for potassium. Some diuretic drugs (used to combat water retention) increase losses of potassium in the urine, and can induce a deficiency. Other diuretics help to retain potassium and can lead to excessively high levels in the blood. A combination of these two different types of diuretic can avoid such problems. If you take diuretics, ask your doctor or pharmacist for advice on this.

Some older people lose more potassium in their urine, and if they are also eating a poor diet based mainly on 'convenience foods', a deficiency of potassium can occur. The symptoms include muscle weakness, confusion and depression, which are easily dismissed as 'just old age'. Potassium supplements may be prescribed, but they do have drawbacks (see p.331).

Potassium and osteoporosis

In a recent study, doctors in California used an artificial source of potassium, known as potassium bicarbonate, to treat women who had gone through the menopause. They measured the loss of calcium and phosphate in the urine, and found that it was greatly reduced by taking potassium bicarbonate. The rate of bone resorption had clearly been reduced. Similar findings have been made with younger people confined to bed, who are at risk of osteoporosis through prolonged inactivity.

This treatment has not yet been tried out on a long term basis, so it is impossible to say if it might have any damaging effects. Until such trials have been carried out, taking potassium bicarbonate cannot be recommended. Within a few years it may have been shown to be safe and introduced as a routine treatment. Until such time, eating plenty of fruit and vegetables is the best protection against calcium loss – these foods also supply valuable antioxidants (see p.339), fibre, Vitamin C, boron and other vital nutrients, which a supplement of potassium bicarbonate does not offer.

Controlling the amount of potassium in the diet

The kidneys are responsible for controlling the composition of the blood, which they do by selectively removing minerals such as potassium and discharging them in the urine. Anyone with kidney damage (such as that sometimes caused by systemic lupus erythematosus, or by the drugs prescribed for inflammatory arthritis) may become less capable of dealing with potassium and therefore have to reduce their intake of this mineral. Your doctor's advice about your diet should be followed closely.

Hazards of potassium supplements

Supplements of potassium are sometimes prescribed for elderly people, but are bulky and difficult to swallow. They can cause ulcers of the stomach, the oesophagus (the tube leading from the mouth to the stomach), or the bowel. If possible, high-potassium foods such as dried fruit, bananas, apricots, rhubarb and blackcurrants should be substituted for part of the supplement. Seek the advice of your doctor or dietitian about this.

· *Manganese* ·

This trace element plays a part in various metabolic reactions, being a vital component of several enzymes. About a quarter of the manganese in the body is found in the bones where it may play a crucial role.

Natural sources of manganese

Like several other minerals, manganese is poorly absorbed when there are large amounts of phytate or oxalate (see p.309–311) in the food. Although green leafy vegetables and whole grains contain manganese they are not good sources because these substances block absorption. Similarly tea is rich in manganese but a very poor source because of all the tannin which binds the mineral and prevents it from being taken up by the body.

Milk, meat and eggs contain smaller amounts of manganese but it is easily absorbed. Some researchers believe that these are the most important sources.

Unfortunately calcium supplements tend to inhibit the absorption of manganese. So too do iron and magnesium supplements. However when milk is used as a source of calcium, the manganese in the milk is absorbed well.

Manganese and osteoporosis

The possible importance of manganese in the prevention of osteoporosis was discovered in a rather dramatic way. A star basketball player, Bill Walton, suffered a series of broken bones, culminating in a broken ankle that would not heal. X-rays of the ankle revealed the astonishing fact that this young, healthy, active male was suffering from osteoporosis – a disease most often associated with housebound elderly women.

Blood tests showed serious mineral imbalances, and a total absence of the mineral manganese. For some time Walton had been following a strict macrobiotic diet, but his doctors now persuaded him to abandon this and prescribed a mineral supplement. Within six weeks, Walton's ankle was well healed and he was back to playing basketball.

A Belgian study of women with osteoporosis apparently confirmed the discovery: compared to women of the same age without osteoporosis, the levels of manganese in their blood were very low. In this particular study there were no significant differences in any other minerals, whereas the average manganese levels were four times higher in the women with healthy bones. (Note that other studies *have* found low levels of other minerals to be linked with osteoporosis – magnesium for example.)

How much manganese is needed?

For anyone depending on supplements, the recommended dose for manganese, according to those at the forefront of research on this mineral, is 4 mg per day.

· Boron ·

The idea that this mineral might be necessary for human health is relatively new. It remains a controversial idea, and there are as yet no estimates of how much might be needed each day.

Natural sources of boron

Natural foodstuffs that are rich in boron include avocado pears, cereal grains, and many fruits and vegetables, although when grown with artificial fertilisers the boron content may be greatly reduced. Organic produce should be a more valuable source. The highest levels are found in honey: 28 gm (1 oz) of honey would supply 6 mg of boron.

Boron and osteoarthritis

In a small pilot study with just 10 patients suffering from osteoarthritis, a supplement of 6 mg of boron per day seemed to produce an improvement in 50% of the patients. This was a double-blind placebo-controlled trial, and only one out of the ten patients in the control group showed any improvement. Although this is an encouraging result, the numbers included in the trial were far too small to be able to draw any firm conclusions. However, if you suffer from osteoarthritis, there would be no harm in increasing your boron intake by eating more organic fruits and vegetables, and eating some honey.

Boron and osteoporosis

One scientific study has looked at the effects of boron on the losses of calcium and magnesium in the urine. The more calcium that is lost, the greater the risk of osteoporosis, and losses of magnesium are also thought to be damaging. Taking 3 mg of boron per day reduced the urinary loss of both calcium and magnesium substantially. This study involved women who were past the menopause and, therefore, at greater risk of osteoporosis. It revealed that a boron supplement also raises the level of natural oestrogen hormone in women of this age. Their oestrogen levels rose as much as if they had been prescribed Hormone Replacement Therapy for menopausal symptoms. The change in oestrogen levels probably accounted for the improved retention of calcium and magnesium. This trial provides good evidence for the usefulness of boron in preventing osteoporosis, and suggests that it should be included in mineral supplements for post-menopausal women. Other recommendations for the avoidance of osteoporosis can be found in Chapter 2.3 (p.161).

Boron supplements

Supplements of boron alone cannot be purchased in many countries because, in much larger doses, boron is a poison: its sale is therefore prohibited. Some multivitamin and mineral supplements may contain boron, and these might be of value, provided that recommended dose is not exceeded. There are some supplements especially designed for osteoporosis prevention, such as one that contains calcium, magnesium and boron.

· *Selenium* ·

This mineral is only needed in the diet in tiny amounts. Selenium is known to have effects on the immune system and it is essential for the action of glutathione peroxidase, a powerful antioxidant (see p.343) which helps to limit the harmful effects of inflammation. It may provide some protection against heart disease, stroke and certain forms of cancer, although the evidence is not conclusive.

Natural sources of selenium

Potential sources of selenium include cereal grains, meat and fish. However, the amounts present in crop plants depend on levels in the soil. Plants will grow perfectly well without selenium so arable farmers are not concerned if it is lacking in their soil – this means that levels in vegetable foods may be low in countries where selenium is naturally scarce, such as China, Finland, Sweden and New Zealand (see below). Animals do not thrive in selenium-deficient conditions, so meat and fish tend to be more reliable sources of this mineral. Liver and kidney are particularly rich in selenium. Those most at risk of selenium deficiency are vegetarians, particularly vegans living in countries whose soil lacks selenium, and relying mainly on local produce.

How much selenium is needed?

Most authorities recommend about 75 µg per day for adult men and 60 µg per day for women, rising to 75 µg per day if breastfeeding. Very low intakes, of about 11 µg per day occur in some parts of China and can cause deficiency diseases mainly among children. In Finland and New Zealand, low intakes of 15–40 µg per day do not cause any obvious symptoms, but blood tests show that giving selenium supplements does improve the performance of glutathione peroxidase. Since this antioxidant could play a role in reducing the damage done by inflammatory arthritis (see p.339), correcting a mild selenium deficiency, if it exists, might be of some value in rheumatoid arthritis. However, there is no evidence that selenium supplements are more generally useful for either rheumatoid arthritis or osteoarthritis (see below).

Selenium and arthritis

Selenium is less abundant in the blood of people with both rheumatoid arthritis and osteoarthritis, compared to healthy individuals. When this discovery was made, it seemed very promising, and there were high hopes that correcting the apparent selenium deficiency with supplements would help patients with rheumatoid arthritis and osteoarthritis.

Trials of selenium supplements were undertaken for both diseases but the results were very disappointing: most trials simply showed no benefit. For example, a trial of selenium, combined with Vitamins A, C and E, ('selenium-ACE') was carried out among patients with osteoarthritis. After six months on the supplement, there were no significant improvements. It seems likely that the low selenium levels are a result of the arthritic disease process, rather than a cause, or that selenium cannot be utilised when given in tablet form.

However, one study with people whose rheumatoid arthritis had begun less than five years earlier did seem to produce some improvement. Unfortunately this study did not include enough patients to produce a truly convincing result. Other more indirect evidence (see p.345) suggests that a high intake of selenium in the diet might be helpful in preventing rheumatoid arthritis, as long as it is combined with plenty of carotenoids and Vitamin E. This possibility deserves further scientific research.

A type of arthritis known as Kashin-Beck disease afflicts children in some parts of China, eastern Siberia, northern Korea and an area near Lake Baikal. Lack of selenium probably plays some part in this disease, but there are other factors involved as well, such as fungus infestations of locally grown crops. Kashin-Beck disease is unlike arthritic diseases found elsewhere in the world, and there is no justification for extrapolating from Kashin-Beck disease to arthritis in general.

Selenium and arthralgia

Swedish doctors have found that some patients with unexplained joint pain (arthralgia) and muscle pain are suffering from a mild selenium deficiency. The patients tend to be vegans eating only local produce grown on selenium-deficient soil (see p.334). A selenium supplement produces striking improvements.

· *Copper* ·

This trace element is widely distributed in the body and plays an important role in many of its chemical reactions.

Natural sources of copper

Beans and lentils, shellfish, liver and nuts are all good sources. In soft-water areas, particularly if the drinking water is slightly acidic, (as when it runs through peaty soil) copper dissolved from pipes can add a little to the daily intake. Phytates in food (see p.309) block the absorption of copper.

Deficiencies of copper

Whether deficiency occurs, except very rarely, is an arguable point. One research study found that the average American diet only contained about 1 mg per day, whereas the recommended amount set by the US authorities is 2 mg per day. However, the recommended intake is only 1.2 mg in Britain and Europe. Certainly, there are no obvious signs of widespread copper deficiency, and in general, copper toxicity (see below) is a greater cause for concern.

High-dose supplements of zinc interfere with the uptake of copper from food and may cause a mild deficiency.

Hazards of copper

Excessive copper in the diet will slowly accumulate in the liver and can cause cirrhosis. It is mainly children who are susceptible. Various other problems have been tentatively linked with excess copper, including schizophrenia.

Copper supplements

Some multivitamin and mineral supplements do contain a small amount of copper and this may be valuable, for example in preventing osteoporosis. As with other minerals, taking a comprehensive supplement guards against the possibility of one mineral, taken in excess, inhibiting the absorption or action of another. No more than 1 mg a day should be taken, as there will invariably be some copper in food and water.

Copper and arthritis

People with rheumatoid arthritis tend to have increased levels of copper in their blood. As far as is known, levels in osteoarthritis are normal. There is certainly no evidence of a deficiency of this mineral for either of the two most common forms of arthritis.

Despite this, copper is widely advocated as an alternative treatment for 'arthritis' – not taken as a tablet, but worn as a bracelet. The copper dissolves in sweat, a tiny amount being lost from the bracelet each day. It seems that this may then be absorbed by the body of the bracelet-wearer.

Whether the copper so absorbed has any benefit in either rheumatoid arthritis or osteoarthritis remains uncertain. The fact that copper combines chemically with substances such as salicylic acid (aspirin) or ascorbic acid (Vitamin C), and that such copper-containing compounds have some anti-inflammatory effects, has prompted speculation that it might. Such chemical reactions between copper and other molecules could occur spontaneously in the body, for example with aspirin taken as a painkiller. If copper is of any benefit, it is acting here as a drug, not as a dietary supplement.

As a result of the existence of a plausible mechanism, there has been some research into whether copper bracelets actually work – but not enough to produce a definitive answer.

A trial carried out in Australia in the 1970s, involving 160 people, produced some interesting results. Copper bracelets were worn for one month, and placebo bracelets which looked like copper were worn for another month. Far more people recorded feeling better while wearing the true copper bracelet, although some people did report benefit from the placebo.

Unfortunately this study had many weaknesses. There were no objective assessments of how patients' arthritis changed during the trial, only their subjective report of feeling better: this is not considered sufficient for a scientific trial. Additionally, no-one checked to see if the patients could tell which bracelet was made of copper. If they could, this might have invalidated the result, assuming that people expected the copper bracelet to succeed, because their expectation could easily influence their perception of how their joints felt.

Confusingly, a survey of over 1,000 arthritis sufferers in the U.S.A. produced the opposite result. Of those surveyed, over 200 had tried a copper bracelet or similar device. Only 6% felt sure it had helped them, and an overwhelming 85% were certain it had not done a thing. Even an entirely inert placebo should produce a better result than this.

How to reconcile these two contradictory results? Are Australians more susceptible to placebo effects than Americans? Or did the fact that the copper bracelets were issued by learned University professors (in the Australian trial) give them greater credibility and thus a more powerful placebo effect? We will never know.

Certainly, the damning verdict of the American survey makes it seem unlikely that there is any real benefit to be had from a copper bracelet. Those surveyed also mentioned unpleasant effects such as a metallic taste in the mouth and green or black skin under the bracelet.

Copper and osteoporosis

If laboratory rats are fed a diet lacking in copper they develop weak bones with inadequate mineral content. Whether this has any relevance to human osteoporosis is unknown, but it suggests that maintaining an adequate intake of copper would be a sensible part of an overall dietary programme to prevent osteoporosis (see Chapter 2.3, p.161).

· *Sulphur* ·

In the 1920s, some doctors thought they had identified a deficiency of sulphur in patients with rheumatoid arthritis and tried dosing them with sulphur. The treatment was always controversial, and research published in 1940 showed it to be of no benefit whatever.

Recently, it has been realised that foods rich in sulphur, such as eggs, meat and cheese, tend to encourage calcium losses from the bones, by affecting the acidity of the blood and urine (see pp.406–7). This may be a contributing factor in osteoporosis, and dietary measures to reduce and/or neutralise sulphur intake are described on pp.164–5.

Chapter 3.4

Antioxidants, Carotenoids, Protein and Amino Acids, Essential Fatty Acids, Fibre and Other Nutrients

This chapter covers the other major nutrients, apart from vitamins and minerals.

· *Antioxidants* ·

Just now there is a great deal of interest among medical researchers in a group of substances that are known collectively as antioxidants. Having adequate levels of antioxidants seems to protect people from some forms of cancer, and from heart disease and cataracts in the eyes. They may also be important in combating Alzheimer's disease, the ageing process, and the secondary effects of diabetes.

Antioxidants counteract the damage caused by inflammation (see p.64), and they are therefore thought to be important in rheumatoid arthritis and other forms of inflammatory arthritis. In these diseases there is rampant inflammation in the affected joints, and the inflammatory reactions may also affect the blood and the body as a whole.

Research has shown that the levels of antioxidants in the blood are altered by the disease process of rheumatoid arthritis, often falling substantially. This does not necessarily mean that restoring antioxidant levels would improve matters for patients with rheumatoid arthritis, but it is possible that it could.

Some of the substances that act as antioxidants are also vitamins, including Vitamin C and Vitamin E. The question of whether eating more of these vitamins might help people with inflammatory arthritis is a difficult one. Before trying to answer answer it, we need to look more closely at what antioxidants actually do.

Fighting free radicals

Antioxidants help to combat some of the worst effects of inflammation by protecting the body from **free radicals**. These are very highly reactive substances – the chemical equivalent of argumentative drunks looking to pick a fight with someone. Free radicals tend to react with any susceptible molecule in the vicinity, often causing damage in the process. (See Glossary pp.412–421 if you are unsure about the exact meaning of words such as 'molecule'.)

The fat molecules that make up the cell membranes are frequent targets for free radicals. These membranes form the outer container and internal partitions of the cell, and are vital elements of its organisation. Any damage caused here is a serious threat to the integrity and smooth running of the cell, and must be prevented if at all possible.

Antioxidants have the job of preventing damage by free radicals. They get their name from the fact that all free radicals are chemically similar to oxygen in their effects, and since free radicals are 'oxidisers', their opponents are 'antioxidants'. Although oxygen is usually thought of as a life-giving substance, it is actually quite dangerous stuff – pure oxygen is lethal, and we only survive undamaged in an oxygenated atmosphere because we are constantly protected by antioxidants.

Antioxidants prevent damage by reacting with atoms of oxygen, or with free radicals, before any other molecule can become a target. In the process the antioxidant molecule itself is changed chemically, and its antioxidant qualities are destroyed, at least temporarily. They can be regenerated, but only at the expense of other antioxidants. If the free radical is an 'argumentative drunk' then the antioxidant molecule is a 'policeman' who successfully prevents a fight – but who invariably gets knocked unconscious in the process. This is an important aspect of the whole process: antioxidants are used up as they do their work. Consequently the more inflammation there is in the body, the lower the level of antioxidants tends to be.

To understand why someone with rheumatoid arthritis generates so many free radicals, we need to consider the way the body fights infectious bacteria. Inflammation of the kind seen in rheumatoid arthritis is not unlike the reaction to infection: it is simply a misplaced and uncontrolled version of the same defensive tactics by the immune systems (see p.416).

When faced with attack by bacteria the immune system uses free radicals such as superoxide and peroxide ions to destroy them. The peroxide is produced by immune cells called phagocytes. These are large cells which first engulf the bacteria, and then, while holding them captive, bombard them with the peroxide and other free radicals. At such close quarters the free radicals can usually kill most kinds of bacteria.

By keeping this aggressive chemical action contained within the phagocyte, the body itself is protected from most of the free radicals. However, some may escape, for example when the phagocyte dies. If peroxide diffuses away from the infection site it can enter the bloodstream and be carried around the body: this is one reason why the blood is well supplied with antioxidants.

Free radicals and rheumatoid factor

Free radicals may be responsible, indirectly, for the appearance of rheumatoid factor (see p.419) in people with rheumatoid arthritis. Recent evidence suggests that free radicals in the joint space cause damage to the IgG antibodies (see p.412) which are present. By changing the chemical structure of IgG slightly they turn it into something which 'looks different' to the immune system, and is no longer seen as a familiar molecule but as something alien. The immune system therefore attacks the changed IgG by forming antibodies against the altered parts of the molecule – these antibodies are rheumatoid factor. When rheumatoid factor is formed, it tends to increase the damage to the joint.

The larger picture

Inflammation is only part of the story however, and we need to look at the larger picture to make proper sense of it all. There are a great many different sources of free radicals, some within the body and some external.

Firstly, free radicals are formed by the body all the time, not just during inflammation. It is simply that the quantity of free radicals increases greatly during inflammation or infection. Normally, free radicals are unwanted by-products of ordinary bodily processes, such as exercise. During a bout of infection it is a different matter – the free radicals have their uses as weapons, and they are deliberately made and deployed as part of the body's defences.

Secondly, although free radicals occur naturally in the body, they are found in the external environment too, and if they enter the body by being eaten or inhaled they are just as damaging. Many modern forms of pollution generate free radicals – there are particularly high levels in traffic fumes for example, and in cigarette smoke (whether actively or passively inhaled). The adulterated olive oil sold in parts of Spain in the early 1980s, which caused widespread and incurable illness, probably owed its effects to a high content of free radicals. Drinking alcohol increases the need for antioxidants, particularly Vitamin E, and so does prolonged exposure to sunlight which generates free radicals in the skin.

A third factor to consider is that intensive exercise generates free radicals in the muscles, and increases the need for antioxidants. This is particularly true of older people who exercise hard. Exercise is not the only healthy activity that increases the need for antioxidants. Eating more polyunsaturated fat, as in margarine and cooking oil, or in oily fish, also boosts the requirement for antioxidants. This is because polyunsaturated fats are particularly vulnerable to the kind of damage that free radicals cause. The word 'unsaturated' describes a type of chemical bond in the fat molecule (see p.357), a bond that can easily be attacked by a free radical.

It is no coincidence that foods such as seeds and nuts, which are naturally rich in polyunsaturated fats, are also rich in Vitamin E: this vitamin acts as an antioxidant for the plant, protecting its seeds. When seeds such as sunflower seeds are crushed to make oil, about half of the Vitamin E present gets into the oil too, because it is fat-soluble. So anyone consuming the oil gets the benefit of its natural Vitamin E at the same time.

Despite this, manufacturers have to add more antioxidants to cooking oil to prevent any chemical damage to the oil while it is in the bottle. The damage in this situation would come from oxygen in the air at the top of the bottle, which would turn the oil rancid. As for the antioxidants, these would usually be synthetic chemical additives approved for use in food, such as BHA or BHT.

Natural antioxidants, such as Vitamin E, can also be used as food additives, but are slightly more expensive. They are most often used in wholefood products which need an antioxidant to prolong shelf life. Manufacturers of fish oil supplements invariably use Vitamin E to preserve their products, something that is relevant to anyone taking fish oil (see p.303).

Within the body, Vitamin E is especially important as an antioxidant precisely because it is fat-soluble. This allows it to come into close contact with cell membranes, which are made largely of fat molecules, and so protect the membranes from free radicals.

Vitamin C is water-soluble and cannot therefore protect membranes so effectively. But Vitamin C can regenerate active Vitamin E from the the incapacitated molecules that are left after an encounter with free radicals. In this way, plentiful supplies of Vitamin C will help Vitamin E in its efforts to protect membranes. Other antioxidants can also work co-operatively with one another in this way.

Many different antioxidants have now been identified, in addition to Vitamin E and Vitamin C. The pigments that make peppers red and carrots orange, known collectively as **carotenoids** (see p.347), are also powerful antioxidants. They are found in all fruits and vegetables with an orange or red colouration, and in green leafy vegetables such as spinach where their colour is masked by the green pigment chlorophyll. Flavonoids (see pp.347–8) may also have some antioxidant properties.

Various substances made by the body itself, rather than consumed as part of the diet, function as antioxidants. One is an enzyme called glutathione peroxidase which needs the mineral selenium to work effectively. (Whether or not this makes selenium supplements of any value in inflammatory arthritis is a question that is considered on pages 334–5.)

Another substance produced in the body which acts as an antioxidant is uric acid. This is, coincidentally, the substance which is deposited as urate crystals in the joints of people with gout and which causes them so much pain. For gout sufferers there is usually a high level of uric acid in the blood, so high that it crystallises out in the joints (see p.104) and provokes severe inflammation. But when uric acid is present at lower levels in the blood this does not usually happen. Indeed, at its normal healthy level, uric acid mops up free radicals in the blood and so protects against the damage that inflammation can cause.

One study has even suggested that, for people with rheumatoid arthritis, uric acid may be the most important antioxidant of all. This study took blood samples from healthy people and from patients with rheumatoid arthritis, then tested the ability of the blood to resist attack by free radicals. The blood from rheumatoid arthritis sufferers did not perform very well, as the researchers expected. More surprisingly, it showed a distinctly different pattern from the other blood samples. Whereas in healthy people the blood's ability to resist free radicals was related to the level of Vitamin E, this was not true of people with rheumatoid arthritis. The ability of their blood to resist free radicals was related to the level of uric acid.

What happens with blood samples in the laboratory does not always correspond well to real life, but in this case there is a striking agreement with other research involving patients with rheumatoid arthritis. A group of 160 patients were studied and their medical records reviewed. These records included measurements of uric acid level in the blood, as well as full assessments of their rheumatoid arthritis symptoms. Twelve patients turned out to have had abnormally high levels of uric acid at some stage in the past year (usually as a result of treatment with diuretic drugs) although none had developed gout. The researchers then discovered that eleven of these patients had experienced a great improvement in their rheumatoid arthritis at the time when their uric acid levels rose, and in eight patients the beginning of this improvement coincided with the rise in uric acid level. Laboratory tests such as the ESR (Erythrocyte Sedimentation Rate), which measures the degree of inflammation, showed striking improvements.

Some patients had been treated for their high uric acid levels: the diuretics were stopped and they were given allopurinol (see p.250). In two cases, as the uric acid level returned to normal values, the rheumatoid arthritis symptoms flared up once again.

Further corroboration comes from the very rare cases of patients who have suffered from both rheumatoid arthritis and gout. In several cases, successfully treating gout with allopurinol provoked the onset of rheumatoid arthritis which had presumably been rumbling away under the surface but was suppressed by the high uric acid level. No patients could be found who actually had gout and rheumatoid arthritis simultaneously.

Antioxidants in the diet

We can now return to the question of whether consuming more of the substances that act as antioxidants could benefit people with inflammatory arthritis.

As regards Vitamin C, the answer is fairly clear cut: although levels of this vitamin in the blood of people with rheumatoid arthritis are often low, as are levels in the affected joints, trials with Vitamin C supplements show no value in rheumatoid arthritis. However, this vitamin is known to increase the clearance of uric acid from the blood and this could cancel out any antioxidant benefits from Vitamin C itself if uric acid is beneficial (see p.345).

Vitamin E is also at low levels in patients with rheumatoid arthritis, according to most researchers. In the case of this vitamin, few good studies of supplements have been carried out. The two trials involving patients with rheumatoid arthritis do not suggest any dramatic benefits (see p.304) but neither do they rule out the possibility of Vitamin E being helpful in a small way. Guidelines for improving intake of Vitamin E are also given on pp.256-7.

No one has yet tested diets rich in carotenoids for patients with rheumatoid arthritis but there is good reason for thinking that they might be relevant. A study in Finland looked at levels of various antioxidants in the blood of over 1,400 people and then waited to see how healthy they were 20 years later. During that 20 years, 14 people developed rheumatoid arthritis. Comparing them with the rest, the antioxidant status of their blood – as measured by a combination of beta-carotene (a common carotenoid), Vitamin E and selenium – was significantly lower. Of the three, beta-carotene was the most strongly linked with risk of rheumatoid arthritis: levels were over 50% higher in those who did not develop the disease compared with those who did. This is an especially valuable piece of research, because it looked at levels of antioxidants *before the onset* of disease. So it is more likely to be measuring a contributory factor in the *cause* of rheumatoid arthritis, rather than the *effects* of the disease in exhausting antioxidant supplies.

Of course, it is possible that the disease process which later emerged as rheumatoid arthritis had already begun, and that it had produced changes in the blood even though there were no obvious symptoms of arthritis – if this were the case, the low levels of antioxidants could have been an effect of the unseen disease, rather than a cause. However, the researchers also showed that, for the group as a whole, the level of beta-carotene in the blood was a good indication of how much beta-carotene people habitually ate: this makes it more likely that low beta-carotene intake led to low levels in the serum and that this then contributed to the development of rheumatoid arthritis.

Note the emphasis on 'contributed to'. There is no question of low antioxidant levels in the diet being the sole cause, or even a major cause of rheumatoid arthritis. Some people in the Finnish study had average or above-average amounts of beta-carotene (and other antioxidants) in their blood, but went on to develop rheumatoid arthritis anyway. Many people who had below-average levels did not develop rheumatoid arthritis. This point needs to be emphasised because some popular books on diet and arthritis claim that all arthritis is a direct result of bad nutrition from a modern westernised diet, and there is a danger that this piece of research will be misused as evidence supporting such a view. What the Finnish study showed was that having low levels of antioxidants in the blood might be a factor that increased the risk of developing rheumatoid arthritis. Those with below-average levels were eight times more likely to develop rheumatoid arthritis during the next 20 years than those with average or above-average levels. But even if the low antioxidant levels were contributing to the development of rheumatoid arthritis (and this is by no means proven) there must have been other causal factors as well.

If the results of the Finnish study described above are a good indication of what might alleviate rheumatoid arthritis, rather than simply prevent it, then consuming more Vitamin E, carotenoids and selenium in combination would seem to be a good plan. However, Finland is one of the countries with very low levels of selenium in the soil, and a mild deficiency of selenium can easily occur, especially among vegetarians (see p.334). This may make the selenium finding less relevant to other countries, compared to the Vitamin E or carotenoid findings. Note that we would advise against taking beta-carotene in supplement form (see p.347) because high doses may be dangerous.

The current enthusiasm for antioxidants has spawned an extraordinary range of new 'food supplements' claiming to offer concentrated antioxidants in tablet or capsule form. They are often rich in carotenoids and flavonoids (see p.347). Some are derived from pine bark, or other equally unlikely sources. We would recommend that you look to real foods for your antioxidant protection, since these are much more likely to be wholesome and non-toxic.

The recent research findings about uric acid and rheumatoid arthritis (see pp.343–4) raise the obvious question: could a high-purine diet be of any help to those with rheumatoid arthritis? No serious consideration has yet been given to this question, and most doctors would be reluctant to have their patients try such a diet. It should be noted that it was diuretic drugs, not diet, that had produced the very high levels of uric acid for those patients whose rheumatoid arthritis went into remission. And although they did not have gout, 50% of them did have unsightly tophi (nodules of urate crystals) in the earlobes and elsewhere on the body. No one knows if the much smaller increases in uric acid that could be achieved by a high-purine diet would have any beneficial effects for rheumatoid arthritis patients, nor whether it would be worth the risk of developing other symptoms, such as tophi.

· *Carotenoids* ·

These are red and orange pigments found in fruit and vegetables. With some exceptions (see below) they are not vitamins in the strict sense of the word, but they are important elements of the diet and they act as antioxidants (see p.359). Their antioxidant properties mean that they may be influential in rheumatoid arthritis and other forms of inflammatory arthritis. Although the evidence gathered so far is rather meagre (see p.345), it does suggest that eating more carotenoids might be helpful in preventing rheumatoid arthritis, or in moderating its effects.

There are different kinds of carotenoids, and some can be converted to Vitamin A by the body. They are known as provitamin A carotenoids, and the principal one is **beta-carotene**. Carrots are the main source of this substance. (There is no risk of Vitamin A toxicity from eating plenty of beta-carotene because the body has its own in-built control mechanisms which stop the conversion of beta-carotene to Vitamin A once the vitamin is present in adequate amounts.)

A good supply of carotenoids can be had from eating fruit and vegetables, which are a useful addition to anyone's diet. Carrots, mangoes and red peppers will provide substantial quantities of carotenoids, as will dark green leafy vegetables such as broccoli. For a complete list of the best sources, see page 258.

We would advise against anyone taking beta-carotene in supplement form, and recommend that food should be used as the source of this and other carotenoids. Trials in which cigarette smokers were given a high-dose supplement of beta-carotene (50 mg per day) showed that, far from preventing lung cancer as was hoped, the beta-carotene appeared to encourage the growth of tumours in some people. Current thinking is that beta-carotene might help to guard against cancer at normal intake – the sort of dose derived from food – but that it has the opposite effect at high doses. The foods that provide your daily beta-carotene will also yield many other useful nutrients, including other carotenoids which may be just as important as beta-carotene for general health – perhaps more important.

· *Flavonoids* ·

The name 'flavonoids' covers an enormous range of substances found in plants. Although they all have a similar chemical unit in their structure, they are in fact very diverse chemically and in their effects on plants and animals. Some are dark purple pigments, such as those which give blackberries and blackcurrants their colour. Others are red, blue or yellow, and some are colourless.

It has been suggested that some of the flavonoids are responsible for the effects of herbal remedies, and they have been studied as potential therapeutic drugs for various diseases. As far as arthritic disorders are concerned, some flavonoids may be anti-inflammatory, while several act as antioxidants in plants. Whether they can be absorbed from food and have a useful role to play as antioxidants in the human body is not entirely certain, but many researchers believe that they do. Anti-inflammatory and antioxidant properties could make them valuable to people with rheumatoid arthritis and other inflammatory forms of arthritis, but this has never been tested.

In the 1930s, Russian scientists identified certain groups of flavonoids as essential nutrients, which they called Vitamin P. Subsequent research has not confirmed the status of flavonoids as true vitamins, but some scientists still consider them to be 'semi-essential' rather like the carotenoids (see p.347).

To obtain an adequate supply of flavonoids, the diet should include plenty of fruit and vegetables. The emphasis should be on diversity as well as quantity, with many different kinds of produce eaten regularly. Herbs and spices are also good sources of flavonoids.

· *Protein and Amino Acids* ·

All living bodies are made up primarily of proteins, and the basic constituents of these must be supplied in the diet. It is essential to eat some protein, although most people in industrialised coutries eat far more than is needed. An intake of 50 gm per day is actually quite adequate, and people can manage on as little as 20 gm per day although this is not advisable except to treat serious medical conditions such as kidney failure. To get an idea of how much protein-containing food is needed to supply 50 gm of protein, refer to Table 21 on page 350.

When extra protein is eaten, it does not produce any nutritional benefits. There may, however, be some incidental benefits, such as the iron and zinc obtained from meat, or A and B vitamins from eggs. Protein also seems to improve the absorption of calcium from food, but on the negative side, protein breakdown products tend to acidify the urine and therefore promote the loss of calcium from the body in the urine (see p.407). This usually far outweighs the improved absorption and may produce a net loss of calcium from the body unless balanced by other foods which neutralise acid (see pp.403–6).

Moderating protein intake and balancing it with vegetable foods may be valuable in preventing osteoporosis (see pp.164–5). Protein restriction is occasionally useful for patients with gout, especially if they also have kidney stones and are not responding well to drugs (see p.246).

Protein quality

Protein quality matters as much as protein quantity, and the smaller the amount of protein eaten, the better the quality needs to be. Understanding the question of protein quality involves knowing about **amino acids**, the basic building blocks from which proteins are made. There are about 20 different kinds of amino acid, and the body must have adequate supplies of all the different kinds: generally speaking, one cannot substitute for another.

Some amino acids we can make for ourselves, while others we must obtain from our food because we cannot make them. The latter are known as essential amino acids.

There is an important difference between animal protein and vegetable protein as regards its amino acid composition. Animal protein is, not surprisingly, much more like the protein in the human body. When we eat eggs, milk, cheese, meat or fish we automatically get the correct proportions of the different amino acids. By contrast, vegetable protein has a different composition, and from the point of view of a human consumer it is usually lacking in one or more of the essential amino acids.

Cereal proteins, such as those in wheat, rice or corn (maize), tend to be short of an essential amino acid called lysine. Beans, peas and lentils (pulses) are deficient in another essential amino acid, methionine, although they are rich in lysine. Fortunately, when these two different kinds of protein are combined, they correct each other's deficiencies.

It is interesting that many traditional dishes from around the world are based on such combinations: rice and peas from the Caribbean, maize tacos with beans from Central America, lentil curry with chapatis or rice from India, and beansprouts or tofu (soyabean curd) with rice from the Far East. In developing their national cuisine, these different regions of the world all seem to have stumbled on the same nutritional principle. It is one that vegans (strict vegetarians who do not eat eggs or dairy produce) also follow to ensure that they get enough protein. Peanuts are pulses, and bread contains wheat protein, so a peanut-butter sandwich also provides a healthy combination of amino acids. So too does that time-honoured convenience meal, baked beans on toast.

Amino acids cannot be stored by the body for more than twenty four hours, so it is necessary to eat the complementary types of vegetable protein on the same day. Ideally the different types of protein should be combined in the same meal. If one of the essential amino acids runs out, protein production cannot continue unless existing body proteins are broken down to yield supplies of the missing amino acid.

If some or all of the amino acids eaten during a meal are not used to build up proteins, they are broken down and disposed of instead. Energy is obtained during this breakdown process.

Table 21: Protein content of foods

Food	Protein
1 egg	6–8 gm, depending on size of egg
Glass of milk, (skimmed or whole), 284 ml (1/2 pint)	9.5 gm
113 gm (4 oz) Cheddar cheese	28 gm
113 gm (4 oz) cottage cheese	16 gm
113 gm (4 oz) cream cheese	4 gm
113 gm (4 oz) wholemilk yoghurt	5.6 gm
113 gm (4 oz) fromage frais	8 gm
1 thin slice white bread (28 gm or 1 oz)	2.4 gm
1 thin slice wholemeal bread (28 gm or 1 oz)	2.5 gm
Portion of white rice (28 gm or 1 oz, dry weight)	2 gm
Portion of pasta (28 gm or 1 oz, dry weight)	4 gm
Portion of potatoes (113 gm or 4 oz, cooked weight)	1.5 gm
170 gm (6 oz) steak, chicken or other lean meat	42 gm
170 gm (6 oz) liver	42 gm
170 gm (6 oz) sausage	28 gm
85 gm (3 oz) bacon	28 gm
170 gm (6 oz) cod	33 gm
170 gm (6 oz) plaice	33 gm
170 gm (6 oz) mackerel	32 gm
170 gm (6 oz) sardines	42 gm
170 gm (6 oz) shrimps	42 gm
2 fish fingers	7 gm

Food	Protein
85 gm (3 oz) lentils (dry weight)	21 gm
85 gm (3 oz) haricot beans (dry weight)	21 gm
170 gm (6 oz) baked beans (tinned)	8 gm
85 gm (3 oz) chick peas (cooked weight)	7 gm
142 gm (5 oz) tofu	11.5 gm
170 gm (6 oz) vegeburger	18–27 gm
227 gm (8 oz) green peas (fresh or frozen)	14 gm
227 gm (8 oz) butter beans/broad beans	16 gm
227 gm (8 oz) other green vegetables	6.5 gm
227 gm (8 oz) lettuce, celery, carrots or cucumber	1.5 gm
113 gm (4 oz) sweetcorn (cooked weight)	4.5 gm
28 gm (1 oz) breakfast cereal	2 gm
1 packet crisps	2 gm
28 gm (1 oz) milk chocolate	2 gm
28 gm (1 oz) plain chocolate	1 gm
57 gm (2 oz) pastry	4 gm
57 gm (2 oz) Yorkshire pudding	4 gm
57 gm (2 oz) oatmeal	8 gm
85 gm (3 oz) peanuts	21 gm
85 gm (3 oz) almonds	14 gm
85 gm (3 oz) Brazil nuts	10 gm
85 gm (3 oz) hazelnuts	7 gm
85 gm (3 oz) chestnuts	2 gm

Foods such as cream, ice cream, marzipan, lemon curd, mousse and some other desserts, jelly, mayonnaise, salad cream, white sauces, batter and creamy soups will also contain some protein. So does the drink Advocaat, as it contains egg.

Amino acids and arthritis

The waste products from amino acid breakdown are characteristic of the individual amino acids, and can be measured in the blood and urine. Such measurements, when carried out on the blood of people with rheumatoid arthritis, show distinct abnormalities for some amino acids.

In the case of the essential amino acid called tryptophan, there are increased levels of several breakdown products in the urine. This is not only the case for people with rheumatoid arthritis, but also for those with systemic sclerosis. Exactly why the breakdown of tryptophan should change in these diseases is unknown, but comparable changes occur in certain other diseases, and in response to some drugs. Diets that are low in tryptophan seem to produce some small improvements for patients with rheumatoid arthritis or systemic sclerosis but there is no scientific certainty about this result.

Much the same story can be told about two other amino acids, phenylalanine and tyrosine. These two are very similar in structure and one can be readily converted to the other. Some researchers have found unusual forms of their breakdown products in the urine of those with rheumatoid arthritis or systemic sclerosis, although this is not a consistent finding. Such shaky evidence would be disregarded but for the fact that Japanese researchers, working in the 1950s, found that giving patients pure tyrosine worsened their arthritis or sclerotis. Such research cannot be repeated, for fear of causing any lasting deterioration in patients, so the original observation cannot be confirmed or refuted.

The same Japanese workers did try out a diet that reduced phenylalanine and tyrosine to the lowest possible level in the diet. They cannot be eliminated entirely because they are essential for making proteins, but most diets contain far more than is needed for this purpose. To achieve the minimal levels of tyrosine and phenylalanine, patients had to rely mainly on a type of refined gelatine for their protein. A little fish and whalemeat was added to this, but the amounts were tiny, and nothing else was allowed apart from a restricted range of fruits and vegetables, and a little oil and margarine. It was not an appetising diet. The researchers claimed benefits in patients with rheumatoid arthritis and patients with systemic sclerosis, but as this was an open trial (rather than a double-blind placebo-controlled trial – see p.27) such results have to be treated cautiously. Because of the strange nature of the diet, and the possibility that it could lead to nutritional deficiencies, it cannot be recommended.

Another essential amino acid, histidine, is frequently found to be at low levels in the blood of people with rheumatoid arthritis. Once again, there is no explanation for this low level. Giving patients histidine supplements does not alleviate their symptoms.

In conclusion, although there are alterations in amino acid metabolism among patients with some arthritic diseases, there is little help to be had from adjusting the amino acid content of the diet. Indeed some of the amino acids sold as supplements, such as tyrosine, could even be damaging to those with rheumatoid arthritis or systemic sclerosis. (Other amino acid supplements, notably tryptophan, are hazardous even to apparently healthy people, and have caused some deaths. There is no evidence that amino acid supplementation serves any useful purpose.)

· *Fibre* ·

Anything found in fruit, vegetables, grains or other plant food, which goes through the digestive tract without being broken down, is referred to as 'dietary fibre'. This is a very mixed bag of substances. A diet based on white bread and white flour, meat, milk, eggs, sugar and fats, with few fruits or vegetables – the typical Western diet – tends to be very low in fibre.

The high incidence, in industrialised countries, of health problems such as diabetes, hardening of the arteries, high blood pressure, and bowel cancer – diseases which are much rarer in poorer countries with higher fibre intakes – has led to the recommendation that more fibre should be eaten. Fibre regulates the absorption and digestion of other food constituents, such as fat and sugar, and is probably responsible for the lower incidence of such diseases in non-industrialised countries.

But there is fibre and fibre – it is not all the same. Adding large amounts of wheat bran to a basic Western diet may do more harm than good by blocking mineral absorption (see p.309–311). The minerals affected include several that are relevant to osteoporosis and arthritis. Rather than eating bran, fruit and vegetables should be eaten regularly to provide the missing fibre.

Elderly people and those with poor appetites should avoid eating a lot of fibre, because it adds bulk to the diet without adding calories or nutrients, and may prevent the intake of enough nourishing food.

· *Essential Fatty Acids* ·

Essential fatty acids (EFAs) are important for good nutrition and are needed by everyone. But they have *no* special relevance in arthritis – which may surprise you if you have read the label on a jar of evening primrose oil, for example. There is a certain amount of inappropriate information given by manufacturers about the oils they are trying to sell: they frequently mention 'essential fatty acids' on labels or in leaflets, which tends to confuse the real issues about why oils can help in rheumatoid arthritis (described in Chapter 1.2, p.46). In this chapter we are simply concerned with essential fatty acids as they apply to anyone aiming for a healthy diet.

Essential fatty acids, like vitamins, are something the body cannot do without because it cannot make them for itself. (At one time they were known as Vitamin F) They are needed to maintain the structure of membranes, and to provide the raw materials for making prostaglandins and similar molecules – important messenger substances in the body. Prostaglandins are central to the question of how oils such as fish oil or evening primrose oil calm inflammation, so they are described in more detail in Chapter 1.2 (p.46).

Essential fatty acids are vital for good health, but when it comes to supplements sold in health food shops the buyer should beware, for things are not what they seem. Statements such as 'this product is a rich source of the principal essential fatty acid, linoleic acid' are correct yet they are also highly misleading. It is rather like selling bath sponges with the slogan 'this product contains a great deal of air which is essential to human life'.

The fact is that you would have to be eating a quite bizarre and unappetising diet to be short of linoleic acid. Everyone in our society gets plenty of linoleic acid, which occurs abundantly in vegetable oils, margarine, milk, butter, lard, meat and eggs, as well as in many other foods. Only a small amount is needed. For someone eating no other fatty foods at all (a very dreary diet that few would undertake) a teaspoonful of sunflower oil would provide the necessary daily intake. Instances of linoleic acid deficiency are immensely rare, and usually occur in severely ill patients being fed artificially on very low-fat diets.

Implying that a product is valuable because it contains linoleic acid is really rather misleading, but there are extenuating circumstances. In all such products there is another ingredient that may be genuinely useful, usually gamma-linolenic acid (GLA, see p.51). But because the oils are not yet licensed as drugs for general usage, the manufacturers are strictly limited in what they can claim for their ingredients, and the labels on the jars can only make very general comments about health-giving properties. It is perhaps understandable that the manufacturers fall back gratefully on impressive sounding phrases such as 'essential fatty acid'.

There are two other essential fatty acids which actually might be in short supply for some people. One is alpha-linolenic acid (note the second 'n' – it is a very different beast from linoleic acid). This is required in even smaller amounts than linoleic acid, but the need is rather more difficult to satisfy because it is far less widespread and abundant in the food we eat. Major sources are soyabean oil and rapeseed oil, with lesser amounts in other vegetable oils. Two teaspoonfuls of soyabean oil would more than fulfil the daily need for this substance. There is also some alpha-linolenic acid in green leafy foods such as lettuce, cabbage and spinach, and this is probably the major dietary source for most people. It would take about 220 gm (8 oz) of lettuce and cabbage to provide the full daily requirement if there was no other source available.

The need for these foods is completely avoided if fish is part of the diet. Fish contains only a little alpha-linolenic acid, but it does contain eicosapentaenoic acid (EPA), which is derived from alpha-linolenic, and is probably the product that the body actually needs.

Exactly how much EPA should be eaten is a complex question. As with several of the vitamins (see p.277–8) there is a well-established minimal dose required to avoid a clearcut deficiency disease, but recent research suggests that taking more than this minimal dose could have additional benefits. In the case of EPA, these additional benefits relate to the prevention of heart disease, and the alleviation of some inflammatory diseases such as rheumatoid arthritis.

A fairly small intake of oily fish is all that is needed to avoid an obvious deficiency state for EPA: one fish dinner a month is adequate, as long as the right kind of fish is eaten (see pp.148–9). Fortunately, EPA can be stored in the body. A serious deficiency of alpha-linolenic acid or of EPA is probably very rare: the only well-documented cases are among hospitalised patients being fed artificially for long periods of time.

To reduce the risk of heart attacks, substantially more EPA is required. Three meals of oily fish per week are commonly recommended, or an equivalent amount of omega-3 fish oil, which is rich in EPA (see p.148). Even more EPA is needed to treat rheumatoid arthritis, as described on pp.58–9. In this instance, EPA is acting as a drug, rather than a nutrient, although no very sharp distinction between the two types of action can be made.

The 'intelligence' nutrient

So much for linoleic acid, alpha-linolenic acid and EPA – although they are 'essential fatty acids', serious deficiencies of these nutrients are very rare. However, there is one essential fatty acid that really might be lacking for a significant number of people: docosahexaenoic acid or DHA. It may be in short supply for strict vegetarians, and this could be a problem if they become pregnant or are breastfeeding. DHA is important for the formation of nerve cells in the baby, and the growth of the brain. This need is supplied by the DHA which is normally found in human breastmilk. The milk of vegetarian mothers is known to contain much less DHA, because they get little from their diet and have little stored in their bodies. The level will probably be lowest in someone who has been a vegetarian for a very long time. There is some concern that this might affect the intellectual development of a vegetarian woman's children. Recent experiments have shown that a shortage of DHA in baby milk leads to significant differences in tests that measure intelligence.

The problem with DHA is that it can probably only be obtained from sea-living fish and shellfish. In theory, DHA can be made from EPA and, as described above, alpha-linolenic acid (found in plant foods) can be converted to EPA. In practice, when vegetarians are given a special supplement containing alpha-linolenic acid, although some of it is turned into EPA, none of this EPA seems to get turned into DHA. No one knows why this should be so, but it is clear that the conversion process is very slow and inefficient.

A vegetarian woman who is about to have a baby should, if she can face it, eat a little oily fish, such as sardines or smoked mackerel, twice a week, to give her the DHA that the baby will need. This is especially important if she has not eaten fish for many years. A teaspoonful of cod-liver oil a day would serve the same purpose, but if vitamin tablets are also being taken it is important to check that the total amount of Vitamins A and D is not excessive (see p.285 and p.300). Omega-3 fish oils (see p.148) have little Vitamin A or D so they are a good alternative.

If a pregnant woman absolutely cannot bring herself to eat fish or take fish oil, the next best thing is to eat a rich source of alpha-linolenic acid and hope that some does get converted to DHA. Linseed oil is one of the richest sources, but it must be *edible* linseed oil, *not* the kind used to oil cricket bats as this is toxic. Alternatively, take rapeseed or soyabean oil (rapeseed oil, if available, is the richer source) and eat plenty of green leafy vegetables, but remember that there is no certainty that enough DHA will be formed from these sources.

Decreasing intake of *linoleic* acid (by eating much less margarine, sunflower oil, safflower oil and maize/corn oil) will probably encourage the body to make its own DHA from alpha-linolenic acid: high intakes of linoleic acid seem to inhibit the conversion process.

If soyabean oil is to be a major part of your diet then a supplement of alpha-tocopherol, the most potent form of Vitamin E, is recommended. The type of Vitamin E found in soyabean oil, gamma-tocopherol, is only 10% as effective as alpha-tocopherol.

Other fatty acids

There are other fatty acids which can act in a drug-like way when taken in fairly large quantities, notably gamma-linolenic acid (GLA), found in evening primrose oil, which seems to have benefits in inflammatory arthritis. This is not an *essential* fatty acid and there is no minimal dose needed to avoid a deficiency state. The drug-like actions of various oils and their constituent fatty acids are discussed in Chapter 1.2 (p.46) and practical advice on taking these oils is given in Chapter 2.2 (p.143).

· *Saturated and Polyunsaturated Fat* ·

Diets rich in animal produce, such as milk, cream, eggs and fatty meat, supply large amounts of saturated fat (as well as some polyunsaturated fat and monounsaturated fat). Diets based on plant foods, such as vegetable oils and nuts, supply mostly polyunsaturated and monounsaturated fat. (An exception is coconut, whose fats are almost entirely saturated fat, although the exact composition is very different from animal fat.)

As is now well known, a diet rich in saturates may increase the risk of heart disease. It is also possible that saturated fat may affect the course of rheumatoid arthritis, although the evidence on this is far from conclusive (see pp.52–3).

The recommendation to replace saturates with polyunsaturates is now being reconsidered in the light of new evidence about the effects of polyunsaturates on factors contributing to heart disease. Current recommendations are to eat plenty of monounsaturated fats, in preference to both saturates and polyunsaturates.

Polyunsaturates tend to be liquid at room temperature – hence their use as cooking oil – whereas saturated fat, such as lard or butter, is solid. Monounsaturated fat is somewhere between the two: generally liquid at room temperature but semi-solid if left in the refrigerator. (Polyunsaturated margarine is solid by virtue of some clever food technology.) The reasons for these differences can be explained in terms of the chemistry of the different fats.

A fatty acid molecule consists of long chains of carbon atoms, each one joined to the next by a chemical bond. (Words such as 'atom' and 'molecule' are explained in the Glossary, pp.412–421.) Carbon atoms can actually make four bonds each, and as only two bonds are involved in joining it to its neighbours, every carbon atom has two bonds to spare.

In a saturated fat, these two spare bonds are joined to two hydrogen atoms. The term 'saturated' actually means 'saturated with hydrogen' – all the spare bonds in the fat molecules are joined to hydrogen.

In a monounsaturated fat, two of the carbon atoms in the chain have only one hydrogen atom each. These two are neighbours, and their spare bond is added to the existing bond between them, to form a 'double bond'. 'Mono' refers to the fact that there is just one double bond in the molecule.

In a polyunsaturated fat, there are two or more of these double bonds in each fat molecule. Each double bond puts a bend into the chain of the fat molecule, so whereas unsaturated fats have straight molecules, those of polyunsaturated fats are kinky. This is what makes them liquid at room temperature: the straight molecules of a saturated fat will pack neatly together to form a solid, as in a block of lard, whereas those of a polyunsaturated fat are too unruly for this. In the same way, polyunsaturated fats make the membranes of cells more fluid, and this accounts for some of their effects on the body.

Trans-fatty acids

All the fatty acids we have been discussing are cis-fatty acids: the 'cis' refers to the detailed architecture of the double bonds (see p.357) in the molecule. Any unsaturated fatty acid can exist in both 'cis' and 'trans' forms: their chemical ingredients are identical but they are arranged in a slightly different way. Most fatty acids found in plants and animals are of the 'cis' variety, although cows and other ruminant animals do produce some 'trans' fatty acids, which they pass into their milk. In fact it is not the cow which produces the trans fatty acids, but the bacteria in the rumen (or second stomach) – bacteria which help the cow digest grass. Milk and milk products are a major source of trans fatty acids in our food, but another source has developed in modern times: hydrogenated vegetable oils. These are fats manufactured in an industrial process, by passing hydrogen gas through a vegetable oil. The hydrogen combines with the polyunsaturated fatty acids in the oil, adding hydrogen to the double bonds, and so turning some of them into saturated fatty acids. Both cis and trans forms are created by this process. The product is a fat that is solid at room temperature, because it contains more saturated fat than the original oil.

Early forms of margarine were made in this way, and hard margarine still is. Hydrogenated vegetable oils are also used widely in bakery products such as biscuits.

Some scientific research has identified trans fatty acids as a potential risk factor for hardening of the arteries and heart disease. The concern about trans fatty acids was fuelled by a general perception of them as 'unnatural', since they were thought of only as the products of a modern industrial process. The more recent realisation that trans fatty acids are also found in milk has allayed such fears to some extent: clearly people have been eating trans fatty acids for thousands of years. Newer research on heart disease suggests that trans fatty acids have about the same level of risk attached to them as saturated fats. Current recommendations are to keep your intake down to the present level.

No one has investigated the effects, if any, of trans fatty acids on inflammation, nor any possible role in arthritis. It seems unlikely that they affect arthritic diseases in any special way, but in the interests of general health it is wise not to consume large amounts.

OTHER DIETS AND SUPPLEMENTS

Chapter 4.1

INTRODUCTION TO THE POPULAR DIETS

There are two main types of popular diet that are advocated for arthritis. Firstly there are 'avoidance diets', in which certain foods are excluded because they are claimed to cause arthritis, or at least make it worse. Secondly there are 'supplemented diets', in which certain foods or food extracts are said to be curative, healing or at least soothing to arthritic joints. Some of the diets have both components and these we describe as 'avoid-and-supplement diets'.

In Section Four we present the best known popular diets and try to assess the probable value of each one. In assessing the value of these diets, we are using information gained from scientific studies of diet and arthritis, plus basic scientific information about bodily processes, nutrition, and the causes of arthritis, plus a ration of 'common sense'. The value of scientific studies is that they include control groups (see p.27), allowing the effects of the diet to be assessed independently of placebo effects (see p.27) and spontaneous remissions (see p.19.)

At the same time we have kept in mind that diets might work in ways which we cannot, as yet, understand or explain. We have tried hard to keep our assessments as open-minded as possible.

One crucial point to remember is that a diet may actually work, but not for the reasons that the originator of the diet suggests. In other words, the diet may have been discovered by chance or developed on a purely pragmatic, trial-and-error basis, until something was found that seemed to help, either for one arthritic patient, or for a number of patients.

Having developed a diet in this way, the originator of the diet naturally speculates about the reasons for its apparent success and develops an explanation that fits in with his or her view of nutrition, on the one hand, and of arthritis on the other. The explanation may not be correct but this does not alter the fact that the diet works. So just because a diet seems to work (for you, or for anyone else) it does not follow that the originator of the diet is right about *how* it works.

Conversely, just because an explanation is simplistic, or lacks any real evidence to support it, this does not mean that the diet itself is without value.

However, when the originator presents an explanation which flies in the face of well established medical knowledge about arthritis, and reveals, as some of the explanations do, a breathtaking indifference to logic and common sense, the question of their objectivity does arise. If they are so cavalier about explanations, how careful have they been to see whether the diet really works for those who try it? Have they really subjected the effects of their diet to any serious scrutiny, or are they just being carried along on a wave of enthusiasm, failing to distinguish the effects of the diet from placebo effect? Before choosing a diet in which you will invest a lot of time and effort, it is worth considering these questions.

For each diet described, the originator's explanation is presented under the heading 'Rationale given for the diet'. Our thoughts on this explanation, and on alternative explanations for the diet's success, are also considered.

A number of the diets or their explanations involve speculation about the same points (eg. 'malnutrition' from food processing, 'poisoning' by food additives, the role of acids, or the calcification of soft tissues) as supposed causes of arthritis. Such explanations are considered in detail in Chapter 4.9 (p.403).

Chapter 4.2

DR DONG'S DIET

This diet is one of the most widely tried, especially in the U.S.A.. It is also one of the few popular diets which has been scientifically tested (see below).

· *The Diet* ·

Dr Dong's Diet is mainly an avoidance diet. The things that are forbidden are meat and fruit of any kind, tomatoes, any type of milk product, egg yolks, vinegar or any other acid, pepper and most spices, chocolate, alcohol and anything containing additives (preservatives, antioxidants, flavour enhancers, flavourings etc.).

There are certain things which are only allowed in small amounts occcasionally, including a little chicken breast and a dash of wine in cooking.

Origins of the diet

Dr Collin H. Dong was a qualified doctor of Chinese extraction, living and working in San Francisco in the U.S.A.. He became ill in 1938, at the age of 35, with a form of inflammatory arthritis accompanied by a widespread rash. He was given various diagnoses, among them rheumatoid arthritis, 'erosive osteoarthritis' and psoriatic arthritis.

He was treated with aspirin, but to little efffect. (In fact, he later concluded that the aspirin had caused the skin disorder.) The illness continued, inexorably, for three years, and his doctors could offer no further help, shaking Dr Dong's faith in the conventional medicine which he had studied and practised. In desperately low spirits, and, in his own words, 'grasping at straws' Dr Dong remembered an old Chinese saying of his father's: 'Sickness enters through the mouth and catastrophe comes out of the mouth'.

He began to think about his diet – by then a conventional American diet – and the extent to which it had changed from the diet of his childhood, when he had eaten simple Chinese food consisting mainly of beef, pork, chicken, fish, vegetables and rice. It also struck him that several members of his family had, in his words, 'allergy to foods'. At that point he decided to change his diet, reverting to the Chinese-style foods of his childhood.

It is worth digressing here to consider the question of 'food allergy' in Dr Dong's family and himself. In his writings, Dr Dong does not specify quite what he means by 'allergies' but it seems clear that he was using the word in a broad sense to mean 'any unusual and adverse reaction to food'. This is one way of using the word, but it blurs the boundaries between two fairly distinct types of reaction, and it adds enormously to the controversy and confusion over food and illness (see p.43). So in this book we make a point of differentiating between true food allergies and food intolerance. It seems most unlikely that all the reactions seen in Dr Dong's family were true food allergies since eight out of his nine brothers and sisters, in addition to his father, are listed as suffering from them. This would be extraordinary, even in the most allergy-prone family. Furthermore, even before the arthritis began, Dr Dong believed that he himself 'was allergic to milk, wheat, eggs and fruit – especially oranges'. Yet he outlines his normal menu at that time and these foods are all included. Someone who has a true allergy to food is made severely ill by a very small amount (see p.83) and could not eat them in the way Dr Dong describes. It seems likely that the sensitivities he described as 'allergy to food' are what we would now call 'food intolerance' or 'food sensitivity'. Even so, it is puzzling that he should have been eating milk products, wheat, eggs and oranges if he knew that these foods disagreed with him.

To return to Dr Dong's account of his illness: the early results of experimenting with his diet, in which he ate meat, vegetables and rice, were not rewarding. However, he persisted, cutting out different foods. Quite quickly he found that he felt better when he avoided meat and ate fish and other seafood instead. Within a few weeks of beginning this diet (seafood, vegetables and rice) he experienced a dramatic improvement. Writing in the mid-1970s he recalled 'I had almost a complete remission from my crippling disease. This remission has miraculously lasted for thirty-four years.'

Once he was well enough to start practising as a doctor again, Dr Dong tried out dietary treatment on his arthritic patients. His written report of this (1973) is very brief: 'In the past thirty years I have treated thousands of cases of rheumatic diseases. The high percentage of remissions from pain and misery with my method is remarkable.' Unfortunately, he does not say how his own very simple and restrictive diet evolved into the published Dong Diet (see above) which also allows bread, egg whites, tea, coffee and a variety of other items. He does allude to 'trial and error' but says little more.

Dr Dong did not try to do any formal research on his diet, because he regarded himself as 'a practising doctor . . . not a research scientist'. As he saw it, to convince the medical establishment, any research would have to answer the question 'How might it work?' not just the question 'Does it work?' (see p.35), and he could not possibly tackle that sort of research. (Many years later, other research scientists did carry out a 'Does it work?' type of trial with the Dong Diet, as described on page 366.)

Dr Dong quietly continued for three decades, putting arthritic patients onto his dietary regime. It was only the enthusiasm of a former patient, Jane Banks, that persuaded him to collaborate in producing a book, *The Arthritic's Cookbook*, published in the U.S.A. in 1973. This was the first time that Dr Dong had publicised his dietary treatment.

When asked why he had been so reticent Dr Dong replied: 'I did not have the courage to fight the medical establishment. We live in a world where it takes many years to build one's professional reputation. My method of treatment is an empirical one. It was not established on a scientific or theoretical basis accepted by the medical world.'

Rationale given for the diet

Dr Dong blamed arthritis on modern forms of food. He based his explanation on the idea that processed food, with additives of various kinds, is damaging to health. He believed that we should return to a simpler and more natural diet, akin to what the rural Chinese have traditionally eaten.

It is rather difficult to reconcile this rationale with various aspects of the diet. Meat is an important part of the Chinese diet, for example, yet it is prohibited. Fruit has been eaten by all mankind (and indeed by the ape-like ancestors of mankind) for millions of years, yet this is disallowed. Furthermore, although rheumatoid arthritis probably is slightly less common in China, this does not seem to be an effect of diet – see p.409.

To expand his original explanation, Dr Dong added the idea of 'allergy' to foods. In his second book he wrote: '. . . the causes of rheumatic diseases are chemical poisoning from the additives and preservatives that are put into our foods, and from allergy to certain foods.' But little emphasis was put on the 'allergy' aspect (see p.371).

Which forms of arthritis is the diet recommended for?

In Dr Dong's first book, no distinction was made between the different forms of arthritis: the diet seemed to be recommended for all kinds. (The one type that was discussed separately was gout, for which the same diet was recommended but further exclusions were made. Oddly enough, these were all vegetables, whereas no mention was made of avoiding some types of fish that are high in purines – the accepted and proven diet for gout.)

In Dr Dong's second book, the different types of arthritis are described separately, but the diet is still recommended for all types. Looking at the case histories given in Dr Dong's second book, eleven are *definitely* cases of rheumatoid arthritis, and another three (including Dr Dong himself) are *probably* rheumatoid arthritis: a total of fourteen. In addition there are seven cases of osteoarthritis and one of polymyositis. Given that osteoarthritis is far more common a problem than rheumatoid arthritis, it seems fair to conclude that Dr Dong's main successes were with rheumatoid arthritis.

. The First Test of Any Treatment: .
Does it Work?

In 1982, eight years after Dr Dong's first book was published, a research team at the University of Florida, headed by Professor Richard S. Panush, tested out the diet on eleven rheumatoid arthritis patients.

This was a double-blind placebo-controlled trial (see p.27). The control group consisted of fifteen patients with rheumatoid arthritis who were put on a placebo diet contrived by the researchers. The placebo diet did not rule out any whole groups of food so it was considered very unlikely to have any effect on arthritis or any other illness: it told patients to avoid certain dietary items such as sour cream, cabbage, margarine, corn flakes, vanilla and turkey. All the patients involved were interviewed to ensure that they had not previously heard of Dr Dong's Diet – this was important because if the patients had known about Dr Dong's alleged successes in advance, those given the Diet might have experienced more placebo effect (see p.27) while those in the control group might have experienced less.

The form of Dr Dong's Diet used was very similar to that in his books, although there were some minor differences. However, Dr Dong himself participated in the study by approving the dietary regime, so it seems that he considered these discrepancies unimportant. The fact that Dr Dong was invited to help the researchers suggests that they wanted to make the trial fair to the diet.

One precaution taken was to allow for the effect of weight loss by patients in both groups. About half those in each group were given a weight-reducing version of their diet, while the others were given a weight-maintaining version. The results showed that there was no difference in effect between those who lost weight and those who did not. (Note that this was with rheumatoid arthritis patients, and the study looked at effects in the short term only. Sustained weight loss is definitely of value in osteoarthritis. It may also help those with rheumatoid arthritis who are overweight and have inflamed knee or hip joints.)

The diet was tried out for ten weeks. Five patients on Dr Dong's Diet (45%) were judged to have improved – but so had six patients on the placebo diet (40%) – a powerful demonstration of the placebo effect operating. All-in-all, Dr Dong's Diet was judged 'no better than placebo' for rheumatoid arthritis, which in medical terms means 'of no intrinsic value'. However, the researchers noted that two patients on Dr Dong's Diet were markedly better, and both of them chose to stay on the diet after the study was over.

One, a 56-year-old woman, had suffered from rheumatoid arthritis for eight years, the other, a 49-year-old man, for eighteen months. They were both positive for rheumatoid factor (see p.419). These two patients remained well for as long as the researchers were in contact with them – nine months and six months respectively. Both deviated from the diet occasionally and suffered ill-effects. The woman noted that she suffered symptoms after eating dairy products, ice cream and chocolate. The man had found more pain and stiffness after 'some meats, spices or alcoholic beverages'.

The researchers were clearly impressed by the large and sustained improvement in these two patients, even though the overall results showed no statistically significant difference between Dr Dong's Diet and the placebo diet.

Initially, the researchers had intended to try the diet out on patients with osteoarthritis as well. Eleven patients with osteoarthritis were entered into the trial but were taken out at an early stage because they did not seem to be benefiting from the diet at all, whereas some with rheumatoid arthritis obviously were: the researchers decided to concentrate their efforts on putting a large number of rheumatoid arthritis patients through the trial, higher numbers being more likely to produce a statistically significant result. It is unfortunate that the osteoarthritis part of the study was abandoned, since the claim that diet can help patients with osteoarthritis is a highly contentious one, and a well-conducted study would have been useful, even if (as seems likely) it merely showed that the diet was of no benefit.

The Second Test of Any Treatment: How Might it Work?

Can we assess Dr Dong's belief that food additives are 'poisoning' arthritis patients? In the elimination diet trials carried out at Epsom, all foods are first tested in their natural, unadulterated form, so if there is a reaction it is clearly to the food itself, not to any additives. Two additives are then tested individually, one being monosodium glutamate, which Dr Dong particularly warns against. The number of patients who have reacted badly to monosodium glutamate is relatively small – only about 3%. Once food testing is complete, patients are then allowed to eat processed foods again and occasionally they do react to these, perhaps indicating a sensitivity to some additives. However, the number of patients affected is, once again, fairly small. If Dr Dong's idea about food additives were correct, large numbers of patients would be expected to relapse at this point, or soon afterwards, but this does not seem to happen. While it seems sensible to eat freshly prepared, home-cooked food whenever possible, and not to eat too many additives, the idea that processed food is 'poisoning' large numbers of people is, to our mind, an exaggeration.

As for the idea that 'allergy to certain foods' might be involved, if one substitutes 'intolerance' or 'sensitivity' for the contentious word 'allergy' (see p.43) then this is, in our opinion, a plausible explanation. But the idea is not carried through logically into Dr Dong's Diet. For example, some of the food items excluded by Dr Dong's Diet are rarely found to cause sensitivity. Fruits are a striking example: although citrus fruits are common offenders in food intolerance, and strawberries are a frequent source of allergy, other fruits are not often a problem. It is unknown for *all* types of fruit to cause someone ill-health, except in those who cannot digest fruit sugar (fructose) and these are rare individuals who are usually aware of the sensitivity from childhood because fruit and sugary food causes an unpleasant sensation in the mouth. Occasionally people who are sensitive to pesticides show a reaction to many different types of fruit because of spray residues, but they are not reacting to the fruit itself, and can eat organically grown fruit.

The possible role of food sensitivity in Dr Dong's Diet is explored more fully in the next section.

· *Our View of Dr Dong's Diet* ·

We believe the successes of Dr Dong's Diet can be readily explained in terms of three factors: food sensitivity (which would produce a prompt benefit for a subgroup of people with rheumatoid arthritis), the anti-inflammatory effects of more fish oil and less saturated fat (which would produce a much more delayed benefit for most people with rheumatoid arthritis), and weight loss (which would produce benefits for those with osteoarthritis who were overweight). The fact that no time limit was set on the expected response to the diet also works in its favour. It allows any spontaneous remissions (or partial remissions) occurring in the months and years after the diet was begun to also be attributed to the diet. Add placebo effect (see p.26) to this, and one would expect a quite reasonable success rate.

Firstly, and perhaps most importantly, Dr Dong's Diet would have produced an effect similar to an elimination diet when tried by patients with rheumatoid arthritis who were sensitive to certain foods. This is particularly likely when the diet was administered by Dr Dong himself, because his patients seem to have begun with a very restricted regime of fish, rice and vegetables, and were then told to introduce other foods (such as bread, chicken, egg white and nuts) at intervals. This is not spelled out in his books, but can be inferred from some of the case histories. We suspect that if reactions were noted to these new foods, they were avoided by that patient thereafter. This is, in effect, an elimination diet.

There are two interesting comments tucked away in the books by Dong and Banks, which support this suspicion. *The Arthritic's Cookbook* says: '. . . everyone's body is different, and one must discover one's own anathemas by experimentation.' In *New Hope for the Arthritic* there is the remark 'Sensitivity to certain foods will vary from person to person; this must be determined by the individual.'

No great emphasis is given to these remarks, however, and there are no instructions in the books on how to test foods. Dr Dong's Diet, in its published form (and as tested at the University of Florida) was essentially a same-for-everyone diet, where patients could eat all the allowed foods from the outset. Even so, the diet was quite restrictive: no milk or milk products, no fruit, no tomatoes, no meat, and quite probably no eggs, since relatively few people would bother to eat the white only. These foods all feature in the 'top twenty' most often identified as culprits by patients going through the elimination diet at Epsom General Hospital (see p.71).

Thus some people with rheumatoid arthritis, who would be helped by an elimination diet, because they have a sensitivity to an item such as milk or oranges, would also do well on Dr Dong's Diet. (But notice that they would probably be avoiding – for the rest of their lives – a number of other foods they could happily eat.) On the other hand, someone with a sensitivity to wheat, corn, oats, rye or coffee – all in the top ten of our league table – would not respond to Dr Dong's Diet nor find out about their problem foods. Their time and effort would have been far better spent on an elimination diet.

Note that the two patients who did really well in the University of Florida study both reported afterwards that their joints flared up in response to *particular foods*, not to everything that Dr Dong disallows.

To take the second factor, Dr Dong's Diet relies heavily on fish to supply protein. Anyone on this diet will probably be eating fish at least once a day, and if they were to choose oily sea-living fish they might be benefiting from the anti-inflammatory effects of fish oil (see Chapter 1.2, p.46). So there could be some modest improvement in the symptoms of inflammatory arthritis through this alone, although it would take months to become evident. This would probably give some help even to those with no food sensitivities, or those whose food sensitivity had not been detected by Dr Dong's Diet.

As for the third factor, weight reduction, many of the case histories in Dr Dong's book describe striking losses, the greatest being 28 kg (63 lb). Of the seven successes with osteoarthritis, four are described as losing weight – between 6 kg (14 lb) and 12 kg (28 lb). This may account for the diet's success with osteoarthritis, although we cannot rule out some other, as yet unknown, effect on osteoarthritis.

To anyone with rheumatoid arthritis considering Dr Dong's Diet we would say that the elimination diet is more likely to be useful. Compare the results of the Epsom studies which produced 36% 'good responders' (see p.29) (and another 40% who benefit to some degree) with those in the University of Florida studies of Dr Dong's Diet which gave only 18% of good responders (two out of eleven patients).

If the elimination diet does not work for you, then you could try some of the dietary changes suggested in Chapter 2.2 (p.143), such as eating more fatty fish and olive oil.

If you have already tried Dr Dong's Diet, and experienced some partial improvement, you may benefit more from trying the full elimination diet as given in Chapter 2.4 (p.170). You should only do this with your doctor's consent, however, and if you are already underweight you should be careful not to lose much more.

Anyone who has tried Dr Dong's Diet and benefited substantially, should consider methodically testing some of the disallowed foods. There may well be items that you can safely eat. Read the instructions for food testing given on pages 182–190. If you have been avoiding the foods for more than six months, then your sensitivity may well have declined, so reintroduce only one food every two weeks. Eat the test food every day for those two weeks, then stop eating it and go on to the next test food.

If you did well on Dr Dong's Diet for a time, but then deteriorated again and returned to your normal menu, consider trying an elimination diet. If you do not improve on the first stage of the diet (the exclusion phase) as described on page 178, you could try a fish-free version: if you have been eating fish daily, then an intolerance might have developed. For a fish-free exclusion phase, substitute turkey and rabbit for the trout, salmon and cod, or see p.182.

In conclusion, there is no doubt that Dr Dong was a sincere and dedicated physician who believed that his diet could help a great many people with arthritis. However, he devised the diet for his own illness, and even before the arthritis began, he considered himself 'allergic to' (we would say 'intolerant of' or 'sensitive to') milk, wheat, eggs, oranges and other fruits. He devised a diet that avoided these foods and was right for himself, though perhaps unduly restrictive. The diet he then gave to his patients was just a slightly expanded version of his own regime, probably with some form of individual food-testing as described on page 369. When he came to publish the diet, however, it was presented as a same-for-everyone diet where patients could eat corn, wheat and other cereals (frequent offenders in food sensitivity) right from the start. In our view Dr Dong had missed the crucial point about food reactions, whether 'allergic' or otherwise, that *everyone is different as regards the culprit foods*. Although he later used the concept of allergy in trying to explain how his diet worked, he did not really apply the essence of that concept in his published diet.

Dr Dong seems to have helped many people with arthritis, but it is sad to think of the many patients who tried the diet and were *not* helped, because of an undisclosed sensitivity to wheat or corn for example. It is also sad to consider thousands of arthritics forever avoiding fruit – one of life's healthiest and simplest pleasures – when they probably had no need to do so.

Chapter 4.3

SISTER HILLS' DIET

Two books by Sister Margaret Hills, *Curing Arthritis the Drug-Free Way* and the *Curing Arthritis Cookbook* have sold extremely well in the U.K.

· *The Diet* ·

This is an 'avoid-and-supplement diet'. The avoidance element involves reducing salt intake and cutting out citrus fruits and various other fruits, and any high-fat milk products (cream, butter, cream cheese, cheese, whole milk). Other forbidden foods are sausages, bacon and other processed meats, alcoholic drinks (although small amounts of brandy or Guinness are allowed), all fried foods, white sugar, white bread, cream cakes, biscuits and 'fruits bottled in syrup' (but not tinned fruits, apparently). Duck, kidney, tomatoes and tinned fish are to be avoided, while eggs are restricted to three or four a week. Tea consumption must be reduced and only decaffeinated coffee is allowed.

The supplementation aspect of the diet advocates vitamin and mineral supplements, taking a teaspoon of honey and a dessertspoon of cider vinegar in hot water three times a day, and taking a teaspoon of black molasses three times a day. Sister Hills also recommends plenty of fish, fresh vegetables and salads.

Sister Hills frequently refers to her diet as an 'acid-free diet', yet it specifically advocates cider vinegar which is very acidic, and it allows items such as apple juice and apricots that are also acidic. (Other foods and drinks that are not acidic she describes as 'being acidic' eg. cream and milk.)

Bathing in hot water containing Epsom salts, three times a week, is also recommended as part of this treatment regime, and gentle exercise is considered important.

Origins of the diet

Margaret Hills was a trainee nurse of 22 when rheumatoid arthritis struck. It was 1947, and the only drug available was aspirin. She was forced to rest in bed for five months, and made a remarkable recovery. Returning to finish her training, she then developed osteoarthritis which got steadily worse over the next sixteen years and caused a lot of pain. Then rheumatoid arthritis struck again, and left her 'totally crippled – locked in every joint'. She had six young children to care for, and again drugs had helped her very little. So she set about developing a treatment for herself: 'I got hold of all the "natural cure" books I could lay my hands on, and eventually hit upon the treatment that was to rid me of all signs of arthritis. That was twenty-two years ago, and I have since had twenty-one years of totally pain-free living.'

In 1982, Margaret Hills read an article on arthritis research in the local newspaper in Coventry, England, where she lives. It spurred her into writing a letter describing her own recovery. The paper ran a story on her, and the response was staggering: an endless stream of phone calls and an avalanche of letters from other arthritics. Sister Hills began producing leaflets on the diet and sending these out, then she opened a private clinic at her home, and later gave talks to large audiences gathered in hotels, in order to reach even more people.

Rationale given for the diet

Sister Hills claims that the underlying cause of both osteoarthritis and rheumatoid arthritis is 'too much uric acid in the body'. This is, quite simply, not true. Gout is caused by excess uric acid (see p.103), but other forms of arthritis are caused in entirely different ways (see Chapter 1.3, p.63).

The rationale given in Sister Hills' book continues as follows (the relevant facts are given in brackets after each quote):

'Acid is taken in over the years in the food we eat, and the liquids we drink' (There is little or no uric acid in food, and the acids that are found in food are different. They do not turn into uric acid in the body. It is purines in food that turn into uric acid – see p.105.)

'If our bodies contain the required nutrients to burn up the acid that we take in, then there is no problem. Unfortunately, the food we eat today is sadly lacking in those nutrients, so we are left with the situation of an undernourished body, full of acid.' (Lack of nutrients would not lead to an accumulation of acid in the body – deficiency diseases caused by lack of vitamins are well documented and this is not among their symptoms. The idea that our bodies are now 'full of acid' is mistaken: the acidity of the blood and body fluids is carefully maintained throughout life, within very tight limits – see pp.404–7.)

Sister Hills justifies the use of cider vinegar (an acid!) in the treatment of arthritis, as follows: 'The hard acid deposits connected with arthritis are very similar in substance to the shell of an egg.' (Eggshells are made of calcium carbonate, the same material as chalk, and definitely not an acid.)

'Cider vinegar has the power to dissolve those acid deposits so they pass out naturally, via the kidneys. The reader can carry out an experiment to show how this works. Place an egg, complete with shell, in a jar or glass. Cover the egg with "neat" cider vinegar and in two days the shell will have completely dissolved, leaving the egg intact.' (Yes, the eggshell will dissolve, but it dissolves because the cider vinegar is *an acid* and the chalky eggshell is attacked by acids!) 'Similarly, when cider vinegar saturates the bloodstream, it gets between the joints, dissolving the acid deposits and passing them away.' (Three spoonfuls of cider vinegar a day would not 'saturate' the bloodstream nor would it 'get between the joints'. And if it did, the effect would very probably be damaging, not beneficial.)

Which forms of arthritis is the diet recommended for?

Sister Hills recommends her treatment for all forms of arthritis, and for a great variety of other diseases.

The supposed 'acid deposits' in various parts of the body are blamed for causing a host of medical conditions incuding head colds, hayfever, acne, pimples, hiccoughs, 'sleeping sickness' (in fact a tropical disease caused by a parasite), dizziness, vertigo, nervous breakdowns, 'mental conditions' and St Vitus's Dance.

. The First Test of Any Treatment: . Does it Work?

No one has ever tested this diet scientifically to see if it has any effect.

The claimed benefits of apple-cider vinegar have been tested and they appear to be non-existent (see pp.399–400). Neither blackstrap molasses nor honey have been tested (see pp.400–401).

The Second Test of Any Treatment: How Might it Work?

The supplement side of the diet – cider vinegar, honey and blackstrap molasses – is discussed in Chapter 4.8 (p.396).

Looking at the avoidance element of the diet, and thinking about it in terms of food sensitivity, there are eight foods from the top-twenty 'frequent offenders' (see p.71) that are totally forbidden by Sister Hills' diet, including two out of the top four. Avoiding these foods might produce significant improvement in a limited number of people with rheumatoid arthritis – those who had a sensitivity to one or more of these foods and not to other foods that are permitted on the diet. This would be a prompt and striking response, and might well explain the remarkable recovery from rheumatoid arthritis that Sister Hills herself experienced, although it is more difficult to understand her recovery from the osteoarthritis (which was already present) in these terms.

The reduction in saturated fat recommended by Sister Hills might also help in rheumatoid arthritis, and so might the increased consumption of fish if oily fish were eaten (see Chapter 2.2, p.143). This would be a slower and less dramatic response. Patients with osteoarthritis would benefit from losing weight on the diet and might also get some small benefit from oily fish (see p.159). Finally, the increased intake of fruits and vegetables might be beneficial in supplying more antioxidants (see p.339). Again this would be a modest and gradual improvement. The unspecified timespan for benefits from the diet could result in any spontaneous remissions or partial remissions that might occur being counted as 'successes' for the diet.

Placebo effect may be playing a large part for some of the people who are helped by Sister Hills. Her book describes some of the cases seen at her clinic:

> 'I find that most people that I see at the clinic think negatively and I am fully convinced that this negative thinking destroys them . . . My patients become my friends, I take a personal interest in each and every one of them . . . Very often a patient will come to my clinic, having lost a spouse recently; he will tell me that he is living alone and trying to adjust to life without his partner. He says his arthritis has got so much worse since his partner passed away. He can see himself ending up in a wheelchair with nobody to look after him, and he projects a picture of hopelessness. I try to tell this patient that there is nothing to fear in life except fear. I ask him to cast out fear and look forward with hope . . . I say that death does not divide,

there is no need to fear separation and death can never separate souls who love . . . . as every healer knows, true healing begins with the spirit.'

One particular case shows that it was the personal contact with Sister Hills, rather than any dietary changes, which helped the patient. As Sister Hills describes it: 'She could not sit on a chair and had been lying on her back for five months . . . She had lost a lot of weight and was very confused. I knelt on the floor beside her and put my hands on her back asking if that was where the trouble was. She said, "Yes, that's it. Please keep your hands there, don't take them away, they're very hot". I realized that my hands were being used to bring warmth and comfort to that patient and I prayed that the pain would go. When I stood up after fifteen minutes, the pain had gone and the patient stood up straight for the first time in five months and cried tears of joy, saying "I'm healed".'

· *Our View of Sister Hills' Diet* ·

Sister Hills is obviously a sincere and well-intentioned person who believes she can help other arthritis sufferers. With her energy, enthusiasm, religious faith and sense of mission, she undoubtedly achieves a great deal simply by encouraging those with arthritis not to give up hope, to keep mobile and to take moderate exercise. There is nothing whatever wrong with healing methods which use psychological and spiritual techniques to hearten the patient, and to activate their own powers of self-healing and pain control. Indeed, conventional doctors giving conventional treatments are also dispensing a little of this form of healing – it is exactly the same as placebo effect (see pp.26–7). For anyone with long-term arthritis, and rather disillusioned with what medicine has to offer them, an inspiring figure such as Sister Hills, promoting an alternative cure, is likely to have a very powerful placebo effect.

Sister Hills' diet and other treatments are unlikely to do anyone harm, and they may encourage a healthier diet with less saturated fat, sugar and alcohol, and more fish and fresh vegetables. The daily need to abide by the rather complex dietary instructions, and to take certain items such as cider vinegar, honey and molasses, might well help in sustaining the original placebo effect.

On the negative side, misinformation about the causes of arthritis and the functioning of the human body is not helpful to patients in the long run. Perhaps the most useful parts of Sister Hills' books are the encouraging words on attitude: 'In your fight for health, keep cheerful and optimistic. The correct mental attitude is a fundamental necessity if you are to have any chance of success.'

Chapter 4.4

THE 'LIVING FOODS' DIET

This diet, devised by Ann Wigmore, has a small but enthusiastic following in the U.S.A. and in Finland.

· *The Diet* ·

No animal foods of any kind are allowed: this is a strictly vegan diet. Foods are eaten raw, although many are blended to make them more digestible; some are dried in a special 'dehydrator', while beans and cereal grains are 'sprouted' (allowed to germinate). Some typical 'living food' dishes are listed on pp.15–16. A great many of the foods in this diet are fermented, including a drink called 'Rejuvelac' which is made by soaking wheat grains in water and allowing them to ferment for two days, then pouring off the liquid. Another drink, which is emphasised as an important part of the diet, is made from the young green leaves of wheat, especially grown in seed trays for the purpose, harvested and then put through a juicer. It has to be drunk within fifteen minutes of being made. Other green leaves, including those of comfrey and various weeds, are treated similarly.

Restrictions are placed on which foods are eaten together: for example, oranges and sunflower seeds must not be combined in one meal, fruits and vegetables cannot be combined, and melons must only ever be eaten alone.

The diet is complicated, it requires an enormous commitment of time and energy, and is socially limiting because almost any food not prepared at home would be disallowed.

Origins of the diet

The diet was developed in the late 1960's by Ann Wigmore, who set up an organisation called the Hippocrates World Health Organisation in Boston in 1970. This has since been renamed the Ann Wigmore

Foundation. Her dietary programme is presented as having a far-reaching beneficial effect on health, and as preventing many different forms of disease. An anti-ageing effect also seems to be hinted at in the name 'Rejuvelac', and benefits for cancer patients are implied in the recipe book published by the Foundation, (*Recipes for Longer Life*) although direct claims are avoided.

Rationale given for the diet

The claims for the 'living foods' diet focus on several different points, including enzymes in food, digestibility of food, vitamins and minerals, chlorophyll, bacteria in food and bacteria in the digestive tract. To deal with each of these in turn:

Enzymes

'Living foods' enthusiasts claim that the enzymes found in plant foods are essential for health, and that they are destroyed by cooking. It is correct that living plants, like other living things, contain enzymes, which control and facilitate all metabolic reactions (see p.415). It is indeed the case that cooking destroys the activity of the enzymes in food. However, the human mouth and stomach both produce large numbers of enzymes that break down the food we eat into smaller fragments; these fragments are then absorbed into the bloodstream. According to conventional scientific understanding, we produce our own enzymes for digestion, and the enzymes contained in the food itself are entirely irrelevant for this process – after all, a plant does not have anything to be gained by being eaten, so why should it have evolved enzymes that aid human digestion?

Indeed, some enzymes found in raw foods are harmful because they attack the fabric of the stomach lining – raw pineapple and papaya (pawpaw) both contain the enzyme papain which can have a damaging effect if eaten on an empty stomach. Papain is rendered inactive by cooking. There are several other rather aggressive chemical substances in food, such as the lectins (also called haemagglutinins) found in raw beans, raw wheatgerm and other plant foods, which bind to the lining of the mouth and digestive tract. Some are absorbed into the blood and can make red blood cells clump together.

Some lectins are harmless, others are toxic (some highly so) but they are largely inactivated by cooking. All these chemical substances are present in plant foods for defensive purposes – to discourage animals from destroying the plant, or its seed. When the earliest human ancestors lived by hunting-and-gathering they selected plants which were relatively non-toxic, and avoided others, as wild animals do. Later, human ancestors mastered the use of fire, and invented cooking. Later still, they became farmers, and it was only then that the consumption of crops such as wheat and beans began. From the first, such foods were cooked, and thorough cooking at high temperature was essential for foods such as beans and lentils, to destroy the toxic lectins they contain. (Fortunately for 'living foods' enthusiasts, sprouting beans and seeds also destroy their lectins, but this takes a few days, and it is important not to eat bean sprouts too soon.)

In short, the idea that natural enzymes found in food can help our own digestive enzymes to fulfil their task seems implausible, but it has never been tested scientifically and we should not dismiss it out-of-hand.

At the same time, it is important to recognise that foods, especially wild foods, are not as benign and cooperative about being eaten as the proponents of 'living food' would suggest. Comfrey leaves, for example, contain some toxic substances, yet this is one of the ingredients advocated for making 'living foods' drinks.

Digestibility

The digestibility argument for 'living foods' is related to the one about enzymes. It suggests that the sprouting of beans and grains, and the fermentation of foods, renders them partially pre-digested and therefore more easily dealt with by the human digestive system. This might be true, to a limited extent, but only for some constituents of the food. It seems unlikely that it would make any greater difference to digestibility than simply cooking the foods, but again this has not been scientifically tested.

Vitamins and minerals

The nutrient content of the diet has been investigated scientifically in Finland, and shown to be adequate in most respects, although it is totally lacking in Vitamin B_{12} (as are all vegan diets – see p.288). The levels of B_{12} in the blood show a sharp decline after just one month on the diet, so a supplement of this vitamin would be necessary for anyone following the diet. The calcium content of the diet could also be inadequate.

On the positive side, the 'living foods' diet supplies more iron, zinc, niacin, Vitamin C and Vitamin E than a typical Finnish diet (which is much like the diet in other industrialised countries). The extra Vitamin E might be of some value in rheumatoid arthritis, but would not make any sudden or substantial difference.

Chlorophyll

This is the green pigment in plants. It is rich in the mineral magnesium, but apart from that, no specific health benefits have been identified. However, this is not something that scientific researchers have investigated. There might be some grounds for looking at the role of chlorophyll in our diet simply because the ape-like ancestors of mankind must have eaten very large amounts of it, whereas we eat relatively little. However, even if chlorophyll is of some special value nutritionally, there are many sources of it in conventional food – a handful of parsley or chives, or a serving of broccoli or spring greens, would provide handsome amounts of chlorophyll without the need to grow wheat plants on the kitchen windowsill or invest in a juicing machine.

Bacteria in food and in the digestive tract

Of all the explanations offered for the effects of the 'living foods' diet, this one has the most in its favour. The topic is dealt with on p.382.

Which forms of arthritis is the diet recommended for?

No specific recommendations are made although the diet is promoted, in a rather vague way, as helpful for all types of disease (see p.379). The objective scientific research on the diet, all carried out in Finland, has focused on rheumatoid arthritis (see below).

. *The First Test of Any Treatment:* . *Does it Work?*

Dr Mikko Nenonen and other Finnish researchers have attempted to test the effects of a 'living foods' diet on patients with rheumatoid arthritis. Unfortunately, it is difficult to conduct a scientific trial of this type of diet, because patients cannot be 'blind' (see p.18) to the type of diet they are receiving, and only those who are already interested in the idea of such a diet would be willing to participate and undertake such a radical change from customary eating habits. Nevertheless, Dr Nenonen has conducted as rigorous a scientific trial as possible.

He found that patients with rheumatoid arthritis experienced some unpleasant symptoms during the first few days of the diet (nausea, headache and digestive problems) but that, over the following weeks, they began to feel better. This subjective improvement was maintained for the 2–3 months that the study lasted, but then disappeared when a normal diet was resumed. More objective measurements, such as the number of tender joints, also showed some improvement, but there was no really striking benefit from the diet, and Dr Nenonen himself suggests that the improvements could be psychogenic (see p.18). Laboratory tests that measure levels of inflammation showed no improvement for the 'living foods' group as a whole, but something interesting emerged when the patients who had followed the dietary rules most carefully, and had drunk 'Rejuvelac', were assessed separately from the others. In the group using 'Rejuvelac', two different laboratory measures of inflammation declined markedly, whereas in the other group (following the 'living foods' diet, but not drinking 'Rejuvelac') these measures either rose or stayed the same.

. *The Second Test of Any Treatment:* . *How Might it Work?*

There is now some evidence that the gut flora (see p.37) of those with rheumatoid arthritis is in some ways different from the normal, healthy gut flora. In the Norwegian study of an elimination diet (see pp.29–30) those who responded well to the diet showed a significant change in their gut flora, as measured by gas-liquid chromatography (see pp.37–8).

Studies in Finland have shown that the 'living foods' diet also changes the composition of the gut flora, introducing far more lactobacilli, which are thought to be generally beneficial. The source of these lactobacilli is probably 'Rejuvelac' which contains very large numbers of living lactobacilli. One researcher found that the patients with the greatest changes in their gut flora were also those with the most notable improvement in their symptoms.

· *Our View of the 'Living Foods' Diet* ·

The scientific evidence in favour of this diet is not particularly strong, but there is enough to encourage further research. It is possible that some of the fermented drinks and other fermented foods have a beneficial effect on the gut flora, and that this effect might influence the symptoms of rheumatoid arthritis, but far more research is needed on these fermented foods before they can be positively recommended. Their effects on the gut flora are clearly temporary – no permanent change is produced. On the basis of the Finnish study, it seems that other aspects of the diet are probably of no particular value.

Chapter 4.5

OTHER POPULAR DIETS

· Dr Campbell's Diet ·

This is described in *A Doctor's Proven New Home Cure for Arthritis* by Dr Giraud W. Campbell, published in the U.S.A. in 1972.

Dr Campbell recommends a complete fast for the first 24 hours. On the second day raw fruits and vegetables are allowed (but not citrus fruits), together with raw or lightly cooked liver, and non-homogenised unpasteurised milk. On the third day, fresh seafood is added. If this is unavailable, then the alternatives are frozen but unprocessed seafood, or offal (organ meats) such as heart, kidney, brain, sweetbread or tripe.

This diet is maintained for three to ten days, during which time, according to Dr Campbell, 'your pain should end and the heat and swelling in the joints should disappear.' Enemas are also recommended during this time.

Thereafter, Dr Campbell instructs his patients to add one new food each day and see if stiffness recurs on the next day. The foods that cause symptoms are then to be avoided.

In fact, the foods to be tested are fairly limited because some foods are never to be eaten again anyway (these are listed below). The foods that need testing include cheese, any meats that have not so far been eaten, any vegetables or fruits not so far eaten, various kinds of nuts, seeds, beans and lentils, potatoes and rice. With fresh citrus fruits, Dr Campbell recommends testing them cautiously, but only when considerable improvement in symptoms has occurred.

Foods that are entirely forbidden include *all* kinds of flour (wheat, corn, rye, soya), coffee, tea, soft drinks, alcoholic drinks, sugar, ice cream, puddings, jams, canned or processed food, frozen fruit and processed breakfast cereals (including things such as quick-cooking oatmeal). Wheat in any form is also forbidden, and is described as being highly damaging to arthritics.

As regards cooking, Dr Campbell believes that meat and vegetables should only be cooked very lightly.

Various dietary supplements are recommended: cod-liver oil (two tablespoons per day – an alarmingly high dose of Vitamins A and D if taken regularly; see p.154); blackstrap molasses (one tablespoon per day); powdered brewer's yeast (one tablespoon per day).

Origins of the diet

The origins of the diet are unknown. Dr Campbell seems to have developed it within his own medical practice.

Rationale given for the diet

Dr Campbell believes that modern food is at fault, firstly in lacking essential nutrients, and secondly in 'poisoning' us with artificial additives. His colourful description of the modern American runs as follows:

'He consumes soft drinks, colas, tea, coffee and alcoholic beverages – trading a few minutes of physical pleasure for years of depleted health. He eats dead food – devitalised, demineralised, devitaminised foods that have been bleached, leached and refined of all nature's goodness, and he susbtitutes instead a few synthetic "enriching" additives and a hundred chemical additives that gradually pollute his entire system.'

Which forms of arthritis is the diet recommended for?

Dr Campbell states that the diet is useful for both osteoarthritis and rheumatoid arthritis. He does not recognise any other forms of arthritis. However, he feels that patients with rheumatoid arthritis who have had prolonged treatment with gold salts, or other 'extensive drug or chemical treatment' do not respond.

The First Test of Any Treatment: Does it Work?

There are many case histories reported in Dr Campbell's book, where patients have apparently done very well on the diet. However, no scientific trial of his diet has ever been carried out.

The Second Test of Any Treatment: . How Might it Work?

In our view, this dietary programme resembles an elimination diet, in that the patient stays on a tightly restricted diet for up to ten days, then tests foods by reintroducing them, one per day.

The resemblance to an elimination diet is strengthened by the fact that Dr Campbell predicts a substantial recovery during the initial ten days of the diet . We would be more cautious and say that *some* people will get substantially better within ten days or so, while others will not respond very much at all. The important point is that the reaction occurs fairly promptly or not at all – it does not require months of sticking to the restricted diet.

We feel that Dr Campbell's diet works by identifying food sensitivity, and the quick response favours that view. (If patients had been 'poisoned' in some way, one would expect a longer interval of time to be neeeded before there was a notable recovery.) As such, the diet is only likely to work for people with rheumatoid arthritis – it is unusual for an elimination diet to help anyone with osteoarthritis.

The idea that arthritis patients are malnourished is a common one among those recommending alternative diets; it is dealt with on p.408. Osteoarthritis was seen in prehistoric man, including the Neanderthals, and there is evidence of rheumatoid arthritis among prehistoric American Indians – none of whom ate processed foods. Both diseases are now found in all races of mankind, eating a wide variety of diets, suggesting that a simple back-to-nature diet of the type that Dr Campbell advocates is not likely to be a panacea for this disorder.

Our View of Dr Campbell's Diet

You would be better off trying an elimination diet as described in Chapter 2.4 (p.170), and following the guidelines for healthy eating in Chapter 2.8 (p.252).

· Norman F. Childers' Diet ·

This is described in *Arthritis – Childers' Diet to Stop It!* by Norman F. Childers, published in the U.S.A. in 1977.

All foods originating from plants of the Solanaceae family are to be strictly avoided. These include tomato, potato, aubergine (eggplant), red, green or yellow sweet peppers (bell peppers, capsicums), pimiento and chilli peppers, plus all spices made from such peppers: paprika, chilli powder, red pepper, cayenne and various 'seasoning mixtures' and curry powders that contain these spices. Another name for the Solanaceae is the 'nightshades family', so this is often referred to as a **no-nightshades diet**.

Tobacco, which comes from the same plant family, is not permitted. Patients are told to avoid contact with the leaves of any nightshade plants.

Sweet potatoes are allowed, because they are unrelated to ordinary potatoes. Similarly, white and black pepper are permitted, since these come from a different plant family, not the nightshades.

The other element in Norman Childers' diet concerns foods that have Vitamins A or D added to them. His advice is to avoid these, or to reduce consumption of them drastically. In the U.S.A, where the diet originated, these foods include milk, cheese and other dairy products, and some brands of margarine. According to Dr Childers, store-bought eggs also have extra doses of Vitamins A and D which are derived from vitamin-enriched feed. Vitamin pills containing Vitamins A or D are prohibited by the diet.

Origins of the diet

At the time he developed the diet, Dr Norman Childers was a horticulturalist working at the University of Florida in the U.S.A. (Note that he is not a medical doctor – the 'Dr' here refers to a research degree in horticulture.) He suffered from diverticulitis (an inflammatory bowel disorder) for many years, along with aching joints. He first suspected that spicy tomato juice had set off the diverticulitis, and tried eliminating this from his diet, with good results. He then began to suspect fresh tomatoes, potatoes and aubergine (eggplant). Removing these from his diet produced further improvement. Being a horticulturalist and therefore knowing about plant relationships, he realised that these were all members of the family Solanaceae – as were sweet peppers and chilli peppers. Having cut out *all* foods from this plant family, Dr Childers' made an excellent recovery.

Several friends of Dr Childers, who also suffered some form of arthritis, then tried the no-nightshades diet and reported good results. They urged him to publicise the diet, which he did, using newspaper advertisements that recruited about 3000 people in six years. (By 1986, the number had doubled to 6000.) Those who replied were asked to try out the diet and report back on the result. Dr Childers named them 'cooperators' and they form an important part of his book.

Based on the response from 'cooperators', Dr Childers added new prohibitions to his diet. He became convinced that synthetic Vitamins A and D added to foods could also cause problems in arthritis.

Sometimes the 'cooperators' reported other foods as causing symptoms, including chocolate, coffee, wines, spirits (liquors), wheat, maize (corn), citrus fruits, pecans, peaches, strawberries, melons, grapes, rhubarb, cherries, peas, asparagus, beets and spinach. Dr Childers generally either dismissed such cases as puzzling anomalies, or sought to explain them by reference to his original ideas. Thus he would explain reactions to chocolate as a result of high Vitamin D content, reactions to peanuts as due to unnoticed paprika in seasoning, and reactions to wheat as a result of the inclusion of potato flour with the wheat flour. The reaction to peas he attributed to contamination by nightshades weeds growing in pea crops, the green nightshade berries being included in the harvest in small amounts. (The latter may sound far-fetched, but one of the 'cooperators' reported working in a pea canning factory and being assigned to pick out the green nightshade berries from among the peas.) Dr Childers also speculated that pesticide residues might be at the root of some reactions to fruit and vegetables.

In time Dr Childers did concede that some people might have their own particular, idiosyncratic reactions to foods other than nightshades. He encouraged his cooperators to track down their individual problem foods. One interesting comment that he made in this context is 'The culprit frequently is something you like very much and are eating or using in excess.' This is in line with the observations frequently made about food intolerance (see p.45).

Rationale given for the diet

Dr Childers believed that natural toxins in the nightshade crops cause chronic poisoning (that is gradual, long-term poisoning, rather than a sudden attack) in some unusually sensitive people. He pointed to the many toxins that are produced by the leaves and other parts of these plants (this is established fact) and concluded that significant amounts remained in the harvested vegetables (this is a more debatable point since plant breeders have worked hard to reduce such toxins to a minimum in the part that is eaten). He believed that these toxins had subtle effects on human health.

In his opinion, arthritis was just one symptom of the nightshade toxins – others might include depression, diarrhoea, dry mouth and eyes, headaches and high blood pressure.

An excess of Vitamins A and D, particularly D, is also blamed by Dr Childers for causing calcium deposits in soft tissues – something that is dealt with on p.410.

Which forms of arthritis is the diet recommended for?

Rheumatoid arthritis, osteoarthritis, systemic lupus erythematosus, ankylosing spondylitis, gout, bursitis and tendinitis. Dr Childers, though not a medical doctor, gains credibility by actually distinguishing these different forms of disease – whereas most of the medically qualified authors discussed in this section of the book group everything together and call it 'arthritis'.

. The First Test of Any Treatment: .
Does it Work?

We only have the reports of Dr Childers' many 'cooperators' to go on, and this is merely anecdotal evidence (see p.20). (However, the fact that Dr Childers was interested to know how many people had *not* responded to the diet, and noted the number in his book, as well as noting the percentage of the original 'cooperators' whom he never heard from again, suggests a willingness to test his diet objectively.)

. The Second Test of Any Treatment: .
How Might it Work?

Firstly, the diet would achieve some successes by picking up patients with food intolerance, although the numbers would be small because, among the foods that Dr Childers originally ruled out, only three – milk, eggs and tomatoes – feature in the top twenty offending foods (see p.71). However, many of the cooperators clearly identified other culprit foods by trial and error (see p.387), reinforcing the impression that this diet, like many other popular diets, works by identifying food intolerance, albeit in a rather inefficient manner.

The first suggested mechanism, that toxins in nightshade plants provoke arthritis, is unproven. The second suggested mechanism, involving excess of Vitamins A and D seems unlikely – indeed doctors have identified some rheumatoid arthritis patients with a Vitamin D deficiency.

Our view of Dr Childers' diet

Most patients would probably benefit just as much, or more, from an elimination diet.

However, there is one other intriguing possibility in relation to Dr Childers' diet. Rheumatoid arthritis may have originated in the Americas, and there is no very convincing evidence for it in Europe before 1800. Most of the nightshade crops – tomatoes, potatoes and peppers – also originated in the Americas, and were brought back to Europe by the early explorers, but not widely cultivated for some time. Could there be something in these crops that, when eaten regularly in large amounts, acts very slowly to provoke rheumatoid arthritis in susceptible people? We know the reaction cannot be a fast one because the nightshades, apart from tomatoes, do not often show up as offending foods in elimination diets: the effect would have to be an insidious one, taking months to develop, and months to clear up when nightshades are avoided – this is indeed the timescale that most of Dr Childers' cooperators report. Some of them say that it took six months for the diet to take effect. One could dismiss this as spontaneous remission (see p.19) except that many of them apparently relapsed again, in an unmistakable way, whenever they went back to eating nightshades. Given their understandable desire to eat favourite foods such as potatoes and tomatoes once again, psychogenic reactions seem an unlikely explanation. All this is highly speculative, and we would not suggest that you try a no-nightshades diet on the strength of it, because this is a very difficult diet to maintain (the nightshades are so often present inconspicuously in prepared foods, as tomato extract, paprika or potato flour). However, it would make an interesting subject for further scientific study.

· *Other Popular Diets* ·

There are at least a dozen other diets recommended for arthritis, some of them variations on those we have already described, others entirely different. However, most of these have not been widely adopted, and there is insufficient space in this book to deal with all of them in detail. None of them is based on a correct understanding of what causes the different kinds of arthritis, and they are unlikely to be of any help.

Chapter 4.6

VEGETARIAN AND VEGAN DIETS

Claims are often made for vegetarian and vegan diets in the treatment of 'arthritis'. Such claims have been tested, but only in relation to rheumatoid arthritis, the most common form of inflammatory arthritis. (Other forms of arthritis are discussed at the end of this chapter.)

Before going any further, we should explain what we mean by 'vegetarian' and 'vegan'. In this book, 'vegetarian' means a diet that includes no meat, fish, shellfish, lard or gelatine, but does include milk, milk products and eggs. (This is sometimes called a 'lacto-ovo-vegetarian' diet.) 'Vegan diet' is a widely accepted term for any diet that excludes absolutely all animal products and relies solely on plant foods.

Most of the medical research into vegetarian diets among patients with rheumatoid arthritis has been carried out in Sweden and Norway. Two Swedish trials have looked at vegan diets, and two at vegetarian diets which also excluded eggs (lacto-vegetarian diets). In all cases the diets were preceded by a period of fasting in which only fruit and vegetable juices were consumed. Patients improved during fasting (see Chapter 4.7) but deteriorated again when eating the lacto-vegetarian or vegan diet. After 1–3 months on the vegetarian/vegan regimes, there were no improvements in rheumatoid arthritis symptoms (compared to those at the outset) which could be objectively measured. In one of the studies of vegan diet, about half the patients did feel subjectively better, but it seems likely that this was placebo effect (see p.27) since there were no changes at all in any standard tests such as grip strength or the number of tender joints.

Although no subgroup of 'good responders' (see p.29) showed up in these studies, one would expect a few rheumatoid arthritis patients embarking on a vegan diet to respond with a prompt and marked improvement similar to that which some people experience in the first phase of an elimination diet (see p.25). This should happen simply because a vegan diet excludes seven items out of the twenty most common offenders (see p.71) identified by an elimination diet (milk, butter, cheese, eggs, beef, pork and lamb). If larger groups had been studied in the trials of vegan diets, perhaps some 'good responders' would have been found.

In the longer term, one might also have expected a moderate improvement on a vegan diet due to the lower intake of saturated fat (see pp.52–3) and the absence of arachidonic acid (see p.55). Some small benefit from the higher intake of antioxidants in fruits, vegetables and vegetable oils would also be expected (see p.339). But no such benefits were seen in these studies – why? We can only speculate that these potential benefits are cancelled out by the lack of EPA (see p.51) due to the absence of fish in a vegan or vegetarian diet. The switch to a vegetarian diet might also lower the levels of uric acid in the blood (see pp.245–6) and this could, just possibly, have an unfavourable effect on rheumatoid arthritis (see pp.343–4) which would help to counteract the potential benefits. However, there is no evidence for any of this, and a proper explanation for the lack of effects of vegan and vegetarian diets will have to await further scientific research.

· *Combined Trials* ·

Various other trials have looked at vegetarian or vegan regimes with some additional dietary change. One of these, described on pp.29–30, was a combination of a vegetarian diet and an elimination diet procedure. It produced a subset of good responders, as elimination diets generally do.

A second study looked at the 'living foods diet' which is an extreme vegan diet, where nothing is cooked and large quantities of sprouted beans and fermented products are consumed – the results of this trial are described in Chapter 4.4 (p.378).

The third trial combined a vegetarian diet with supplements of omega-3 fish oil, comparing a group of rheumatoid arthritis patients on this regime, with a control group eating a non-vegetarian diet plus omega-3 fish oil. The control group improved on the omega-3 fish oil, as expected, with less morning stiffness, fewer painful and swollen joints, and increased grip strength, but the group eating the vegetarian diet as well as taking omega-3s did even better, with more substantial improvements in all these symptoms and tests. It seems as if the fish oil had a greater impact against the background of a vegetarian diet than it did normally. Unfortunately, the methods and assessment procedures used in this trial have not been published in full, and without such details it is difficult to assesss its scientific value. Nevertheless it is an interesting study. The author suggests that it may be the lower levels of arachidonic acid in the vegetarian diet that allowed the omega-3 fish oil to produce greater benefits, a conclusion that seems plausible, given other evidence about arachidonic acid (see p.55).

. Nutrition on a Vegetarian or . Vegan Diet

Even if they have little effect on rheumatoid arthritis, vegetarian diets are beneficial in terms of lowering blood pressure and preventing heart disease; they may also reduce the risk of certain different forms of cancer. If you do decide to follow a vegetarian or vegan diet, or have already been following one, ensure that you are getting enough nutrients.

Vegans have no source of Vitamin B_{12} in their diet (claims made for seaweed and yeast are mistaken – see p.288) and must take supplements. The lack of the essential fatty acid DHA may also be a problem, particularly during pregnancy and breastfeeding (see p.355). Vegans may also be short of protein (see pp.348–350), iron (see p.320), calcium (see pp.315–7), zinc (see p.323) manganese (see p.331), and (if not exposed to much sunlight) Vitamin D (see p.297).

Vegetarians are mainly at risk of iron deficiency, and Vitamin D deficiency in some cases.

Vegetarian and vegan children need special nutritional care, and you should seek the advice of a dietician (your doctor can refer you), or that of a reputable organisation such as The Vegan Society or The Vegetarian Society (addresses on p.431).

Chapter 4.7

FASTING

There have been a number of scientific studies of fasting, either total fasts where only water is allowed, or 'juice fasts' in which fruit and vegetable juices are allowed, supplying about 200–500 calories per day.

Such studies consistently report a good response to fasting, which begins to be apparent within about three days. Symptoms improve considerably, and there are also changes for the better in laboratory tests which measure inflammation. Immune cells taken from fasting patients are generally less reactive than before the fast.

Fasting would be an excellent treatment for rheumatoid arthritis, if it were not so very fatal! Unfortunately, the good effects of the fast vanish within a few days of returning to a normal diet (or returning to a vegetarian or vegan diet – see Chapter 4.6).

Some patients with rheumatoid arthritis use fasting as an occasional treatment when they would like to be more fit and able for some important event, such as a family wedding. Unfortunately there is the 'fasting trap' which some patients with rheumatoid arthritis easily fall into: they engage in repeated fasts until they become severely malnourished and underweight, with devastating effects on their general health. Because fasting depresses the activity of the immune system, there is a greater risk of infections with repeated fasting. For this reason we cannot recommend fasting as a treatment.

However, there will probably be readers with rheumatoid arthritis who have already tried fasting for special occasions, who know that they can use it sparingly and with discretion, and not allow it to get out of control. If this applies to you, and as long as you are not underweight, and you have your doctor's agreement, there is probably no harm in continuing with the (very) occasional fast. But you must be cautious. A fast should not be undertaken more than once a year, and *never for more than seven days*. The fast can begin about four days before the event, and end on the 'big day' – the benefits will persist for at least another 24 hours. A juice fast is less arduous than a total fast, and provides some calories. Whether you take juice or water, be sure to consume plenty of liquids.

How exactly does fasting work? For some patients, the fast is having the same beneficial effect as the exclusion phase of an elimination diet (see p.25): these are the subgroup of patients whose rheumatoid arthritis is related to specific food sensitivities (see Chapter 1.1). Clearly, they will show striking improvement when their culprit foods are cut out of the diet. (Even a juice fast will be likely to cut out most of the common offending foods, and a mineral water fast will obviously exclude them all.) If you have experienced good effects from short-term fasts then you may want to try an elimination diet (see Chapter 2.4) to see if you can identify culprit foods.

From a theoretical point of view, for those of us trying to understand the interactions between diet and rheumatoid arthritis, it is interesting that whereas the elimination diet produces these marked benefits for a sub-group of 'good responders', fasting produces a temporary improvement for almost everyone with rheumatoid arthritis. Why?

First and foremost, fasting has a suppressive effect on several different parts of the immune system. One way in which lack of food may suppress immune responses is by inhibiting the production of prostaglandins, which are localised messengers for many bodily systems including the immune system (see pp.48–9). Prostaglandins are made from fatty substances that we obtain from our food. An interesting experiment required patients to fast completely and then consume either vegetable oil or a non-oily diet supplying the same number of calories. Prostaglandin production rose again, but *only* in the group fed vegetable oil. This could explain why a juice fast is as good as a total fast: it contains virtually no fat or oil, and it may therefore suppress prostaglandin production. If this is correct, then a totally fat-free diet should produce benefits comparable with fasting, as one medical researcher claims to have shown (see p.57). Unfortunately, a totally fat-free diet is very damaging, in the long run, because it lacks essential fatty acids (see p.353).

Although prostaglandin production might be an important mechanism behind the good effects of fasting, it is probably just one effect among many. Fasting is known to alter a great many other processes in the body, and to affect the hormonal and nervous systems in fundamental ways which could influence pain perception, for example.

Finally, if the gut flora (see pp.39–40) does play a part in causing rheumatoid arthritis, then fasting could produce benefits in two additional ways. On the one hand, it would reduce the activity of the gut flora by depriving the bacteria of food – this will reduce the output of bacterial products, including bacterial antigens (see p.413) which may influence the disease process in rheumatoid arthritis. On the other hand, fasting is known to make the gut wall less permeable, so that fewer bacterial products would pass through into the bloodstream.

Fasting is not recommended for those with osteoarthritis. In the absence of food, protein has to be withdrawn from the muscles for use elsewhere in the body, and this has many different consequences. One may be a reduction in the rate at which collagen is made, and since collagen is the main ingredient in the articular cartilage (see p.413) which lines the joints, this effect might be damaging, especially for those with osteoarthritis, whose cartilage is breaking down more quickly than it can be repaired.

Anyone with gout should never undertake a fast. The blood becomes very slightly more acidic when fasting and this can provoke an acute attack of gout (see p.244).

Chapter 4.8

CIDER VINEGAR, MOLASSES, SHARK CARTILAGE AND OTHER 'FOOD SUPPLEMENTS'

Alongside the vitamins and minerals, most health food shops have a bewildering array of other 'food supplements', such as Devil's claw, extract of New Zealand green-lipped mussel, shark cartilage and yucca.

What is the truth about these products? Can any of them help you? Or are they a waste of money? And are there any potential dangers in taking them?

These products are not, in most cases, common items of the diet, but they are included in this book for two reasons. Firstly, many are derived from plant or animal sources. Secondly, the products are described as 'dietary supplements', the implication of the word 'supplement' being that something essential is lacking in the diet which needs to be provided in tablet or capsule form.

The fact is that these products are, for the most part, not supplying any nutrients that you could not get more easily and cheaply elsewhere. What they actually offer are unproven drug treatments under the guise of 'supplements', because a loophole in the law allows 'supplements' to be sold without the same stringent testing required for drugs. You will notice that no claims at all are made on the jar or packet – such claims are forbidden under the regulations. These products rely on magazine or newspaper articles to announce the discovery of an exciting new 'treatment' for arthritis. If you follow such news stories about arthritis over the years, you will discover that these 'miracle cures' crop up regularly. All those products on the health food shop shelf have had their moment of glory, when they were heralded with a fanfare of publicity, as the wonder cure for arthritis.

Unfortunately, most of them have never been tested in any way – the evidence for them is purely anecdotal (see p.20) – individual patients believing that the product has helped them. There are various ways in which such beliefs can be generated, even by a product with no intrinsic value, including placebo effect (see p.27) and spontaneous remission (see p.19) coinciding with taking the supplement.

In this chapter we will describe the few scientific trials which have been carried out on these 'food supplement' products.

The other type of product that may be on offer in health food shops, and in some chemists, is the herbal remedy: again, these can be sold without the careful testing required of drugs.

Devil's Claw

This is the root of a plant whose scientific name is *Harpagophytum procumbens*. Claims have been made that extracts of the root have an anti-inflammatory action and can improve symptoms in rheumatoid arthritis. Three teams of medical researchers have studied Devil's claw, using standard screening methods applied to any anti-arthritic drug. There seems to be no benefit whatever from Devil's claw.

New-Zealand green-lipped mussel

There have been several scientific trials of this substance, which is extracted from a shellfish found in the waters around New Zealand. One study was a double-blind placebo-controlled trial (see p.27) involving 66 patients in all, some with rheumatoid arthritis, others with osteoarthritis. The researchers claimed significant benefits for 68% of those with rheumatoid arthritis and 39% of those with osteoarthritis, but the way in which they analysed their results has been heavily criticised by other researchers, who question the validity of their findings. The side-effects reported in this trial, such as nausea, were few and mild, except in one patient who suffered from water retention: this resolved when the mussel extract was stopped for a week, then reintroduced at a lower dose.

Some patients reported a worsening of their symptoms 2–4 weeks after starting the treatment. This deterioration usually lasted for only 1–2 weeks, and the patients then seemed to improve. There did not seem to be any serious ill-effects when the extract was taken for six months.

All the patients involved in this trial were elderly, and had been suffering from arthritis for over ten years, so if there were genuine improvements this would be an impressive response.

However, other research teams have not found the same benefits when treating rheumatoid arthritis patients with the mussel extract. Despite this, three different research trials have produced evidence that New Zealand green-lipped mussel does contain substances that are potentially anti-inflammatory. At present, 'the jury is still out' on this particular product. If you do decide to try it, remember that extract of New Zealand green-lipped mussel is almost certainly having a drug-like action, rather than being a 'food supplement'. For this reason, and because one patient in the study described above had a side effect that would require medical supervision, you must seek your doctor's advice about taking this product.

Shark cartilage, Arthro-vite and other cartilage preparations

These may be of some limited value to certain patients with rheumatoid arthritis. It is known that about 25–40% of rheumatoid arthritis sufferers begin producing antibodies to collagen, the basic constituent of cartilage (see p.130). This probably adds to the inflammation in their joints.

Feeding patients cartilage preparations might reduce the production of these anti-collagen antibodies. If it works – and this is far from certain – it would do so by means of something called 'oral tolerance' (see p.37). This is the basic mechanism that stops us from mounting an immune attack against food: the immune system is programmed to 'turn itself off' as regards food molecules. 'Oral tolerance' usually works well, although it clearly breaks down in cases of true food allergy (see p.36).

Collagen preparations are used to treat arthritis in dogs, and several trials in patients with rheumatoid arthritis have suggested that there might be some benefits, but these are very small. Currently, there is no agreement among researchers about the optimum dose of collagen.

Antibodies against collagen are probably not a feature of osteoarthritis, so the collagen preparations are unlikely, in theory, to be useful in this disease.

Glucosamine sulphate

Unlike most of the products in this chapter, this substance has been extensively tested, mainly by researchers in Italy, Portugal and Germany. It is believed to relieve pain and stiffness in osteoarthritis, and the research studies do seem to suggest a significant benefit. In most studies it has proved at least as good as NSAIDs (see p.418) – a family of drugs often prescribed for osteoarthritis – but with fewer side-effects. Glucosamine sulphate may also have some protective effect on the cartilage, similar to that of chondroprotective drugs (see p.117).

Glucosamine sulphate (also called glycosamine sulphate) is in no sense a 'food'. It acts as a drug, and should be treated as a drug – so if you are interested in taking it please consult your doctor first.

Lactobacillus acidophilus capsules, live yoghurt and Yakult

Given the possibility that the gut flora might somehow be involved in rheumatoid arthritis (see pp.39–40), it is reasonable to ask if treatments that claim to produce beneficial changes in the gut flora might be helpful to patients with this disease. This is all highly speculative, because the role of the gut flora has not been convincingly demonstrated. Even if it were to prove important in rheumatoid arthritis, these treatments would not necessarily be of any value. It is extremely difficult to get live bacteria (such as those in *Lactobacillus acidophilus* capsules, or in live yoghurt) through the stomach and into the intestine, without the bacteria being killed by the stomach acid.

Most of the products sold do not actually introduce significant numbers of live bacteria into the intestine, despite their claims. One new product that may be able to achieve a useful change in the gut flora is a yoghurt-type drink called Yakult. The scientific evidence in its favour is not very strong, but it may work, and it is unlikely to be harmful, so this might be worth trying.

Note that no treatment of this kind can achieve a *permanent* change in the gut flora without continued use of the treatment: if you stop taking the product, your gut flora will quickly revert to its previous composition.

Cider vinegar

This owes its popularity to the late Dr D C Jarvis of Vermont, author of *Arthritis and Folk Medicine*. His book lovingly describes Vermont as an earthly paradise where all ills are dispelled by cider vinegar: as well as curing *all* forms of arthritis, cider vinegar will apparently calm angry bulls, prevent influenza, cure haemorrhoids and make children more placid and manageable. Dr Jarvis recommended adding honey to the cider vinegar, although he clearly felt the vinegar was the most important element, and would work well alone. He believed that the body was lacking in acids and that the vinegar corrected this deficit.

A survey of over a thousand arthritis sufferers in the U.S.A. asked about the remedies they had tried. The survey found that only sixteen people had tried apple-cider vinegar, either with or without honey. Out of the sixteen, only one person felt that it had helped – incidentally, she had taken it with honey. This level of response is much *less* than a placebo response (see pp.26–7).

One group of medical researchers has tested cider vinegar to see if it might produce any improvement in inflammatory arthritis, but there was none. A dentist has reported serious damage to tooth enamel from habitually drinking cider vinegar mixed with honey, as many arthritis sufferers do: in some cases, the acid vinegar had so damaged their teeth that they all had to be removed and replaced with dentures.

Honey

This is frequently recommended to arthritis sufferers, either taken alone or in combination with cider vinegar. No scientific studies have been undertaken, but a survey carried out in the U.S.A. found that, of those who had tried honey, about one third felt it had been beneficial. This is not an impressive response, and could probably be accounted for by placebo effect (see pp.26–7).

On the other hand, honey is a good source of boron, a mineral that might be valuable in the prevention of osteoporosis (see p.333) and might also help with osteoarthritis (see p.333). Honey is unlikely to do any harm if you reduce other sugary foods to compensate for the extra calories.

Alfalfa tablets

These are sometimes suggested for those with arthritis, and for more general health promotion. It seems likely that they can be very damaging to people with systemic lupus erythematosus (see pp.138–9). We would not recommend anyone to take alfalfa.

Propolis

This is a resinous substance produced by bees which apparently protects their young from certain infections. Some claims have been made that it might encourage regeneration of cartilage. There is no evidence that this is the case. Some studies suggest that it may have anti-inflammatory activity, but this has never been tested scientifically.

Ginger

This is used in traditional Indian medicine as a treatment for arthritis. It is claimed to have some anti-inflammatory effects, but these have not been demonstrated in a scientific trial. There is no good evidence that ginger actually works.

Yucca

One study has been made of yucca, a desert plant from the southwestern U.S.A. This was a placebo-controlled study, but it would probably not withstand close scientific scrutiny. It is impossible to say if yucca has any benefits for arthritic patients.

Blackstrap molasses and kelp

No scientific trials, nor any other studies, have been done with these substances.

· Hazards of Food Supplements ·

Several 'food supplements' marketed as being generally good for health (rather than being cures for arthritis) deserve a special mention here because they are potentially hazardous.

Two supplements, germanium and tryptophan have caused several deaths in Japan and the U.S.A., and have now been withdrawn from sale in most countries.

Alfalfa should not be taken (see p.400). Omega-3 fish oils should be avoided by some patients (see p.152) and evening primrose oil is inadvisable for anyone with epilepsy.

· Herbal Remedies for Arthritis ·

No information is available on the effectiveness of most of these products, which generally contain a mixture of herbs.

BG–104

BG–104 is a mixture of Chinese herbs which has been tested in Japan for its ability to reduce the action of free radicals (see p.340) in inflammatory disorders. It apparently produced good effects for patients with Sjörgren's syndrome and patients with Behçet's syndrome. However, comparable results were obtained by taking Vitamin E.

To the best of our knowledge, BG-104 is not yet on general sale, but we have included mention of it here because it is the type of 'herbal remedy' that may be found on the shelves of health food shops in the near future. Although it might be of some help in Behçet's or Sjörgren's syndrome, or in other forms of inflammatory arthritis, simply taking a supplement of Vitamin E might be just as effective.

Hazards of herbal remedies

Note that some herbal remedies for arthritis include comfrey leaves, which contain toxins that can cause a potentially fatal liver disease. Other herbal remedies for arthritis contain large amounts of celery seed: this can provoke an allergic reaction to sunlight.

See p.400 for the hazards of alfalfa tablets.

Chapter 4.9

SCIENCE FACT AND SCIENCE FICTION – ACIDS AND OTHER ARTHRITIS MYTHS

· *Acids – Fact and Fiction* ·

Mention diet and arthritis to people and very often the reply comes back: 'Ah yes, it's all to do with acids isn't it?'.

Looking at the popular books on the market, it is easy to see how this idea has taken root so firmly, because the notion of acidic foods being linked to arthritis is proposed again and again, though in strikingly different forms. Sister Margaret Hills (see p.372) blames all forms of arthritis on an accumulation of 'acid deposits' in the joints which are in turn due to acids in the diet, whereas Dr D C Jarvis (see p.399) attributes all arthritis to insufficient acid in the diet. (Despite this fundamental difference of opinion, they both recommend apple-cider vinegar – an acid – as a remedy!)

These and other popular books on arthritis include a great deal of information about 'acids', most of it highly inaccurate. We will try to correct some of those errors, as well as explaining how some foods really do affect the acidity of the urine, and the importance of this, not to arthritis but to osteoporosis, a common disease of the elderly, especially women, in which the bones become weaker and easily broken.

Acids and their opposites

Everyone is familiar with acids – they are found in lemon juice, other fruits and fruit juices, wine and vinegar. Our taste buds tell us that such foods are acidic. We also produce acid in our stomachs in order to digest food: in this case hydrochloric acid, a much stronger acid than any found in food.

Slightly less familiar is the word '**alkali**' (also called a 'base'). An alkali is, in chemical terms, the very opposite of an acid. When an alkali is added to an acid, they 'neutralise' each other. That is, they react chemically and the alkali cancels out some or all of the acidity. Most people have experienced this chemical reaction when taking sodium bicarbonate (also called bicarbonate-of-soda or baking soda) to alleviate acid indigestion. The sodium bicarbonate is a mild alkali which reduces the acidity of the stomach contents. You can feel the chemical reaction between the acid and alkali actually taking place in the stomach – the reaction produces gas, which is why a large and sudden burp follows.

There are a great many different kinds of acid, some strong acids, others weak acids. In the course of this book you will find mention of amino acids, fatty acids and several others. All these are very weak acids, but they are also quite large and complex molecules with many other chemical properties besides acidity. (Words such as molecule and atom are explained in the glossary on pages 412–421.) Whatever effect fatty acids or amino acids may have on arthritis – good, bad or neutral – is nothing to do with the fact that they are acids, but is related to other far more complex chemical characteristics. The same is also true of uric acid which is the immediate cause of gouty arthritis: it causes problems because of its tendency to form crystals of urate in the joints (see p.104), not because it is an acid.

This point needs to be emphasised because so many popular books lump all acids together, as if they were a single type of substance – in fact they are enormously diverse.

One other fundamental point needs to be made before we can look at what happens to the acids in foods. A system of measurement known as pH is used to denote acidity or alkalinity. Acid liquids have a pH below 7.0, and the more acidic they are the lower the pH. Alkaline liquids have a pH above 7.0, and the more alkaline they are the higher the pH. Neutral liquids have a pH of exactly 7.

The fate of acids in food

What happens to the acids in foods such as oranges or tomatoes after they are eaten? Do they pass straight into the bloodstream and then into the joints, making both acidic, as some authors suggest? They most certainly do not.

Firstly, the citric acid in an orange is far weaker than the naturally occurring hydrochloric acid in the stomach – so eating an orange makes only a slight difference to the acidity of the stomach. As for the bloodstream, if any citric acid is absorbed from the food its acidity is cancelled out almost immediately, because the blood has its own powerful defences against any change in its pH.

The blood and other body fluids have to be kept at a steady pH of 7.4 come what may. To keep the pH stable, these fluids contain a mixture of substances which automatically adjust to any influx of acid or alkali and bring the pH back to 7.4. The substances that achieve this extraordinary chemical stability are known as **buffers**, and the blood is described as being 'buffered'.

This sophisticated system of pH control is not there to deal with our appetite for oranges. Its main function is to cope with the large volume of acid created by breathing. When we breathe we take in oxygen and combine this with carbon (ultimately obtained from food) to form carbon dioxide. Both the oxygen and the carbon dioxide are carried around the body in the bloodstream. Oxygen enters the body via the lungs and is taken up by the blood. In its circular journey around the body, this oxygen meets up with waste carbon and thus forms carbon dioxide. The blood carries this carbon dioxide back to the lungs where it escapes from the bloodstream into the lung cavity and then out into the atmosphere.

The problem, from a pH point of view, is that carbon dioxide forms an acid (carbonic acid) in the blood. Were it not for the buffers, the pH of the blood would fall drastically as the oxygen turned to carbon dioxide, then rise again as the carbon dioxide was offloaded into the lung space. The pH of the blood would yo-yo up and down with every breath. Fortunately for us, the buffers in the blood successfully cope with this constant and substantial acid challenge, and the pH scarcely changes.

Clearly, if the buffers in the blood can achieve this, they are unlikely to be defeated by the relatively trivial amount of weak citric acid in an orange, or even a large glass of juice.

While it does not affect the blood, orange juice can affect the pH of the urine – but the irony is that it will make it slightly *more alkaline*, not more acidic. To understand this we need to look more closely at what is in the juice, and how it is digested by the body.

Breakdown products
Once in the bloodstream, a substance such as citric acid will be broken down into smaller parts, as will other food molecules. In the process their chemical properties will be fundamentally changed. What matters at this stage is the number and type of atoms which the molecules contain — these may have an acidic or alkaline potential which was not achieved when the atoms were bound up in a much larger molecule.

For example, the proteins in an egg are neutral (neither acid nor alkaline), but these proteins are rich in sulphur. When the egg protein is digested and the sulphur released, it creates a small amount of sulphuric acid (or, to be more precise, sulphate ions) in the blood. Thus the egg protein, although it is neutral itself, generates acids in the blood. Other high-protein foods, particularly hard cheeses, also generate acid when broken down. So too do many cereal grains. These acids do not actually change the pH of the blood, of course, because the buffers prevent any such change.

But while the buffers can cancel out the immediate effect of such acid, they cannot destroy it entirely. No further breakdown of the sulphuric acid by the body is possible – it is as small as it can be. So the acid has to be disposed of somehow, and this is done by flushing it out of the body in the urine. As a result, the pH of the urine falls – it becomes more acidic. (Disposal of this acid in the urine has important consequences for anyone prone to osteoporosis, which we will come back to later. First we need to look at what happens to the citric acid.)

Because citric acid contains no sulphur, nor any phosphorous or chlorine – the other elements with acidic potential – its breakdown products will not have any acidifying effect on the urine. (The main product is carbon dioxide, which is breathed out through the lung; see p.405.) Other components of orange juice do contain a little sulphur, phosphorous and chlorine, but they also contain potassium, and in far larger amounts. When released from the molecules that contain it, potassium has an alkaline effect – it would raise the pH of the blood, were it not for the action of the buffers, and it does raise the pH of the urine.

Thanks to the high potassium content, the combined effect of all the breakdown products of oranges and orange juice is an alkaline one. When you drink orange juice, your urine becomes more alkaline. The same is true of most other fruits and vegetables, although the extent to which they will raise the pH of the urine varies.

A few fruits prove to be exceptions to the rule: they contain unusual acids which are only partially broken down by the body. The only commonly eaten fruits to contain such acids are cranberries and plums. (Since prunes are dried plums they possess the same acids.)

The acids concerned are benzoic acid and quinic acid, which the body breaks down into hippuric acid, a very weak acid that circulates in the blood and is passed out unchanged in the urine. While in the bloodstream, its acidifying effects are cancelled out by the buffers, but hippuric acid does make the urine more acid. (This fact has been utilised medically, by giving cranberry juice to patients with urinary tract infections, where increased acidity of the urine is often helpful.)

Acidifying the blood

There are some unusul circumstances in which the buffering capacity of the blood is overwhelmed and the blood does become slightly more acidic. Kidney disease, in its more advanced stages, can lead to an acidification of the blood, known as acidosis. This occurs because the kidneys are losing their ability to move acid out of the blood, or their ability to retain buffers. Severe lung diseases can also lower the pH of the blood because carbon dioxide (see p.405) is not extracted efficiently. Liver disease and diabetes can also lead to acidosis. These are all serious medical conditions, and you would be severely ill if affected in this way.

Dieting, if it involves sudden and drastic weight loss, can also make the blood very slightly more acid. Lack of food compels the body to break down its fat reserves very quickly and this produces a change in the body chemistry known as ketosis. During ketosis the pH of the blood falls a little. Such a change in pH can affect people with gout (see p.244), but has no other impact on arthritis.

Losing calcium

The more acid our urine, the more calcium it contains. The reasons for this are complex, and beyond the scope of this book to explain, but the facts of calcium loss are vitally important to those at risk of osteoporosis, in which there is thinning of the bones (see p.120). Many people in the industrialised countries lose more calcium in their urine than they absorb from their food – and the difference is made up by calcium extracted from the skeleton.

The amount of calcium removed from the skeleton in a single day will be miniscule, but when this is added up over weeks, months and years, it can amount to a steady erosion of the bones. The high protein and cereal intake and meagre vegetable consumption of many people in Western societies tends to make the urine more acid, and may well be contributing to the continuing problem of osteoporosis among older people. Practical advice about avoiding osteoporosis can be found in Chapter 2.3 (p.161).

Do acids cause arthritis?

The short answer is 'no'. Acids derived from the breakdown products of cheese, eggs, meat, fish and cereal grains, probably do contribute to osteoporosis, but osteoporosis is a disease of the bones, not the joints –

it is not a form of arthritis. Furthermore, these are not the 'acid foods' so often prohibited by popular diets.

Gout is directly associated with high uric acid levels in the blood, which leads to urate crystals forming in the joint space (see p.104). However, the problems created by uric acid are unrelated to its acidity, which is in any case quite weak. The uric acid is derived from foods such as liver, kidneys and anchovies, not from the acidic fruits that are banned by Sister Hills, Dr Dong and other such authors. Gout is a distinctive type of arthritis, unrelated to conditions such as rheumatoid arthritis or osteoarthritis where urate crystals play no part (see p.69).

No other form of arthritis is caused by any type of acid, certainly not by the weak acids found in fruit and vegetables. If they were, one would expect arthritics to deteriorate if eating a diet very rich in fruit. Such diets were tried out in the 1930s, when vitamin therapy was all the rage (see p.282). While these high-fruit diets did not help arthritics, they did not harm them either.

If you have tried cutting out acid foods and felt much better, this improvement is probably indicative of food intolerance (see p.43) to a specific item, such as citrus fruits (common offenders in food intolerance). Avoiding all fruit and acid vegetables is almost certainly unnecessary, and is probably depriving you of important minerals and vitamins. You could undoubtedly broaden your diet without making your symptoms worse, by testing individual foods and discovering which ones cause problems. More detailed suggestions for such testing are given on pages 182–190.

· *Modern food* ·

Among those advocating special diets for arthritis, many attribute all arthritic diseases to malnutrition, as a result of modern processed food, or poisoning by synthetic food additives – or both combined. This is a popular explanation among authors such as Dr Campbell (see p.383), Dr Dong and Sister Hills. If it were correct, we could make certain predictions about the occurrence of arthritis:

1. There would be no signs of arthritis in skeletons excavated by archaeologists from prehistoric and ancient sites. There would be no records of arthritis before the mid-19th century.

2. The would be no arthritis among peasant populations growing all their own food – still a common way of life in many parts of the world.

3. Arthritis would be most common among people relying solely on processed food.

This is what we actually find:

1. The signs of osteoarthritis are commonly seen in prehistoric skeletons, and in other human remains, throughout history, and in every part of the world.

   The signs of rheumatoid arthritis are also seen in prehistoric skeletons of American Indians, and many tribes were so badly affected that they manufactured crutches from the long branches of trees: these have been found by archaeologists in parts of New Mexico. None of these people were eating processed food.

   However, there is no convincing evidence of rheumatoid arthritis in Europe or Asia before 1800. This is a puzzle to researchers, and some believe that the disease may have come from the Americas, but there is certainly no case here for modern processed foods being responsible. Few processed foods, in the modern sense of the word, were being eaten in 1800, or 1900 for that matter. (Bread, cheese, beer and wine are all 'processed foods' in a sense, but then these had been consumed for many centuries before 1800.)

   Clearly, both osteoarthritis and rheumatoid arthritis precede the introduction of highly processed, mass-manufactured, packeted food.

2. The rates of osteoarthritis are much the same the world over, although hard physical labour tends to produce more cases (see p.114). Rheumatoid arthritis does not vary a great deal either: the rates are about 1% in most parts of the world. The rates may be slightly lower in some areas, such as China, where typical rates are about 0.3%. But the same rates are seen among rural Chinese and the urbanised Chinese living in Hong Kong – whose diet would be substantially more modern and processed.

   By contrast, the rates of hip fracture, a symptom of osteoporosis (thinning of the bones) vary enormously between industrialised countries and developing countries, where the problem is very rare. This suggests that a modern Westernised diet really *is* at fault in this disease. The distribution pattern worldwide for osteoporosis illustrates what we would expect to see for arthritic diseases if they really were a result of 'modern processed foods'.

   It does seem plausible that a diet low in fruits, vegetables and vegetable oils (and therefore low in antioxidants) may lead to a more severe form of rheumatoid arthritis, and may even promote the development of rheumatoid arthritis in susceptible individuals. But such a diet is not the major cause, by any means (see pp.345–6), and certainly not the sole cause as some popular diet books suggest.

3. There are some people who live *entirely* on canned and packeted foods – do they suffer arthritis any more than the rest of the population? The answer is 'no'. Middle-aged and elderly men living alone sometimes fall into such eating habits. They usually come to medical attention when they develop 'bachelor's scurvy' through a lack of Vitamin C. Scurvy causes a variety of symptoms, notably easy bruising, bleeding and swollen gums, and a dry scaly skin. Sometimes those with scurvy also have joint pain, but this is caused by the rupture of tiny blood vessels, with consequent bleeding into the joint space. This has nothing in common with osteoarthritis, rheumatoid arthritis or other common forms of arthritis. Once the scurvy is treated with Vitamin C supplements, the joints of these patients recover – and they are no more likley to get rheumatoid arthritis or osteoarthritis than anyone else.

· *Calcification* ·

The idea that arthritis is caused by deposits of calcium in the joints, or in soft tissues where calcium does not belong, crops up frequently in explanations for popular diets.

The facts are as follows:
Abnormal calcification does occur in certain arthritic conditions. One is ankylosing spondylitis where it affects the intervertebral discs and the ligaments around the spine (see p.86), and another is pseudogout (see p.123) where calcium pyrophosphate crystals form in the cartilage. In neither case is diet considered to be responsible for producing this abnormal calcification.

In the most common form of arthritis, osteoarthritis, abnormal calcification is not a significant part of the disease process. Although there are osteophytes (small bony outgrowths around the edge of the damaged joint), these are a secondary effect, and not responsible for the main symptoms of osteoarthritis (see p.115). Again, diet is not known to play any role in producing osteophytes.

In rheumatoid arthritis, the second most common form of arthritis, there is no abnormal calcification.

In certain other rheumatic diseases there is sometimes abnormal calcification of soft tissues, as in sarcoidosis (see pp.300–301) where there may be calcification of the kidney. Long-term treatment with high doses of Vitamin D, as for refractory rickets, osteomalacia or some cases of systemic lupus erythematosus, can also lead to calcification of the kidney. High-dose Vitamin D treatment must be closely monitored to avoid this. Cod-liver oil and supplements of Vitamin D should always be used with caution (see p.300) but most ordinary diets do not involve any risk of abnormal calcification.

GLOSSARY

Abdomen The central part of the body, below the chest.

Allergen Any antigen (see p.413) that stimulates an allergic reaction.

Allergic reaction A reaction by the immune system against an inoffensive substance such as pollen or food. See p.82.

Ankylosing Producing stiffness.

Antibody Antibodies are molecules made by the immune system and their usual role is to bind to disease-causing microbes in the fight against infection. The structure of an antibody is shown in Figure 2. Antibodies are always highly specific, and most bind to only one type of target molecule (called an antigen). However, antibodies sometimes bind to molecules that are chemically similar to their antigen, a phenomenon known as cross-reactivity. Antibodies belong to different classes and subclasses; IgE and IgG are two of the classes. These different classes and subclasses provoke different reactions by the immune system. For example, IgE antibodies to egg proteins will provoke an allergic reaction to egg, and so will one

Figure 2

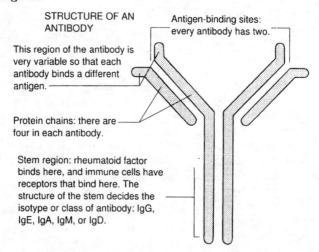

STRUCTURE OF AN ANTIBODY

Antigen-binding sites: every antibody has two.

This region of the antibody is very variable so that each antibody binds a different antigen.

Protein chains: there are four in each antibody.

Stem region: rheumatoid factor binds here, and immune cells have receptors that bind here. The structure of the stem decides the isotype or class of antibody: IgG, IgE, IgA, IgM, or IgD.

of the subclasses of IgG, called IgG4, whereas antibodies to egg belonging to other subclasses of IgG will bind egg proteins but will not provoke an allergic reaction to egg.

Antigen A distinctive chemical marker that sparks off an immune response. It is a molecule, usually a protein molecule, part of which has a distinctive shape and chemical profile. These characteristics are 'recognised' by antibodies, or by receptors on immune cells that function in a similar way to antibodies. The antibody or receptor binds chemically to the distinctive area.

Anti-DNA antibody An auto-antibody which binds to the genetic material, DNA (see p.415). One form of anti-DNA antibody, which binds only to double-stranded DNA (DNA that is coiled in the double-helix arrangement) is particularly characteristic of systemic lupus erythematosus. If found in significant quantity, it helps to confirm the diagnosis of this disease.

Antinuclear antibody Antinuclear antibodies are autoantibodies (see below) which bind to various constituents of the cell nucleus (see p.419). These antibodies are useful in the diagnosis of systemic lupus erythematosus, systemic sclerosis and mixed connective tissue disease. However, they are also seen in 20–40% of patients with rheumatoid arthritis, and many apparently healthy people: about 8% of the normal population are high enough to score a positive test.

Arthritis An inflammatory joint condition. See p.90.

Arthropathy A disease of the joints. See p.91.

Articular cartilage A layer of material that covers the ends of the bones. See synovial joint (p.421).

Aspiration A medical procedure that involves removing fluid from a joint where excess synovial fluid (see p.420) has accumulated and is contributing to pain and stiffness.

Atom See **Molecules and atoms** (p.418).

Autoantibody An antibody which, rather than binding to a microbe or other invader, binds to 'self' – that is, to some part of the body. Autoantibodies include rheumatoid factor (see p.419) and antinuclear antibodies (see above). If a disease is primarily caused by the action of autoantibodies, then it is known as an auto-immune disease.

Auto-immune disease A disease in which the immune system turns against the body itself and attacks some part of it.

B cell A type of immune cell (see p.416). It produces antibodies in response to particular antigens.

Biopsy The removal of a tiny amount of body tissue (eg. the synovial membrane or the lining of the gut) for inspection under a microscope or other investigations. A biopsy can help in diagnosis, or be used to check how the disease is progressing.

C-reactive protein (CRP) A protein found in the blood whose level rises with increasing inflammation.

Capsule Around most joints there is a complex ball of ligaments, attached to the bones at points above and below the joint. Known as the joint capsule, these ligaments form a tough but elastic 'bandage' that holds everything together.

In a healthy joint these ligaments provide both stability and control over movements of the joint. But it is a precise piece of engineering, geared to the exact size of the healthy joint. If the joint space narrows, due to arthritic changes, then there may be capsular laxity – see p.115.

Cartilage A rubbery material, made of the protein **collagen**. As articular cartilage it covers the ends of bones within the joint; see Synovial joint (p.421).

Cell Our bodies are made up of small individual units, called cells, each surrounded by a barrier known as a cell membrane. Most cells have a nucleus which contains the hereditary material, DNA. Some cells in the body are tightly packed together with others of their kind, such as muscle cells and skin cells. Others occur singly in the blood, and some of these are free to leave the blood stream and roam about the body, such as the macrophages and neutrophils, important types of immune cell. Some cells, such as the chondrocytes of cartilage, occur singly but do not move about much, being embedded in a matrix of collagen. All cells die and are replaced regularly, some having a life-time of only a few days.

Circulating immune complexes See **Immune complexes** (p.416).

Collagen The rubbery material of which cartilage is made.

Corticosteroids Drugs that are prescribed to quell inflammation; they have nothing whatever to do with the 'anabolic steroids' taken by some sportsmen and women to build up their muscles. Corticosteroid drugs mimic the effects of hormones produced by the adrenal glands. The main hormone produced is hydrocortisone (cortisol), which has various effects on the body besides suppressing inflammation, such as moving protein out of the muscles and bones, and influencing the way fat is deposited. Corticosteroid drugs are designed to have fewer of these other effects, while retaining the ability to suppress inflammation.

Cytokines Chemical messenger molecules, released by the immune system (see p.416). Cytokines play various roles in the immune response. They stimulate or suppress, as required, the action of the many different types of immune cells. Three particular cytokines are over-abundant in the joints of someone with rheumatoid arthritis: TNF (Tumour Necrosis Factor), and IL-1 and IL-6 (Interleukin 1 and Interleukin 6).

DNA The chemical substance which carries the hereditary information. It is found in the chromosomes which are in the nucleus of cells (see p.414).

Enzymes These chemicals are the 'skilled workers' of the body: they make particular chemical reactions happen in the body. One enzyme controls one chemical reaction – this is the general rule. There are tens of thousands of different enzymes in the body, acting in concert with one another. Because enzymes regulate chemical reactions they regulate the entire metabolism of the body.

All enzymes are proteins. Some require the presence of a **coenzyme** molecule to fulfil their role. This coenzyme often contains a mineral, such as copper or selenium, and without sufficient intake of the mineral concerned, the enzyme may not work efficiently.

ESR Erythrocyte Sedimentation Rate is the most frequently used of all the blood tests. The blood is prevented from clotting and allowed to stand. The rate at which the red blood cells (the erythrocytes) settle out from the liquid part of the blood is observed.

When there is inflammation (see p.64) in the body, this affects the blood in various ways and one consequence is that the red cells tend to cling together and, therefore, settle out more quickly than usual. The more active the inflammation, the faster the red cells settle and the higher the ESR.

Fatty acid A molecule consisting of a long chain of carbon atoms (the 'fatty' section) attached to an acidic section. They are very weak acids. Fatty acids, combined into larger molecules, are important components of cell membranes (see p.414). See also p.353.

Food allergy A reaction to food in which the immune system is demonstrably involved. The main type of food allergy is a true allergy, involving the allergy antibody, IgE.

Food intolerance Any unpleasant and unusual reaction to food (other than psychogenic reactions) in which a direct reaction by the immune system against the food does not appear to be the major cause of symptoms. See pp.43–5 and p.83.

Food sensitivity Any adverse and idiosyncratic reaction to food other than a psychogenic reaction. The term embraces food allergy and food intolerance but it does not include psychological reactions to food.

Grip strength A test that is frequently used to assess the hand. It shows how badly the finger and knuckle joints are affected by arthritis.

Gut flora The bacteria and yeasts that live naturally in the gut. (See p.37.)

Hyperostosis Overgrowth of bone.

IgG A type of antibody (see p.412). It is one of the most abundant antibodies in the body.

IgE A type of antibody (see p.412) that is responsible for producing true allergic reactions (see p.82). This type of antibody binds to immune cells called mast cells and, if then bound by its allergen, it stimulates the mast cells to release chemical mediators (molecules that have powerful effects on the body) such as histamine.

Immune cell Any cell that forms part of the immune system, the defensive force which protects the body against infections and tumours. Many of these cells move freely around the body in the blood and the lymphatic fluid (see p.417). Concentrations of stationary immune cells are found in the lymph nodes. Immune cells are very diverse; they include T cells and B cells (also called lymphocytes), neutrophils, macrophages and antigen-presenting cells.

Immune complexes A dense, tangled cluster of molecules, made up of numerous antibodies bound to numbers of their antigens (see Figure 3). When they occur in the blood they are known as circulating immune complexes or CICs. These are found in some patients with rheumatoid arthritis, systemic lupus erythematosus, and other forms of inflammatory arthritis.

Immune complexes tend to provoke inflammation wherever they are deposited. Because the blood vessels in the tissues around a joint are very small, and immune complexes can be fairly large, it often happens that immune complexes deposit in the joints. They can cause, or add to, inflammation in the joints.

Immune system The body's defensive system, which protects against infectious diseases, by killing or incapacitating disease-causing bacteria, viruses and other microbes. It also guards against the development of tumours. Poorly controlled reactions by the immune system can lead to diseases such as allergies, auto-immune diseases, inflammatory arthritis or reactive arthritis.

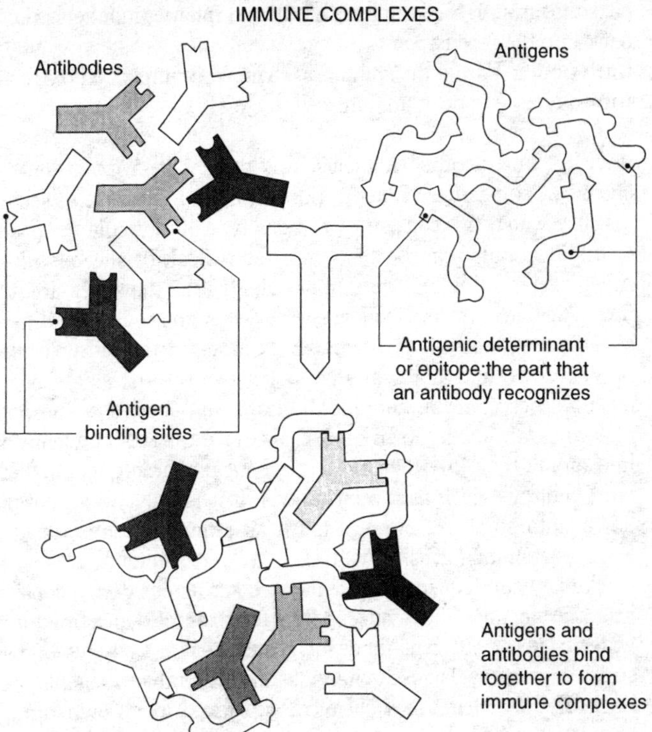

IMMUNE COMPLEXES

Figure 3

Inflammation A concerted reaction by the immune system – See p.64.

Inflammatory arthritis Those forms of arthritis in which there is a strong inflammatory reaction in the synovial membranes of the joints (see p.421), without any infection provoking the inflammation, nor any crystal formation (as in gout). See p.65.

Joint A point where two bones meet. Most of the joints in the body are synovial joints (see p.421).

Joint capsule See **Capsule**.

Lymphatic fluid A clear white fluid, derived from the blood and rich in immune cells (see p.416). It bathes all the tissues of the body, and collects in the vessels of the lymphatic system. These vessels lead to lymph nodes, small swollen areas which are rich in immune cells, and have an important role in the fight against infection. After passing through the lymph nodes, the lymphatic fluid is channelled back into the bloodstream.

Lymph nodes Part of the immune system. See Lymphatic fluid (p.417).

Lymphocyte A type of immune cell (see p.416).

Molecules and atoms A molecule is the smallest intact unit of a chemical substance. Take a pure chemical substance such as distilled water: this consists of just one type of molecule. A spoonful of distilled water can be thought of as a flock of sheep, with one sheep representing one water molecule. Just as the sheep are made up of fleece, meat and bones, so the water molecule has different constituents, known as atoms. But once the water molecule is broken down into atoms it is no longer 'water', just as a sheep cut up into fleece, meat, fat and bones is no longer a sheep. All molecules are made up of atoms, but once they are broken down into atoms they lose their unique chemical characteristics. With a large molecule such as a protein, even if it is only *partially* broken down, into smaller molecules (such as individual amino acids) it loses most of its intrinsic qualities.

Unlike water, most of the items we come across do not consist of just one chemical substance. Milk, for example, is a mixture of water, several different kinds of proteins, various types of fat, a sugar known as lactose, vitamins and several other substances. Each of these items is a chemical substance in its own right, so there are many different kinds of molecules in the milk – more like a 'chemical Noah's ark' than a flock of sheep.

When we speak of a 'food molecule' we mean one type of molecule from this assortment, such as a molecule of lactose, or a molecule of the milk protein, lactalbumin.

Morning stiffness The length of time, after waking up, during which someone with rheumatoid arthritis suffers from stiffness of the joints, greater than that experienced later in the day.

NSAIDs (non-steroidal anti-inflammatory drugs) A large family of drugs, commonly prescribed for several different kinds of arthritis, NSAIDs will reduce inflammation (see p.64) and so control symptoms such as pain, swelling and stiffness. They appear to act by affecting one chemical – an enzyme called cyclo-oxygenase, prostaglandin synthetase or PGHS – which produces messenger molecules called prostaglandins, prostacyclins and thromboxanes. These messengers control a variety of responses in the body, including some aspects of inflammation (see pp.48–49).

The NSAID that is best known is aspirin, which belongs to a group of drugs called salicylates. (Note that aspirin only has an anti-inflammatory effect at high doses.) There are many other NSAIDs, and they are very varied chemically, the only common factor being their effect on prostaglandin synthesis.

Examples of NSAIDs, include Ibuprofen (Brufen), Naproxen (Naprosyn), Flurbiprofen (Froben), Fenoprofen (Fenopron), Ketoprofen (Oruvail), Fenbufen (Lederfen), Diclofenac (Voltarol), Piroxicam (Feldene), Tiaprofenic acid (Surgam), Diflunisal (Dolobid), Benorylate (Benoral), Indomethacin (Indocid), Sulindac (Clinoril), Phenylbutazone (Butacote), Azapropazone (Rheumox), Nabumetone (Relifex), Mefenamic acid (Ponstan), and Etodolac (Lodine).

Nucleus A structure found in most cells, which contains the hereditary material, DNA, as well as many other substances.

Platelets These are tiny cell-like structures found in the blood. Platelets are responsible for helping the blood to clot, but they also play a part in immune responses by releasing chemical messengers which activate immune cells or affect the blood vessels. Platelet counts tend to be very high during active phases of rheumatoid arthritis. They are low in Felty's syndrome (see p.103) and, occasionally, in patients who have an adverse reaction to certain drugs.

Prostacyclins and prostaglandins See pp.48–9.

Psychogenic reaction A reaction that is purely psychological in origin.

Rheumatoid factor An antibody found at high levels in some patients with rheumatoid arthritis; it may also occur in Sjögrens syndrome and systemic lupus erythematosus. A great many people, including the healthy, have some small amount of rheumatoid factor in their blood. Many rheumatoid arthritis patients have levels that are no higher than this, especially in the early stages of the disease. If a low level is found, the patient is described as 'seronegative' or 'RF negative'. Where the level is higher the patient is described as 'seropositive'. Those who are seronegative generally have a milder disease which progresses more slowly and is relatively uncomplicated. A rather arbitrary dividing line has to be set below which the blood is seronegative and above which it is seropositive. It has been set at a level that includes as many rheumatoid arthritis patients as possible in the seropositive group while excluding most healthy people.

Rheumatoid factor is a type of antibody (see p.412) that is targeted at other antibodies: it binds to a class of antibodies called

IgG. Because it binds to the stem region of the IgG (see Figure 2 on p.412) it does not stop the IgG from binding its own antigen. Thus rheumatoid factor can become part of immune complexes (see p.417) making them even larger.

Rheumatoid factor (at levels high enough to be designated seropositive) is also found in long-term infections such as tuberculosis, 'glandular fever', malaria, leprosy and syphilis. Diseases of the liver may be associated with rheumatoid factor, and some healthy people – about 4-5% of the population – have levels of rheumatoid factor high enough to fall in the seropositive range. This percentage increases in older people: among those over 75 years, 25% are seropositive. Smokers tend to have higher levels of rheumatoid factor, as do people exposed to air pollution, and workers in prolonged contact with silica or asbestos. However, very high levels of rheumatoid factor are fairly specific for rheumatoid arthritis.

It is now widely believed that rheumatoid factor is probably not a primary cause of rheumatoid arthritis, but a development that occurs during the disease, perhaps as a response to the presence of unusually large numbers of IgG antibodies in the blood. This would explain why it also appears in long-term infections. There could also be chemical damage to the IgG molecules which made them more susceptible to auto-immune attack (see p.341).

Seropositive/seronegative When used in relation to someone with rheumatoid arthritis, these terms refer to the results of tests for rheumatoid factor (see p.420).

Skin-prick test A test in which a drop of food extract (or extract of any other suspected allergen) is placed on the skin, and the skin gently pricked so that a small amount of the extract penetrates. Skin-prick tests detect true food allergy (although they are not foolproof) but are ineffective for other forms of food sensitivity. They do not usually work for people with rheumatoid arthritis who are sensitive to food. This has been shown with patients whose food reaction is proven by double-blind capsule tests (see p.27) of the food – these capsule tests may be positive every time, but the skin-prick test is either negative or shows a very weak reaction. For this reason, skin-prick testing is of little use for detecting culprit foods in rheumatoid arthritis.

Synovial fluid A clear liquid with the consistency of egg white, which fills the narrow joint space between two bones. The synovial fluid lubricates the joint and nourishes the articular cartilage. It is derived from blood, with certain items, such as the red blood cells,

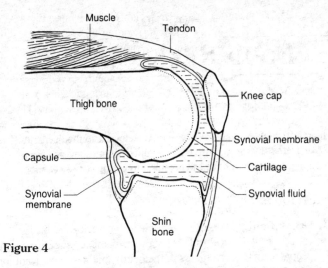

Muscle

Tendon

Thigh bone

Knee cap

Synovial membrane

Capsule

Cartilage

Synovial
membrane

Synovial fluid

Shin
bone

Figure 4

being removed. The conversion of blood to synovial fluid takes place in the synovial membrane, which has many tiny blood vessels known as capillaries running through it.

Synovial joint Any joint that has a synovial membrane (see below). Most of the joints in the body are synovial joints. It is synovial joints that are affected by arthritis.

The basic structure of a synovial joint is shown in Figure 4. The ends of both the bones are covered by articular cartilage. In a healthy joint, this cartilage is very smooth, to reduce friction in the joint, resilient and slightly rubbery to cushion the bones against shocks, yet alive and self-renovating so that damage can be repaired. There are no pain-receiving nerves in the cartilage. The joint space is filled by synovial fluid (see p.420) which lubricates the joint. The whole joint is enclosed by a joint capsule (see p.414).

Synovial membrane Also called the **synovium**, this membrane lines the joint space in all synovial joints. In rheumatoid arthritis and other forms of inflammatory arthritis, the synovium is the site of inflammation. There are no pain-receiving nerves in the synovium.

Synovitis Inflammation of the synovial membrane.

T cell A type of immune cell (see p.416).

True food allergy An allergy to food that involves IgE antibodies. (See p.43 and pp.82–3.)

White blood cell A blood cell which does not contain the red pigment haemoglobin. Most of these are immune cells (see p.416).

Appendix I

FOOD RELATIONSHIPS

The relationships given below are often relevant to food sensitivity (see p.000). Herbs and spices are only included where they are likely to be eaten in quantity and have the potential to cause a cross-reaction.

Plant foods

1. **Grass family, Gramineae:** wheat, rye, triticale, barley, oats, corn, rice, wild rice, millet, sorghum, bamboo, sugarcane. Some people react to all members of the family, but most on a traditional Western diet are sensitive to wheat and its close relatives, or to corn (maize). The subfamilies are often more relevant. They are:
   Pooidae: wheat, rye, barley, oats
   Panicoideae: corn (maize), sorghum, sugarcane, bulrush, or pearl millet
   Bambusoideae: rice, wild rice
   Chloridoideae: finger millet

2. **Nightshade family, Solanaceae:** potato (but not sweet potato), tomato, aubergine (eggplant), sweet peppers (green, red, and yellow peppers), paprika, chilli peppers, tobacco, cape gooseberry (Physalis).

3. **Pea, lentil and bean family, Leguminosae:** peas, haricot beans (kidney beans, whether white-, red-, brown- or black-skinned, also baked beans and flageolets), peanuts, soyabeans, lentils, split peas, broad beans, butter beans, mung beans, lima beans, chick-peas, black-eyed peas, carob, runner beans, green beans, snap beans, string beans, mangetout peas. The various kinds of haricot beans and their green forms (snap beans, string beans, and green beans, including those sold as a frozen vegetable) are all the same species and should be regarded as the same food. Peanuts belong to a separate tribe from other members of the family, and experience with patients who are allergic to peanuts suggests that cross-reactivity with other legumes is generally low, but peanut-sensitive people may react to soyabeans. Patients

sensitive to soyabeans are likely to react to a wide range of legumes. Anyone with these sensitivities is usually advised to avoid peanut and soyabean oils as well.

4. **Cabbage family, Cruciferae:** many foods in this family are actually products of the same species, which means that they are very closely related indeed. They are cabbage, cauliflower, Brussels sprouts, broccoli, calabrese, 'spring greens', kohlrabi, and kale. Other members of the family are turnip, oilseed rape, Chinese leaves, horseradish, radish, rutabaga, cress, watercress, and mustard. Rapeseed oil might cross-react with other cabbage-family foods.

5. **Carrot family, Umbelliferae:** carrot, parsnip, celery, celeriac, fennel, parsley, aniseed, caraway, dill, cumin, coriander.

6. **Cucumber family, Cucurbitaceae:** cucumber, melon, watermelon, marrow, courgette (zucchini), squash, pumpkin.

7. **Onion family, Liliaceae:** onion, leek, shallot, garlic, chives, asparagus.

8. **Sunflower family, Compositae:** lettuce, chicory, endive, globe artichoke, Jerusalem artichoke, salsify, sunflower, safflower, chamomile, sunflower oil, safflower oil.

9. **Spinach family, Chenopodiaceae:** spinach, spinach beet, Swiss chard, chard, beetroot, sugar beet.

10. **Walnut family, Juglandaceae:** walnuts, pecans. *See also the general section on nuts, page 426.*

11. **Palm family, Palmaceae:** coconut, dates, sago, palm oil.

12. **Banana family, Musaceae:** banana, plantain, one form of arrowroot (Musa arrowroot).

13. **Mulberry family, Moraceae:** mulberry, fig, hops (and, therefore, beer).

14. **Buckwheat family, Polygonaceae:** buckwheat, rhubarb.

15. **Currant family, Saxifragaceae:** blackcurrant, red currant, white currant, gooseberry. (The 'currants' used in buns and cakes are actually dried grapes).

16. **Rose family, Rosaceae:** The groups most relevant to cross-reactions are the sub-families:

Rosoideae: blackberry, raspberry, wineberry, cloudberry, loganberry (all in the same genus, so quite closely related); also strawberry and rosehip.

Prunoideae: plum, prune, apricot, greengage, cherry, peach, nectarine, sloe (all in the same genus, so quite closely related); also almond.

Maloideae: apple, pear, quince, medlar, loquat.

17. **Citrus family, Rutaceae;** orange, lemon, tangerine, clementine, grapefruit, lime, citron, kumquats. These are all members of the same genus, and therefore very closely related, so cross-reactions are likely.

18. **Cashew family, Anacardiaceae:** cashew, pistachio, mango.

19. **Grape family, Vitaceae:** grapes, muscatels, raisins, sultanas, currants ie. the dried fruits – not blackcurrants or redcurrants.

20. **Bilberry family, Ericaceae:** bilberry (also called blueberry or whortleberry), cranberry, cowberry.

21. **Mint family, Labiatae:** mint, basil, marjoram, oregano, rosemary, sage, thyme, savory.

22. **Fungi kingdom:** mushrooms, puffballs, truffles, morels, chanterelles, yeast, 'mycoprotein', Quorn.

Poultry and eggs

23. **Pheasant subfamily, Phasianinae;** chicken, pheasant, quail, partridge.

24. **Grouse subfamily, Tetraoninae:** grouse, turkey, guineafowl.

25. **Duck family, Anatidae:** all types of duck and goose.

26. **Pigeon family, Columbidae:** pigeon, squab, dove.

27. **Snipe family, Scolopacidae;** snipe, woodcock.

28. **Eggs:** all birds' eggs are very similar in the proteins they contain, and are best regarded as a single food item.

Fish and shellfish

29. **Fish:** the family concept is irrelevant with respect to fish, because all the fish in the main group eaten (the bony fish) share a

particular type of protein known as a parvalbumin. The parvalbumins are known to provoke allergic reactions, and they probably account for the fact that many people are sensitive to *all* the types of fish they have tried. It is uncertain whether parvalbumins are found in the other main group of fish, the sharks, rays, skates, and dogfish (cartilaginous fish). The two groups are only very distantly related, and it is possible that people sensitive to bony fish could tolerate cartilaginous fish. (However, no one who has a true allergy to fish should test cartilaginous fish except under close medical supervision.)

30. **Crustaceans, Phylum Crustacea;** crab, lobster, crayfish, shrimp, prawn. A very large group, including many different families. Many patients react to all forms of crustacea, so the family concept does not seem relevant here. There may be some common allergen in all of them, as in fish. *See also the section on shellfish on p.426.*

31. **Molluscs, Phylum Mollusca:** mussels, cockles, winkles, oysters, clams, scallops, squid, cuttlefish, octopus, snails, (*escargots*). Again, this is a very broad group, but the family concept does not seem to be relevant here, because people who are sensitive to one type are usually sensitive to them all. *See also the section on shellfish on p.426.*

Meat and milk

32. **Cattle family, Bovidae:** cows (beef, veal), sheep (lamb, mutton), goats. The sheep and goats are grouped in one subfamily, the cows in another, so cross-reactions are most likely between lamb/mutton and goat meat. Cross-reactions between the milk of these three species defy the taxonomic groups: those sensitive to cow's milk quite often react to goat's milk but less often to sheep milk. Why this should be so is unknown.

33. **Pig family, Suidae:** pig (pork, ham, bacon).

34. **Deer family, Cervidae:** venison.

35. **Rabbit family, Leporidae:** rabbit, hare.

· *Unexpected Cross-Reactions* ·

Nuts

People who are allergic to one type of nut are often allergic to others, despite the fact that most nuts are not at all closely related. Apart from those in the walnut family (family 10 in the list above) and the cashew family (family 18) every nut is an individualist – in all, there are at least eight families of plants that supply us with edible nuts. So why should there be this apparent cross-reaction between them? One can only assume that their common 'way of life' requires certain chemical constituents (to prevent rotting for example – most nuts are carried off and stored by animals). Perhaps the different nuts have evolved similar chemicals for this purpose.

Whether this cross-reaction between different types of nuts occurs in food intolerance as well as food allergy is unknown. One problem here is that both physicians and patients tend to refer to them rather vaguely as 'nuts,' instead of specifying which type.

Shellfish

Some people seem to be sensitive to both crustacean shellfish and molluscan shellfish (families 30 and 31). Why this should be is a mystery – it is unlikely to be a cross-reaction, in the conventional sense, since the two groups are not at all closely related. Biologically speaking, they are as similar to humans or birds as they are to each other. Again, the use of an imprecise name for both groups – 'shellfish' – is a confusing factor.

For certain people, it may be something other than the shellfish themselves causing the problem. Toxins acquired from their food, or the preservatives that are liberally added to shellfish might be to blame. This could explain the apparent cross-reaction.

· *Index of Foods* ·

A number following the food shows the group it belongs to in the list on pages 422–5. An 'S' shows that it is the only commonly eaten member of its family. A 'U' shows that it may be involved in some unexpected cross-reactions.

alfalfa 3
almond 16
aniseed 5
apple 16
apricot 16
arrowroot (Musa) 12
arrowroot S
asparagus 7
aubergine 2
avocado S

bacon 33
baked beans 3
bamboo 1
banana 12
barley 1
basil 21
beans 3
beef 32
beetroot 9
beet sugar 9
bilberry 20
black-eyed peas 3
blackberry 16
blackcurrant 15
blueberry 20
Brazil nut S
broad beans 3
broccoli 4
Brussels sprouts 4
buckwheat 14
butter beans 3

cabbage 4
calabrese 4
cane sugar 1
cape gooseberry 2
caraway 5
carob 3
carrot 5
cashew 18
cassava (tapioca) S
cauliflower 4
celeriac 5
celery 5
chamomile 8

chanterelles 22
chard 9
cherry 16
chestnut S, U
chicken 23
chick-peas 3
chicory 8
chilli peppers 2
Chinese gooseberry S
Chinese leaves 4
chives 7
chocolate S
chow-chow S
citron 17
clams 31
clementine 17
cloudberry 16
cockles 31
coconut 11
coriander 5
corn 1
courgette 6
cowberry 20
crab 30
cranberry 20
crayfish 30
cucumber 6
cumin 5
currants 15, 19
cuttlefish 31

dates 11
dill 5
duck 25

eggplant 2
eggs 29
elderberry S
endive 8
escargots 31

fennel 5
fish 29
fig 13
flageolets 3
frogs S

garlic 7
globe artichoke 8
goat 32
goose 25
gooseberry 15
grapefruit 17
grapes 19
green peppers 2
greengage 16
green beans 3
grouse 24
guava S
guineafowl 24

ham 33
hare 35
haricot beans 3
hazelnut (cobnut) S, U
hops 13
horseradish 4

Jerusalem artichoke 8

kale 4
kidney beans 3
kiwi fruit S
kohlrabi 4
kumquat 17

ladies' fingers S
lamb 32
leek 7
lemon 17
lentils 3
lettuce 8
lima beans 3
lime 17
lobster 30
loganberry 16
loquat 16
lychee S

macadamia nut S, U
mangetout peas 3
mango 18
maple syrup S

marjoram 21
marrow 6
maté S
medlar 16
melon 6
milk 32
millet 1
mint 21
morels 22
mulberry 13
mung beans 3
muscatels 19
mushrooms 22
mussels 31
mustard 4
mutton 32

nectarine 16
New Zealand spinach S

oats 1
octopus 31
okra S
olive S
onion 7
orange 17
oregano 21
oysters 31

palm oil 11
papaya S
parsley 5
parsnip 5
partridge 23
passion fruit S
pawpaw S
peach 16
peanuts 3
pear 16
peas 3
pecans 10
pepper (black/white) S
persimmon S
pheasant 23
pigeon 26
pine nut S, U

pineapple S
pistachio 18
plantain 12
plum 16
pomegranate S
pork 33
prawn 30
prickly pear S
prune 16
puffballs 22
pumpkin 6

quail 23
quince 16

rabbit 35
radish 4
raisins 19
rape 4
raspberry 16
red currant 15
red peppers 2
rhubarb 14
rice 1
rosehip 16
rosemary 21
runner beans 3
rutabaga 4
rye 1

safflower 8
sage 21
sago 11
salsify 8
savory 21
scallops 31
sesame S
shallot 7
shrimp 30
sloe 16
snails 31
snap beans 3
snipe 27
sorghum 1
soya beans 3
spinach 9

spinach beet 9
split peas 3
spring greens 4
squab 26
squash 6
squid 31
strawberry 16
string beans 3
sugar, (*see* beet, cane)
sultanas 19
sunflower 8
sweet potato S
sweet peppers 2

tangerine 17
tapioca (cassava) S
tea S
thyme 21
tobacco 2
tomato 2
triticale 1
truffles 22
turkey 24
turnip 4

veal 32
venison 34

walnuts 10
water chestnut S
watercress 4
watermelon 6
wheat 1
white currant 15
whortleberry 20
wild rice 1
wineberry 16
winkles 31
woodcock 27

yam S
yeast 22

zucchini 6

Appendix II

RECIPE BOOKS

The Essential Olive Oil Companion, Anne Dolamore, published by Grub Street, London, 1988

An excellent compendium of Mediterranean recipes featuring olive oil.

The Foodwatch Alternative Cookbook, Honor J. Campbell, published by Ashgrove Press, 1992

Hundreds of useful recipes for those avoiding staple foods such as wheat, eggs or milk.

The Allergy Diet, Elizabeth Workman, Dr John Hunter and Dr Virginia Alun Jones, published by Martin Dunitz, 1984.

An illustrated recipe book for those cooking without basic ingredients such as eggs, milk or wheat.

Appendix III

SOCIAL SECURITY BENEFITS

This appendix only relates to the U.K., and does not deal with all the Social Security benefits that may be available to those with arthritis, only benefits that are directly relevant to shopping and cooking. The principal benefits of this kind, at the time of writing (July 1996), are classified as Disability Living Allowances. There are two categories: 'help with getting around' and 'help with personal care'.

You qualify for 'help with getting around' if you can only walk a short distance before you feel severe discomfort. The current rate is £32.65 per week. You can qualify for 'help with personal care' on several grounds, but the one most relevant here relates to cooking: you would qualify if you needed help to prepare a main meal for yourself, despite having everything you needed to hand. The rate for this is £12.40 each week. (If, however, you also need help with washing, dressing or using the toilet, then a higher rate is payable, up to £46.70 per week.)

To find out more about Disability Living Allowance, you can telephone 0800 882 200; the call is free. This help-line also offers advice about other benefits for people with disabilities.

Under Care in the Community Legislation your local Social Services Dept has responsibility for offering 'assistance in kind' to people in their own homes. For example this may include aids and adaptations to make it easier to get around your home and to prepare food. Services vary from one area to another, you should contact your local office to find out how they can help.

Local self-help and support groups (sometimes affiliated to national organisations such as Arthritis Care; see p.431 for addresses) can be an invaluable source of information and advice about benefits and services in your area.

Appendix IV

USEFUL ADDRESSES

Arthritis Care, 5 Grosvenor Crescent, London SW1X 7ER. Tel: 0171 235 0902.

National Osteoporosis Society, PO Box 10, Radstock, Bath, BA3 3YB.

The Vegan Society, 7 Battle Road, St Leonards-on-Sea, East Sussex TN37 7AA.

The Vegetarian Society, Parkdale, Dunham Road, Altrincham, Cheshire WA14 4QG.

This organisation provides information to consumers on nutritional value of foods and publishes a useful newsletter on food and nutrition issues:

The Food Commission, 102 Gloucester Place, London WC1. Tel: 0171 935 9078.

The following companies produce a wide range of kitchen implements, kettles, teapots, crockery, cutlery and other aids that are specially designed for those affected by arthritis in their wrists, hands and fingers:

Nottingham Rehab Ltd, Ludlow Hill Road, West Bridgford, Nottingham NG2 6HD. Tel: 0115 9452345; Fax: 0115 9452124.

Llewellyn – SML Health Care Services, 1 Regent Road, City Liverpool L3 7BX. Tel: 0151 2365311

Peta Scissorcraft, Marks Hall, Marks Hall Lane, Margaret Roding, Dunmow, Essex CM6 14T. Tel/Fax: 01245 231811

Homecraft Supplies Ltd, Sidings Road, Lowsmore Estate, Kirkby, Ashfield, Notts NG17 7J2. Tel: 01623 754047; Fax: 01623 755585.

The following organisations provide advice for those needing special equipment, and on other disability problems:

The Disability Information Trust, Mary Marlborough Lodge, Nuffield Orthopaedic Centre, Headington, Oxford OX3 7LD. Tel: 01865 227592.

Disabled Living Foundation, 380–384 Harrow Road, London W9 2HU.
   Tel: 0171 289 6111.

Ready-made meals

The following company delivers inexpensive ready-made frozen meals
that are easily reheated:

Wiltshire Farm Foods, Ladydown, Trowbridge, Wiltshire BA14 8RJ.
   Tel: 01225 753636 Fax: 01225 777084

Foods by post or delivery

Inclusion of an organisation in this list does not necessarily mean that
the authors agree with all the policies or opinions advanced by that
organisation. In the same way, we give no general endorsement of the
commercial companies included – they may sell other items, besides
those for which they are listed here, which we believe to be ineffectual,
or even damaging if used wrongly. Readers are advised to be sceptical
about the claims made for some products.

Natural Foods Ltd, Unit 14, Hainault Industrial Estate, Hainault Road,
   Leytonstone, London E11. Tel: 0181 539 1034.
      Home delivery service of a huge range of food and beverages,
   many organic, and many useful to those with specific food
   sensitivities.
Foodwatch International Ltd, 9 Corporation Street, Taunton, Somerset
   TA1 4AJ. Tel: 01823 325022.
      Foodwatch specialises in supplying foods for those with food
   sensitivity. Their extensive stock includes most of the standard
   alternative foods, plus many ususual items not generally available
   elsewhere.
Nutricia Dietary Products Ltd, 494–496 Honeypot Lane, Stanmore,
   Middlesex HA7 1JH. Tel: 0181 9515155.
      Nutricia produces a variety of gluten-free and low-protein
   products under the Glutafin, Loprofin and Rite Diet brand names.
   They also provide products which are free of wheat starch, milk,
   lactose, egg and soya. These products are available from pharmacies
   and many health food shops. A mail-order service is also available.
The Cantassium Company, 225 Putney Bridge Road, London SW15
   2PY. Tel: 0181 874 1130; Fax: 0181 871 0066
      Sell a range of gluten-free, lactose-free flours, under the name
   Trufree. Some of the flours are free of all cereal grains. They also
   produce a free leaflet showing the ingredients of all flours, and a
   recipe book.

Country Harvest Products, 2A/23 Koornang Road, Carnegie, Victoria
   3163, Australia. Tel: 03 563 6538
       Country Harvest manufacture and supply gluten-free foods
   ('Country Harvest') and other products suitable for those with food
   sensitivity; by mail order and to retailers. Product list available.
National Dietary Supplies, 2A/23 Koornang Road, Carnegie, Victora
   3163, Australia. Tel: 03 563 6538.
       Supply gluten-free foods and other products suitable for those
   with food sensitivity. Product list and mail-order form available.
Allergy Aid Centre, 1st Floor, Pran Central, 325 Chapel Street, Prahran,
   Victoria 3181, Australia. Tel: 03 529 7348.
       Allergy Aid can supply foods suitable for those with food
   sensitivity.

Supplements by post
Health Plus Ltd, Dolphin House, 30 Lushington Rd, Eastbourne,
   E.Sussex BN21 4LL. Tel: 01323 737374; Fax: 01323 737375
       Health Plus sell a high-strength evening primrose oil which can
   be taken at a maximum dose of 500 mg of GLA per day (see p.156)
   and a high-strength 'starflower' oil, which can be taken at a
   maximum dose of 660 mg GLA per day.

INDEX